MODERN MATERNITIES

Modern Maternities: Medical Advice about Breastfeeding in Colonial Calcutta brings to light rare textual and visual materials on medical opinions about breastfeeding by memsahibs (European women), *dais* (indigenous midwives and/or wet nurses) and the *bhadramahila* (here the focus is on 'respectable' Bengali-Hindu women). With the help of archival resources, the author discusses themes like:

- modernity, maternities and medicine
- intersections of 'race', gender, class, caste, community and age in diet
- artificial foods versus wet nursing
- 'cleanliness', corporeality and culture
- 'clean midwifery' versus 'dirty midwifery'
- customary breastfeeding practices
- child-mothers and childcare
- breastfeeding, mothercraft and modern clocks
- exhibitions, baby shows and baby weeks
- colonialism and anti-colonial nation-building

The book offers critical insights into social histories of medicine, motherhood and childcare in nineteenth and early twentieth century colonial Calcutta. It is intended for anyone interested in the book's interdisciplinary focus on the regional, national and global resonances of childrearing advice. In particular, it will interest scholars and researchers from modern Indian history, global history, health history, medical anthropology, gender studies and South Asian studies.

Ranjana Saha is a postdoctoral teaching fellow (History Faculty) at the Manipal Centre for Humanities (MCH), Manipal Academy of Higher Education, Manipal. Prior to joining MCH, she was a two-year postdoctoral research fellow at the Indian Institute of Science Education and Research (IISER), Mohali. She completed her PhD from the Department of History, University of Delhi, Delhi. Her research has been published in national and international journals such as *The Indian Economic and Social History Review*, *Women's Studies International Forum* and *South Asia Research*.

MODERN MATERNITIES

Medical Advice about Breastfeeding in Colonial Calcutta

Ranjana Saha

Routledge
Taylor & Francis Group
LONDON AND NEW YORK

First published 2024
by Routledge
4 Park Square, Milton Park, Abingdon, Oxon OX14 4RN

and by Routledge
605 Third Avenue, New York, NY 10158

Routledge is an imprint of the Taylor & Francis Group, an informa business

British Library Cataloguing-in-Publication Data
A catalogue record for this book is available from the British Library

ISBN: 978-1-032-06619-6 (hbk)
ISBN: 978-1-032-35648-8 (pbk)
ISBN: 978-1-003-32783-7 (ebk)

DOI: 10.4324/9781003327837

Typeset in Sabon
by Apex CoVantage, LLC

For Dr Pati (Sir)

CONTENTS

TABLES

FIGURES

PREFACE

This journey began from one footnote in my MPhil dissertation that I decided to pursue. Reading Anja Müller's *Fashioning Childhood in the Eighteenth Century* and Anna Davin's arguments on 'Imperialism and Motherhood' together with a particular article on mothering of infants by Kabiraj Srijukta Girijabhushan Ray Sengupta from a Bengali periodical got me thinking about tracing the transnational traffic in ideas about breastfeeding and child character formation. The journey, however, actually began in the lobby of the Nehru Memorial Museum and Library in New Delhi as Dr. Biswamoy Pati (endearingly called Sir by all his students) and I discussed my preliminary ideas on medical advice about breastfeeding and motherhood in colonial Bengal. Sir's guidance and patience turned my ideas into a doctoral project and this book.

Late nineteenth and early twentieth century childcare manuals featuring anxieties about high infant mortality rates, medical instruction about clocked infant feeding, and various maternal and child welfare measures were globally connected. These were associated with medicalised motherhood as 'mothercraft' which was intimately related to imperial, colonial and nationalist discourses on motherhood aimed to create 'good' wives and mothers who would produce patriotic sons as model future citizens. In the context of colonial Bengal, regular breastfeeding of infants by the clock was central to the nationalist medical repertoire about dutiful mothers and the creation of pious and patriotic sons needed to rescue the motherland from foreigners. Medical print media also provided fascinating lists of dos and don'ts about 'proper' maternal breastfeeding, wet nursing and artificial feeding of infants, particularly in colonial Calcutta. Yet, besides brief scholarly references on the subject, I have found that this particular area presents itself as a lacuna in the existing historiography on medicine, motherhood and nationalism.

My study focuses on medical advice on breastfeeding and motherhood in colonial Calcutta. It also touches upon how medical advice and statistical data on maternal and infant morbidity and mortality became tied to concerns about the differential growth rates of communities. It is argued that medical instruction and propaganda about what was 'good' nursing of infants was a politically and culturally mediated discursive practice aimed at a 'scientific' refashioning of the everyday lives of individual families and communities.

ACKNOWLEDGEMENTS

Dr. Biswamoy Pati's kindness and efforts made my doctoral thesis possible. He was always very supportive with words of encouragement and an understanding smile, while his very perceptive, invaluable insights along with constructive criticism whenever necessary made my work better at every step. Not only in academic matters but also in moments of personal crisis, both Sir and his wife and my advisor, Dr. Indrani Sen, have been my pillars of strength and shown me the way to be strong and fight it out. Due to unfortunate circumstances, Sir is not with us anymore. His sad demise has left an irreplaceable void. I would like to express my deepest gratitude to Sir – my supervisor, mentor, father figure and friend. You had said that you were thinking of my book, not thesis. I am grateful to the universe that I am finally able to transform your inspiring words into reality. Without you, my PhD and book would have just remained a dream.

I am indebted to Sir's close friend and colleague, Professor Amar Farooqui, for kindly agreeing to supervise my PhD thesis in its final stages during this most difficult period. His kindness, humility, insightful guidance and meticulous attention to detail have been enormously helpful and pulled me through the final submission of my PhD thesis which led to the completion of the book.

In the course of my postdoctoral journey (2020–present), I would like to express my gratitude to the Manipal Academy of Higher Education (MAHE), Manipal, which provides a vibrant academic environment. I am first and foremost grateful to my students at the MCH for their enthusiasm for learning and support, which inspires me enormously. I am indebted to our Head of Institute at the Manipal Centre for Humanities (MCH), MAHE, Professor Nikhil Govind, for his guidance and insightful suggestions. I am very grateful to Dr. Gayathri Prabhu, Associate Professor, MCH, MAHE, who has been exceptionally kind and generous. I would like to thank Dr. Emma Dawson Varughese, Senior Fellow, MCH, MAHE, for always being very encouraging. I would like to say a huge thank you to my dear colleagues, Dr. Anubhav Sengupta, Dr. Ashokan Nambiar C., Dr. Jagriti Gangopadhyay, Dr. Ketaki Chowkhani, Dr. Mohamed Shafeeq Karinkurayil, Dr. Neha Chatterji, Dr. Prabodhan Pol and Dr. Shining Star Lyngdoh, for all their support, patience and for making MCH feel like home. I am indebted for my postdoctoral research fellowship for a two-year period at the Humanities and Social Sciences Department (HSS), Indian Institute of Science Education and Research (IISER, Mohali) from 2018 to 2020 under the supervision of Dr. V. Rajesh, Associate Professor and Head of the Department. I would like to express my gratitude to the faculty members, particularly Dr. Adrene Freeda D'Cruz, Professor Anu Sabhlok, Dr. Parth Chauhan and Dr. Ritajyoti Bandyopadhyay, for engaging discussions and insightful suggestions. I am grateful to the scholars namely: Ankur Parashar, Anubhav Preet Kaur, Akash Srinivas, Ansad C, Manisha Kushwaha, Nidhin Johny, Navdeep, Rajesh Poojary, Shashi Mehra, Shriya Raina, Swapnil Chaudhary, Vaibhav Pathak and Yezad Pardiwalla, from a wide range of disciplines at the HSS at IISER, Mohali, for their enormous support. I am indebted for the Junior Research Fellowship (JRF, 2013–2015) and the Foreign Travel Grant of airfare (2015) from the Indian Council of Historical Research (ICHR), New Delhi, and the Charles Wallace India Trust UK Short-Term Research Grant (2015). I would also like to thank the Indian Institute of Science Education and Research (IISER, Mohali, India) for funding my postdoctoral research trip to the U.K. in 2018. I would like to express my gratitude for funding and invaluable feedback from the Doctoral and Early Career Workshop at the University of Warwick, 2018, and the Archival Workshop (Marbourg and Berlin, 2019) funded by the Indian Council of Historical Research (ICHR) and Deutsche Forschungsgemeinschaft German Research Foundation (DFG).

I have also incurred the debt of many wonderful, warm and inspiring teachers who have been kind, understanding and helpful in so many ways. I would like to thank my PhD advisor, Professor Anshu Malhotra, currently Professor in the Department of Global Studies and Kundan Kaur Kapany Professor and Chair of Sikh Studies at the University of California, as her warmth, encouragement and guidance have had an enormous impact on my work. I would like to express my deepest gratitude to Professor Sunil Kumar for his unwavering support and kindness throughout my doctoral and postdoctoral research. I am very grateful for the PhD Fellowship for the duration of one year from February 2016 to February 2017 by the CSDS (Centre for the Study of Developing Societies), Delhi, under the supervision of Dr. Awadhendra Sharan, Director, CSDS. The Fellowship grant also allowed me the opportunity to complete the writing of my chapters and revisit the libraries in both Kolkata and New Delhi. I am indebted to Dr. Sharan for our interesting discussions and his detailed comments on the chapter drafts in their nascent stage which have enormously influenced and improved my writing and the main arguments of my thesis. At the Department of History, University of Delhi, Dr. Arup Banerji, my MPhil supervisor, has been very helpful with suggestions when I was beginning research on this topic. I am very grateful for his guidance and our friendship. Dr. Prabhu Mohapatra has always been very warm and helpful with suggestions. In the course of my MPhil and PhD, Professor Mahesh Rangarajan, Professor Upinder Singh and

Professor B. P. Sahu have always been very kind and supportive. A detailed discussion on my topic with Dr. Yasser Arafat was immensely beneficial. Dr. Raizuddin Aquil has kindly given very useful comments on my work, and he has always greeted us students with a smile and provided warm support. Dr. Shalini Jain has been very kind to me. Dr. Charu Gupta's works on gender and caste have been very helpful in shaping the main arguments of my thesis and this book. I had the invaluable opportunity to briefly be a PhD candidate and TA at Queen's University, Kingston, Ontario, Canada (2009–10, 2011–12). I was unable to complete my doctoral studies there. I am very grateful to Professor Sandra den Otter, Professor Ishita Pande, Professor Karen Dubinsky, Dr. Gordon Dueck, Professor Jeffrey L. McNairn, and Dr. Marisha Caswell for their enormous support and understanding. Yvonne T. Place was kind to me and her words stayed with me.

I have also been enormously influenced by the rigorous Master's programme at the Centre for Historical Studies (CHS), Jawaharlal Nehru University, New Delhi. I remain indebted to our very generous and enormously influential teachers, especially Professor Mridula Mukherjee, Professor Sucheta Mahajan, Professor Aditya Mukherjee, Professor Bhagwan Josh, Professor Kumkum Roy, Professor Tanika Sarkar, Professor Neeladri Bhattacharya, Professor Rajat Datta and Professor Indivar Kamtekar. Professor Ranabir Chakravarti has been very kind and helpful always. Professor Chakravarti's suggestion to read Rahul Peter Das' book, *The Origin of the Life of a Human Being*, has been immensely useful. Dr. Mary E. John's Women's Studies course at the School of Social Sciences has been very enlightening and enjoyable. I remain indebted to Professor Tanika Sarkar for her insightful comments on my paper presented at the Nehru Memorial Museum and Library workshop 'Re-Contextualizing Social Histories of Health and Medicine in Colonial India' on August 23, 2013 and at the 'Between & Beyond: Transnational Networks & the British Empire Ca. 18–20th Centuries, Doctoral and Early Career Workshop', University of Warwick, U.K., June 23–24, 2018. She has always been verykind, supportive and inspiring. I would also like to express my gratitude to Dr. Samiksha Sehrawat, Newcastle University, Newcastle (U.K.), Professor Deepak Kumar, Jawaharlal Nehru University, New Delhi, Professor Denys Leighton at the Ambedkar University, Delhi, Dr. Partho Dutta at the Zakir Hussain College, University of Delhi, Delhi and Dr. Debjani Das at the Vidyasagar University in Medinipur who have provided immensely helpful comments. At the Vidyasagar University, Associate Professor Gautam Chando Roy has always been warm and supportive. Dr. Pati kindly introduced me to Dr. Amitava Chatterjee, currently at the Kazi Nazrul University, who gave me the wonderful opportunity to present a paper at the UGC Sponsored Two Day National Seminar on 'Gendering Modernity' in Kolkata in January 2014. Dr. Saurabh Mishra at The University of Sheffield continues to provide enormous support and helpful guidance. In 2015, Dr. Elizabeth Rahman and Dr. Kaveri Qureshi at the University of Oxford were immensely helpful with their kind suggestions during the writing stages of my paper for the *Women's Studies International Forum* (2017). Dr. Kaveri Qureshi, currently Senior Lecturer at The University of Edinburgh, was very kind to me during my U.K. research trip in 2015. She got packed lunch and she was so warm and wonderful in the middle of a rainy, freezing afternoon at Oxford. I am very grateful to Dr. Qureshi, as she continues to be very warm, inspiring and supportive. I am indebted to Professor Emeritus of Maternal and Infant Health at the University of Central Lancashire, Professor Fiona Dykes, for helping me formulate core arguments around breastfeeding. I am also indebted to Professor Mrinalini Sinha at the University of Michigan for our chance meeting at the British Library which turned into a very productive and interesting discussion over a cup of coffee about my work and so many interesting issues. I am very grateful to my BA (Hons) dissertation supervisor at the Department of History, Lancaster University, Professor Deborah Sutton, whose warm support first gave me the confidence to do field work. A chance meeting with Professor Sutton and Dr. Aparna Balachandran, History Faculty, University of Delhi, while at the the Archival Workshop (Marbourg and Berlin, 2019) was a delightful treat. I will remain indebted to my teachers Professor Ruth Henig and Professor Martin Blinkhorn at Lancaster University as they provided a very educative, interactive and enjoyable learning environment.

This book is primarily focused on materials available at the various repositories in India. I would like to thank the staff at the National Archives of India, and the Nehru Memorial Museum and Library in New Delhi, and the Central Research Library at the University of Delhi, Delhi; and the West Bengal State Archives, the National Library, Hitesranjan Sanyal Archives at the Centre for Studies in Social Sciences Calcutta (CSSSC), and the Bangiya Sahitya Parishad, Kolkata, West Bengal. I am also indebted to the very helpful and kind staff, especially Ankita Ma'am, at the Department of History, University of Delhi. At the West Bengal State Archives, in particular, Dr. Sarmistha De (Sarmisthadi) has been very warm and helpful. Dr. Partha Sarthi Das and Ashim Mukhopadhyay at the National Library have been always very kind with immensely helpful suggestions. I also had the wonderful opportunity to conduct part of my doctoral and postdoctoral research in the U.K. I would like to thank the staff at the British Library, Wellcome Library, London, and Highgate Literary & Scientific Institution, London; and the Radcliffe Science Library, University of Oxford, for their kindness and support. The research trips were very productive, and I was able to locate many rare sources. Furthermore, as the West Bengal State Archives was also closed for renovation for some time during a crucial period of archival research for my doctoral studies, I also benefitted immensely from consulting necessary archival materials at the British Library. I would also like to express my gratitude to the staff at the British Council, Kolkata and New Delhi, for their support. I am grateful especially to Richard Alford at the Charles Wallace India Trust (U.K.) for his kindness. I will always remember his helpful suggestions and our enjoyable discussions at the British Library over a warm cup of coffee. I would also like to thank the CWIT Fellows who provided a home away from home in the U.K. My research trip was also very productive, because I lived near the British Library and the Wellcome Library at the International Lutheran Students Centre and Dinwiddy House, London. I have met some really wonderful people there.

I am deeply indebted to my friends who have always been honest, warm and supportive. I would particularly like to express my gratitude to Shilpi Rajpal for always having been my pillar of strength. Suchitra Choudhury is a close friend and often the voice in my head which does not let me give up. Ruth Amelia Pluckrose is a dear friend and an elder sister. Emily Marie Thomas is like a breath of fresh air – always an honest friend. Vibhuti Sharma and I have been close friends and neighbours in MA and PhD days – feel truly blessed, as she showed me the way forward always. Nikhil Pandey's friendship and sense of humour have been a healthy respite. Chirojit Dutta is a family friend and he has always been like family. Peter Price's sincerity and friendship have been very influential. Somak Biswas has been a good friend and a very kind host in Warwick, U.K. Besides our discussions at Delhi University and the lobby of the International Lutheran Students Centre in the U.K., Sarath Pillai has been exceptionally kind to download and send articles whenever I was unable to avail them in India. I was also blessed with MPhil and PhD batchmates and friends Heeral Chhabra, Radha Kapuria, Sonia Wigh, Robert Rahman Raman, Vibha Tayal and Prachi Sharma, who have always been very kind, supportive and helpful from discussing and reading drafts to a friendly banter once in a while. Blessy Abraham and Achintya also helped me enormously by taking pains to obtain the technological apparatus to support my PhD pre-submission PowerPoint presentation, and I will always remain indebted. I would like to thank my parents for their love and for believing in me. I wish my mother could have seen this book. She taught me that we are capable of doing anything as long as we have an imaginary tin with an endless supply of 'I cans'. From a very young age, she gave me the freedom and courage to think beyond gender stereotypes. My father continues to give me immense support and love. Jethu and Jethun always provide warmth and a home away from home. I will remain indebted to my brother Rupak Saha for his big heart and for taking on the responsibility of funding my undergraduate studies. I would like to express that I feel truly blessed and very grateful to have a very supportive family. Thank you Mamma and Baba for your blessings and love. I do not think there are any words that can fully express my deepest gratitude to my husband and friend, Prithvi, for his perceptive comments, sense of discipline, love and support. You made this book possible.

I will remain indebted to Dr. Pati for his kindness and understanding at every step. Sir, you will always be terribly missed.

INTRODUCTION

Motherhood defined a woman's identity to a very large extent in colonial India. Women were variously educated in order to become 'good' wives and mothers to ensure a brighter future for the community, 'race' and/or nation. My book will be one of the first to focus entirely on breastfeeding advice in colonial Bengal, mainly Calcutta. As the title suggests, medical advice about breastfeeding is analysed here as central to the very making of so-called scientific and modern maternities in colonial Calcutta. This study explores nursing of infants as a site integral to the very definition of as well as the pathologisation, 'medicalization'[1] and modernisation of different kinds of maternities. It problematises and analyses medical opinion about breastfeeding by the Bengali-Hindu *bhadramahila*[2] as the 'immature' child-wife and mother, and the 'mature', goddess-like mother, memsahibs[3] and *dais*[4] in the 'tropical' environment. It primarily focuses on the centrality of medical print media in shaping motherhood and infant feeding in nineteenth and early twentieth century colonial Calcutta. The main argument is that lactation, breast milk, maternal breastfeeding, wet nursing and the associated problem of artificial feeding of infants are discursive entities and biocultural[5] experiences that were socially constructed by imperial, colonial, and nationalist, reformist and revivalist, medicalised discourses about motherhood, manhood and nationhood to revive community, 'racial' and national health and virility.

These are further located within the broader historical context of 'global domesticity'[6] across transnational borders as well as the interrelated areas of the medicalisation of midwifery, childbirth, motherhood as 'mothercraft', and maternal and child welfare.[7] By the early twentieth century, maternities were usually characterised by age, bodily and emotional 'maturity', culture and socioeconomic backgrounds of the mother and wet nurse, various infant feeding methods like breastfeeding, wet nursing and artificial feeding; customary and socio-religious birthing and infant feeding beliefs and practices; and guidelines on medicalised motherhood popularised as 'mothercraft' central to the global infant welfare movement. '[C]lean midwifery',[8] encompassing antenatal and postpartum care by trained midwives and medical

DOI: 10.4324/9781003327837-1

practitioners in domestic and hospital settings, and 'mothercraft' which included elaborate guidelines about breastfeeding and artificial feeding of infants learned by the mother under medical supervision were imbued with moralising and 'scientific' rhetoric aimed at remodelling maternal and infant welfare. Effective breastfeeding was a central aspect of 'mothercraft' which was promoted as a 'modern' and 'scientific' taught/learnt duty to rejuvenate the family, community and nation requiring expert medical knowledge and surveillance. European and indigenous medical practitioners mainly blamed the 'ignorance' and lack of hygiene of mothers, *dais* or untrained midwives and wet nurses for the high infant and/or maternal morbidity and mortality rates which justified the modernisation and medicalisation of antenatal and postnatal maternal and childcare.[9] This study analyses how ideas about 'dirt'/'pollution',[10] 'purity'/'cleanliness', corporeality and culture figured in the historical construction of lactation and breast milk as the bearers of racialised, gendered, classed and caste-ridden biocultural qualities.

Historiography

Georges Canguilhem argues that there is 'no biological science of the normal' as normality is context-specific or 'situated in action'.[11] Michel Foucault, Canguilhem's doctoral student and a profound philosopher who has influenced the study of almost every discipline, furthers Canguilhem's arguments on the normal and the pathological.[12] Foucault guides our understanding of the crucial role of modern 'science' in the normalisation and standardisation of the anatomical body and disease causation by biological agents inaugurated by the transition from eighteenth- and nineteenth-century Galenic humoral medicine, including ideas about miasma (noxious vapours from decaying surroundings) and miasmic theory, to anatomical pathology and 'germ theory' by the late nineteenth century.[13] In the case of colonial India, particularly Bengal, the most recent study by Ambalika Guha argues that anatomic dissection and clinical anatomy were the main driving epistemic shifts leading to the emergence of a new medical culture which involved the professionalisation, institutionalisation and hierarchisation of the doctor-patient relationship.[14] Health science with detailed instructions about the care of self and body were internalised, reconfigured and disseminated widely by the Bengali midwifery and maternal and infant care manuals as well as women's magazines from the mid-nineteenth century onwards.[15]

My research particularly builds on Foucault's arguments, from the 1970s, about discourses (generally implying formal/informal and personal/institutional writings, speeches, confessions and exchanges on various subjects) and bodily discipline. To begin with, he argues that meanings are derived from the location of a particular subject within the matrix of discourses and more crucially, the differentiation between the pathological and the normal occurred within the field of medical discourses and interventions.[16]

He points out that power and knowledge are entangled together in discourse.[17] He argues that 'we must not imagine a world of discourse divided between accepted discourse and excluded discourse, or between the dominant discourse and the dominated one; but as a multiplicity of discursive elements that can come into play in various strategies'.[18] He explains further that '[d]iscourse transmits and produces power; it reinforces it, but also undermines and exposes it. . . . There is not, on the one side, a discourse of power, and opposite it, another discourse that runs counter to it'.[19]

Edward Said's engagement with Foucauldian notions of discourse in a colonial setting is pertinent as it points out that 'without examining Orientalism as a discourse one cannot possibly understand the enormously systematic discipline by which European culture was able to manage—and even produce—the Orient politically, sociologically, militarily, ideologically, scientifically, and imaginatively during the post-Enlightenment period'.[20] He argues that Orientalism was Europe's 'way of coming to terms' with the Orient's 'special place' in the West. He points out that the Orient was not only located next to Europe but it was also Europe's 'Other' – the colonies – which provided its civilizations and cultural contestants. The Orient, therefore, defines the West often in the form of a contest between the European Self versus the Other as its 'contrasting image, idea, personality, experience'. He warns, however, that the Orient is not just a figment of European imagination as it is as much an integral part of European material culture and civilisation. Orientalism as a form of discourse is also supported by 'institutions, vocabulary, scholarship, imagery, doctrines, even colonial bureaucracies and colonial styles'.[21]

Foucault's theory about how Benthamite surveillance, discipline and industrial time exercise power and control over the body from his *Discipline and Punish* is also enormously useful in understanding breastfeeding as a biocultural experience.[22] As also discussed in Chapter 5 of this book, Robbie P. Kahn explains that the Greek word 'maia', meaning 'mother or nurse' from Indo-European 'ma' derived from the child's cry for the breast, as *The American Heritage Dictionary* points out, is both 'a linguistic universal', and 'a speaking voice' in 'demand feeding' which is opposed to clocked feeding.[23] Fiona Dykes draws from Kahn's notion of 'maialogical time', that is, the 'cyclical time'/time of mother-child 'mutuality'/a 'period of the woman's life when she bears children, and lactates', as an attempt at separating 'time spent' on mothering (bearing and rearing of children) from the control of 'industrial' or 'linear time' on our bodies, dividing of bodies into 'productive'/'working' and 'not working' parts,[24] although both often coexist. She reinterprets Foucault's arguments by highlighting that, unlike clocked breastfeeding, 'maialogical time' restores 'time for women to engage in breastfeeding their baby in a more fulfilling way'.[25]

In the context of colonial Bengal, this also relates with Tanika Sarkar's argument based on Julia Kristeva's notions about 'cyclical'/'monumental'/

'women's time' to explain the oppressiveness of colonialism as 'a radically new civilisation' and an 'axiomatically superior one'. Among the intelligentsia, it brought about 'a simultaneous attraction' for and 'a need to escape from it to one's own past'. Westernised ideas of progress and civilisation together with teleological linear time created 'intolerable anxieties' and a 'violent desire to break out of its iron frame' by returning 'to a past, to one's mother, a reversion to the womb, to a state of innocence, of pleasure, where the infant is as yet undifferentiated from the mother, as yet unaware of his own distinct self'.[26]

About the harshness and humiliation of office work or '*chakri*'[27] together with clock time and print culture,[28] which gave rise to 'diverse ways of thinking about time'[29] – Sumit Sarkar highlights that it was the trope of Kaliyuga which was used to denote the 'eternally repeated four-*yuga* cycle, the epochs distinguished from each other by their moral qualities'.[30] He emphasised that 'Kaliyuga normally is the most degenerate of times, when Shudras (low-castes) dominate over high-castes and hierarchies of gender and age are reversed'.[31] Sarkar emphasises that clock time was mostly internalised by upper-caste middle-class 'patriotic *bhadralok*' who invested a high premium on 'moving forward in harmony with time'.[32] However, like the frequent references made to Kaliyuga by the Bengali lower middle class unable to benefit from English education and clock time – 'the narrative of high-bhadralok activism would be repeatedly punctuated by gaps, relapses into passivity, inward-turning moods, doubts, mordant autocritiques'.[33] The 'tonalities of Kaliyuga', as Sarkar points out, fascinated the high *bhadralok* in their 'darker moods' since colonial exploitation kept the 'self-image of the successful enterprising male always fragile, unstable, open to racist humiliation'.[34]

My research builds on and extends this existing scholarship about time and discipline to argue that 'scientific' clocked breastfeeding was central to the colonial and indigenous medical manuals, based on medical supervision, discipline, and precision – given by the clock – often paralleling workforce discipline and surveillance. It was an instance of introducing clock time into the inner spaces of the home as well as anti-colonial nation-building through identity formation of the Bengali middle class by discoursing about the modern and medicalised self-disciplining regimen in the Bengali maternal and infant care manuals.[35]

Moreover, besides the pervasiveness of medical discursive power, modern clocks and discipline, this study is also, first and foremost, about the problematisation and analysis of the 'doctrine of maternal ignorance', a recurring theme which was central to medical print media about maternal and infant care in colonial Bengal. Anna Davin highlights that discourses about 'maternal ignorance' were crucial to 'mothercraft' – the driving force behind the global infant welfare movement. Underlying the British anxieties concerning census figures of infant mortality and the infant welfare movement in the early twentieth century were eugenicist imperialist concerns that '[i]f the British population did not increase fast enough to fill the empty spaces of the empire, others would'. 'The threat was not from the indigenous populations' but 'from rival master-races'.[36] Thus, the mothercraft movement translates as the 'authority of state over individual, of professional over amateur, of science over tradition, of male over female, of ruling class over working class . . . all involved in the redefining of motherhood'[37] ensuring that the mothers of the 'Imperial race'[38] would be carefully educated. Similarly, Milton Lewis argues that the figure of the 'ignorant' mother and the popular 'doctrine of maternal ignorance'[39] were central to the infant welfare movement in early twentieth-century Britain and across the British empire. This argument on maternal ignorance, which often took on racialist overtones in a colonial framework, was recently redeployed by Manisha Lal in the context of colonial North India pointing out that both western and indigenous medicine targeted to educate 'ignorant' Indian mothers, often blamed as the 'house of illness'.[40]

Lewis explains that the 'doctrine of maternal ignorance' meant that the 'ignorant' mother was usually held responsible for the contemporary high infant mortality rates, resulting mainly from diarrhoeal deaths. Arthur Newsholme, medical officer of health for Brighton in 1899 and also medical officer of the Local Government Board between 1908 and 1918,[41] enormously influenced the emergence of the infant welfare movement in England through his observation that the source of infection was usually in the home thereby emphasising the central role of the mother in infant welfare, mainly 'proper feeding and hygienic care'.[42] His writings reinforced the importance of breastfeeding and mothercraft in childcare, which were also catchphrases of the worldwide infant welfare movement.[43] Lewis also highlights that gone were the days when high infant mortality and declining birth rates were considered 'inevitable hardships in a Malthusian world of scarcity'[44] as imperial rivalries together with anxieties about national efficiency were intimately related with the question of the '[q]uantity and quality of population'.[45] The British authorities were primarily alarmed by the 'physical deterioration of the race' as evident from the poor physical fitness of working class recruits to fight the Boer War in South Africa which ultimately transformed 'the problem of infant health into a national and imperial issue'.[46] Similarly, in settler colonies like Australia, infant health was considered the 'health of the race' and integral to the 'population question' to survive as a 'white British nation'.[47]

Daniel R. Headrick argues that the goal of imperialism, the establishment of political and economic control on colonies, was achieved through technological innovations like the steamer or quinine prophylaxis which ultimately hardened racist attitudes based on blurred ideas about colonial backwardness in technology/culture/biological capacity.[48] Headrick points out '[e]asy conquests' due to technological prowess had 'warped the judgement of even the scientific elites'.[49] Building on Foucault's arguments on discourse and governmentality,

Ishita Pande points out that the idea of medicine simply as a 'tool of empire' has been overtaken by historiographical shifts focused on the discursive power of liberal racialism[50] and medicine, as in David Arnold's *Colonizing the Body*. Arnold points out the colonising nature of medicine itself in both the metropolis and the colony.[51] However, he emphasises that while 'the violence of the climate and the extreme effects of heat and humidity were held largely to blame for this tropical aggravation of disease'[52] – in a colonial context, 'the career of Western medicine in India showed the importance of different and often opposing "readings" of the body'.[53] His emphasis on the 'importance of the body as a site of colonizing power and of contestation between the colonized and the colonizer' located amidst the 'corporality of colonialism in India'[54] is central to this study. He highlights that colonialism operated through 'an enormous battery of texts and discursive practices' is intimately associated with the 'physical being of the colonized'.[55] Colonial rule was mainly built on knowledge/power concerning the body.[56] Arnold argues that medicine cannot be regarded just as a matter of scientific curiosity and research as 'even in its moments of criticism and dissent, it remained integral to colonialism's political concerns, its economic intents, and its cultural preoccupations'.[57]

> As Western medicine grew in confidence and political authority, as it freed itself from the humoral pathology which had earlier kept it in touch with the principles of Ayurvedic and Yunani medicine, and as it began to take responsibility for Indian as well as European health and thus to see indigenous medicine more clearly as its rival, it also exhibited a growing tendency to dismiss indigenous medicine and its practitioners, almost without qualification.[58]

Far from being a source of comfort and healing to the sick, Indian medicine was represented as confused, dangerous, and anachronistic, even, like *thagi*, a barbarous crime against the individuals on whom it was practiced from the mid-nineteenth century.[59] However, unlike Arnold's focus on state medicine, epidemics and public health measures, this study builds on Pande's arguments on colonial and modern western medicine as a discursive practice which also allowed the subject formation of the colonised for anti-colonial purposes.[60]

In this regard, my research highlights that Ayurveda was also refashioned as a 'traditional' yet 'modern' and 'scientific' nationalist challenge to colonial western medicine and other medical systems through the 'vernacularization'[61] or translation of Sanskrit Ayurvedic texts into the vernacular as easily readable guidelines for everyday life.[62] Projit Bihari Mukharji argues that an integrated Hindu medical system of Ayurveda with communal and national ties was an early nineteenth-century Orientalist phenomenon while, by the mid-nineteenth century, various *daktari* or Bengali vernacular treatises which 'provincialized' western medicine also multiplied.[63] European and indigenous maternal and childcare manuals provided an enormous amount of advice related to the twin processes of the pathologisation and medicalisation of 'Indian mothers' and *dais* and their ways of nursing infants. *Daktars*, and later *'ledi daktars'*, were indigenous western medical practitioners at hospitals and dispensaries or in private practice, with different medical qualifications,[64] who wrote on various aspects of family health, especially midwifery which was often inclusive of issues related to maternal and child health management.[65]

The 'women's question' was intimately tied with the nationalist 'new patriarchy' and their 'glorification of motherhood'.[66] Key arguments by Partha Chatterjee include specific symbolisms of the 'uncolonized' spaces of the home/inner/spiritual world as opposed to the colonised/materialist/public sphere, and the conceptualisation of the *bhadramahila* as the guardian of traditional values as the 'good' wife and mother (*sugrihini*) as well as reader and/or author of Bengali magazines and manuals rearing strong, patriotic sons devoted to the motherland. These neatly fit the central focus of this book on textual analysis of official and vernacular, English and Bengali medical literature concerning maternal and infant care in colonial Calcutta.[67] Chatterjee also argues that

> because of the way in which the history of our modernity has been intertwined with the history of colonialism, we have never quite been able to believe that there exists a universal domain of free discourse, unfettered by differences of race or nationality.[68]

He explains that due to 'the close complicity between modern knowledges and modern regimes of power' – 'we have tried, for over a hundred years, to take our eyes away from this chimera of universal modernity and clear up a space where we might become the creators of our own modernity'.[69] Yet Chatterjee stops short of analysing how 'race' and these 'universal' discursive 'modern regimes of power' became central to the identity formation of the Bengali middle class.[70]

As medical writings were situated amidst a wider context of 'science' as a 'civilising mission' and the 'trope of the tropics', significant in an understanding of both the European 'Self' and the colonised 'Other'[71] – my research builds on Margaret Jolly's arguments on the roles of gender, 'race' and class in the interrelated terrain of maternities and modernities. She begins by pointing out that it is not just an 'alliterative conjunction' between two pluralised concepts – maternities and modernities.[72] There were different Asian and Pacific indigenous forms of mothering of infants which were variously challenged by colonial and postcolonial projects of 'civilization, modernity and scientific medicine'.[73] She argues that '[t]he embodied maternal subject is pervaded by a profound tension, perhaps even a split, as the mother is sundered in contests between "tradition" and "modernity" '.[74] The 'seemingly natural processes of swelling, bearing and suckling, the flows of blood, semen and milk are constituted and fixed not just by the force of cultural conception but by coagulations of power'.[75] She explains that indigenous mothers were accused of 'lacking a maternal instinct' or being 'incompetent mothers'. 'Perhaps most predictably there were concerted attacks on indigenous forms of contraception, abortion and infanticide'.[76] Indigenous mother love was either insufficient or 'too indulgent'.[77]

I also build on Meredith Borthwick and Supriya Guha's arguments that medicine is a cultural practice. Borthwick points out that a 'continuing stream of mother and child care manuals, based generally on English prototypes' appeared in Bengali from the 1850s onwards. She argues that doctors often perpetuated or rejected traditional customary beliefs and practices related to childbirth and infant feeding while medical advice on infant care was not always penned by medical practitioners alone.[78] Guha also highlights that 'the break between medical and popular ideas was not always sharp'.[79] In late nineteenth- and early twentieth-century colonial Bengal, myriad forms of advice on the age of consent for sexual intercourse, conjugality, women's reproductive health and childrearing became increasingly visible. It also included meticulous medical advice to the *bhadramahila* mother on pregnancy, childbirth, and infant feeding as a disciplined and regulated activity by the modern clock and 'humanisation' of animal milk (a recurring term used in European and Bengali medical manuals to imply making animal milk 'akin' to breast milk often by adding sugar, water, etc). These were voiced by people from different walks of life ranging from medical practitioners, administrators, ethnographers, lawyers, teachers, women members of various organisations, and so on. My research probes medical advice on infant feeding and its myriad, underlying cultural and political leanings to contribute towards the social histories of motherhood and childrearing in colonial Bengal, mainly Calcutta.

Judith E. Walsh argues that there was not a single aspect of domestic life which was inconsequential enough to have been left out of debates concerning the family, and especially the 'women's question' in relation to the so-called respectable Bengali-Hindu women, in the Bengali domestic manuals in late nineteenth and early twentieth century colonial Bengal.[80] She categorises nineteenth-century Bengali domestic manuals as 'hybrid' in nature situated within the broader genre of advice literature steeped in the 'transnational, hegemonic discourse' of an apparently 'natural', 'modern' and 'civilised' 'global domesticity'.[81] 'Global domesticity saw the "natural" order of human relations as a patriarchal family system' and 'imprinted with Enlightenment themes of order, reason and science: system, order, efficiency were essential for daily home life'.[82] Walsh also points out similarities between English, American, Anglo-Indian and Bengali domestic manuals and highlights the importance of the everyday lives of memsahibs displayed as 'public domesticity' in the colonies.[83] My research builds on and furthers her arguments on Bengali domestic manuals which incorporated advice for lactating mothers, for example, her translation of Nagendrabala Dasi's *Nārīdharma* (Woman's Dharma) which argued that, like ancient Hindu women, modern Indian women were like a 'race of mothers'.[84] They needed to possess goddess-like qualities to become *grhlaksmi* (goddess of the home) like Lakshmi, the goddess of wealth and prosperity.[85] Women needed to be educated to become dutiful mothers. A mother who assigned her breastfeeding duties to her 'loudly wailing infant' to a wet nurse, while she was for example 'confounded by her card game', was criticised.[86] Unlike Walsh's arguments favouring the opinion that there had been a 'resolution' of the 'women's question'[87] from early twentieth century onwards, however, this study locates this issue amidst the highly volatile medical and medico-legal age of consent debates of the 1890s to 1920s, and maternal and child welfare in the early twentieth century.

This study is ultimately about the centrality of print in shaping and articulating the main debates concerning the 'women's question' and the medicalisation of maternal and infant care in nineteenth- and early twentieth-century colonial Calcutta. It has benefitted from Tapti Roy's excellent background on the vernacular publishing industry in Bengal. She points out that, from the mid-nineteenth century onwards, the publishing industry was most probably the second largest indigenous enterprise, after jute industry, in Calcutta.[88] In the 1860s, as Bengali books kept flooding the market, the government decided to keep them under surveillance. The Act XXV of 1867 was put in place 'for the regulation of printing-presses and Newspapers, for the preservation of copies of books printed in British India, and for the registration of such books'.[89] In effect, it meant that any book printed in India was supposed to be officially registered.[90] From 1868 onwards, the Bengal Library Catalogue was underway and a copy of each book listed there was packed off to the India Office Library (London) and the Imperial Library (Calcutta).[91] Around the same time, 'the *Calcutta Gazette* listed, every quarter, all books and periodicals published by the native Bengali press'.[92] Furthermore, she points out that the worldviews of the Bengali intellectual elite coincided with the motives of colonial surveillance from 'a position of externality'[93] as both voiced similar problems 'of taste, of public decency, and of the waste – the 'frittering away' – of a powerful instrument of education and cultural improvement'.[94] She argues, however, that, unlike early nineteenth-century Bengali social reformers who desired colonial intervention, the late nineteenth-century Bengali intellectual elite usually delimited 'a cultural zone' that would be run by governing beliefs and practices enforced by institutions set up most often by 'the dominant practitioners of that culture, not by an external colonial government'.[95] In short, they sought 'to discipline' the printed text 'from within' through the creation of a select set of 'normative literary practices'.[96]

Finally, a brief look at the colonial machinery of surveillance in order to also decipher the problematic affinities between colonial 'scientific' ethnography and medicine which enormously influenced the categorisations of the 'manly Englishman', the 'effeminate Bengali' and the 'martial races' of northern India.[97] My research builds on Bernard S. Cohn's main argument and methodology that the metropole and the colony form 'a unitary field of analysis'.[98] Colonial administrative power stemmed from control over 'a territory' and an 'epistemological space'.[99] Knowledge was power when it was collected through specific 'investigative modalities' and then turned into 'facts' within the wider colonial regime.[100] He explains:

> [A]n investigative modality includes the definition of a body of information that is needed, the procedures by which appropriate knowledge is gathered, its ordering and classification, and then how it is transformed into useable forms such as published reports, statistical returns, histories, gazetteers, legal codes, and encyclopedias.[101]

He adds that most investigative modalities were constructed in close association with institutions and administrative sites with a fixed regimen. These together lent authority and credibility and thereby transformed many of them into 'sciences' like ethnology and tropical medicine and 'their practitioners became professionals'.[102]

The ethnographic 'essentialization and somaticization of group differences'[103] or holistic representations of Indian populations through certain physical or cultural characteristics neatly differentiating 'races' and the various racialised castes and tribes were grounded in the 'science' of anthropometry.[104] Anthropometry[105] was the 'scientific' methodology of measuring living bodies behind the ethnographic information in the censuses of late nineteenth- and early twentieth-century India.[106] As Nicholas Dirks also points out, building on Cohn's arguments, that the Indian subject was imprisoned in a 'typecast role' by the British rulers.[107] Dirks emphasises that anthropometry incorporated 'the determination of everything from average height and weight' to 'detailed measurements of the shape and size of the skull, the face, and the nasal index (breadth × 100/height); the relation of head size to body size; and the relative sizes of different body parts'.[108] He highlights that '[t]he history of the nineteenth century in India is the history of desperate attempts to fix an inchoate and uncolonizable place in textual form . . . [e]thnographic citation produced colonial conviction, the reality effect of context'.[109] Dirks also explains the 'modernity of caste'[110] as a part of a history that chose caste as the major 'systematic category to name, and thereby contain, the Indian social order'.[111] Thus, the census represented 'colonial science', 'conversion of barbarism into civilized data' and the 'transformation of moral condemnation into the moral basis of both science and state'.[112] It is pertinent to note, however, that also relevant as a kind of counter argument to the belief in the infallibility of anthropometry at the time, for example, was a bunch of texts circulated at the time of the Census of 1911 by E. A. Gait Census Commissioner for

India – *Summaries of some essays, etc. relating to census and caste* (1911). This mainly included an essay titled 'Brief précis of an article in the Muenchener Medizinische Wochenschrift, dated January 17, 1911, by Walcher, on the subject of artificial changes in the shape of the skull' which mentioned that sleeping patterns and pillows are often responsible for such changes.[113]

Primarily in the context of late nineteenth and early twentieth century colonial India, ethnographic empirical data was an odd combination of pseudo-scientific and 'brahminized' Darwinist evolutionary ideas.[114] Meena Radhakrishna argues that the authenticity and authority of such supposedly expert knowledge was based on the 'circularity of information' or the blurred and 'circular nature' of information as authors often cited each other unquestioningly across genres from fiction to ethnography.[115] She explains that this is how evolutionary theories about the supposed animality and backwardness of the dark-skinned 'races' and tribes located in the lower ranks of the 'scale of civilization' were circulated and justified.[116] She highlights that there was an inherent basic contradiction between anthropology and the '*doctrine of evolution*' however – between the ethnographer's belief in the 'static nature of indigenous societies' and the '*doctrine of the civilizing mission of imperialism*'.[117]

The scheme for a systematic ethnographic survey of the whole of India was announced by the Government of India in 1901.[118] It was clearly outlined that a Director for the entire Ethnographic Survey of India as well as several of the Superintendent of Ethnography for each Province or Presidency would be appointed as they would carry out both their official duties and the survey. Herbert Hope Risley, colonial administrator, became the Director of the Ethnographic Survey of the whole of India (officially undertaken between 1901 and 1908) and Superintendent of the Ethnographic Survey of Northern India. He authored the anthology *The People of India* (1908) and contributed significantly to the *Census of India* (1901). He carried out anthropometric studies approved by Sir William Flower, (1831–1899) museologist and eventually Director of the Natural History Department of the British Museum, London and with the help of Paul Topinard's (1830–1911, French anthropometrist and anthropologist) anthropometric instruments and instructions.[119] According to Risley, if *varna* translates into distinctions of colour and physique, then scientific classification was necessary in order to determine the tangible, fixed, 'definite', 'anthropometric characters' of the 'castes' and 'tribes' of India in order to contribute towards 'a *final* classification of the people of India on the basis of their physical characters' (emphasis added).[120] For Risley, 'caste' was the cohesive principle keeping together the entire social fabric of India:

> We should rather conceive of it as a congenital instinct, an all-pervading principle of attraction and repulsion entering into and shaping every relation of life. For Hindus caste is bound up with

> their religion, and its observance is enforced by the authority of the priests; its influence is conspicuous in the social usages of most Indian Muhammadans; and it extends even to the relatively small communities of Christians. Thus it forms the cement that holds together the myriad units of Indian society.[121]

In colonial Bengal, the lying-in room represented ritual pollution and impurity associated with childbirth and caste-related beliefs together with problematic issues like traditional 'dirty midwifery' and unhygienic birthing and customary breastfeeding practices.[122] This study explores the role of medical literature in bringing Bengali maternal and infant bodies and domestic spaces (mainly the lying-in room) under medical scrutiny for promoting effective breastfeeding. It is relevant to note that even the Victoria Memorial Scholarships Fund meant to restrict untrained *dais* from practising their trade and thereby creating 'trained midwives' out of them[123]:

> bore the imprint of H H Risley, a member of the committee established to make recommendations for the Fund. Risley, as a Bengal Civilian, had written a comprehensive ethnography of the tribes and castes of greater Bengal, which included detailed accounts of customs of childbirth. As with many scholars, his knowledge was to provide certain *idées fixes*, chiefly relating to the immutability of caste-related practices. There was also political sensitivity to the question of domestic or ritual customs.[124]

Methodology and Sources

Medical and medico-legal, along with ethnographical and popular, representations of mothering of infants, imbued with 'scientific' and moralising rhetoric, are my entry points into the social histories of motherhood and childcare in colonial Bengal, mainly Calcutta. In the late nineteenth and early twentieth centuries, 'scientific' midwifery and medicalised motherhood as 'mothercraft' were influenced by imperial, colonial and nationalist ideals of manly vigour, motherhood and nationhood. Debates about infant feeding and associated character formation and bodily growth of the child amidst prevalent high infant and maternal mortality rates were, therefore, heated discursive exchanges. Anti-colonial ideals also became 'marketing strategies'[125] for products related to 'proper' infant feeding. The analytical categories of gender, 'race', class, caste, community, and age, alongside biological/cultural and 'pure'/'polluting' qualities often believed to have been transmissible through blood and milk are central to my interrogation of the crisscrossing perceptions of modernity, colonial medicine and motherhood. This study about breastfeeding primarily aims to contribute towards a better understanding of 'what was colonial about colonial medicine?'[126]

My research aims to highlight that the so-called universal western medicine was not always imposed on, or a matter of objectifying, the colonised. It emphasises that western medicine also allowed opportunities for subject formation of the colonised, both men and women, by their internalisation and deployment for various purposes, primarily anti-colonial nation-building.[127] My analytical methodology also coincides with the Foucauldian approach of Pande which goes beyond the 'Said-inflected critique of colonial power/knowledge'.[128] It focuses on the 'biopolitical basis of the colonized subjects' self-representation' through dialogue and resistance in the course of conversations between medical practitioners belonging to divergent medical systems.[129] Pande argues that the colonial state was an always already racialised and modern colonial state.[130] She points out that the colonial state was the 'entwinement of politics and medicine, power and knowledge, in the age of empire'.[131] The 'creation of racialized medicine' occurred through 'a dialogue between doctors and colonial administrators, which provided a potent justification for a liberal empire: as a cure for native pathologies'.[132] However, she highlights that instead of focusing on 'colonial difference' as the impossibility of internalising colonial knowledge as self-knowledge by the colonised middle class – which marked the need to nationalise and indigenise modernity with the help of Hindu science as argued by Gyan Prakash[133] – a reinterpretation of the Foucauldian notion of 'biopower' following Said's *Orientalism* is necessary.[134] As nationalist medicalised prescriptions and proscriptions on the 'proper' nurturing of infants were about creating a 'traditional' and/or 'modern', 'scientific' and 'respectable' domesticity and motherhood – it depended on the subject formation of the colonised elite, usually the upper and middle class and/or caste mainly male and gradually female populations, who 'attempts to write itself into history'[135] by discoursing on 'modernity' and 'hygiene' to improve individual, family, community and national health.

Source materials primarily include Bengali and English medical and popular manuals and periodicals discussing different medical systems, mainly western medicine. Medical books by (male) *daktars*, on the subject of maternal and child welfare include allopathic practitioner Jodu Nath Mukerje's, *Dhatri Sikkha*, and homeopathic and allopathic *daktar* and Assistant Surgeon, Annada Charan Khastagir's, *A Treatise on the Science and Practice of Midwifery with Diseases of Children and Women*,[136] among others. These are indicative of the fact that *daktars* were actively part and parcel of the discourse on ignorance, pollutants, and superstitions which needed 'scientific' sanitisation. Ayurvedic treatises on midwifery, for example, Kabiraj Sri Harimohan Dasgupta's *Ayurvediyo Dhatribidya sangraha Pratam Khando* [An Anthology of Ayurvedic Midwifery Part 1],[137] and Ayurvedic and allopathic practitioner, Surendranath Goswami's *Arya Dhatrividya: a treatise on the Ayurvedic system of midwifery, with Sanskrit text and English translation,*[138] highlight the significance of '*Ayurvediyo*' *dhatribidya*, which often implies indigenous Ayurvedic treatises on midwifery usually invoking the 'scientific' practices of the ancient Aryans and Hindus. These writings usually had an undercurrent of fears around 'degenerating' Hinduism, Ayurveda and Hindu populations. My research also emphasises that medical knowledge systems were often combined and hybridised in their application in anti-colonial nation-building. A detailed analysis of Brahmo and nationalist *daktar* Sundari Mohan Das' works on childcare reveals that he brought together 'tradition' and 'modernity' as he combined western medicine, Ayurveda and Hinduism in his deification of the breastfeeding 'Indian mother' figure as well as her pathologisation and medicalisation with the help of modern clocks as anti-colonial nation-building.[139] The study aims to illustrate that western medicine and Ayurveda were markedly visible in alternating confrontation, competition and alignment with each other in the process of educating the 'ignorant' mother and midwife in 'proper' maternal and infant care.

Besides these medical handbooks, it examines various reports associated with the quasi-governmental 'civilising missions' like the National Association for Supplying Female Medical Aid to the Women of India, founded by Lady Dufferin in 1885 and popularly known as the Countess of Dufferin's Fund; the Victoria Memorial Scholarships Fund (V.M.S.F) established in 1903 by Lady Curzon, the Women's Medical Service (WMS) from 1913, and the Lady Chelmsford All-India League for Maternity and Child Welfare established in 1920 by Lady Chelmsford. Official documents mainly include governmental judicial and medical branch proceedings, sanitary commissioners and public health reports, municipal administration reports, censuses, and native newspaper reports, alongside various national and international infant welfare exhibition and conference papers like the *Proceedings of the English-Speaking Conference on Infant Mortality* held in England in 1913, and the report of the Health and Child Welfare Exhibition held in Calcutta in 1920. The study also explores a wide range of official and vernacular medical periodicals: *The Lancet, Indian Medical Gazette, Calcutta Journal of Medicine, Chikitsa Sammilani, Chikitsa-Prokash, Chikitsak Bandhab, Swasthya Samachar, and Ayurved,* among others, discussing different medical systems and their infant feeding methods; and women's magazines like *Bamabodhini Patrika* famous for 'home tutoring'[140] of the *bhadramahila*. Personal papers, correspondence, memoirs, illustrations, and advertisements are also explored as these provide a treasure trove of information on maternal and infant care. My research was conducted at various repositories in India, mainly the National Archives of India (New Delhi), Nehru Memorial Museum and Library (New Delhi), Central Research Library, University of Delhi (Delhi), West Bengal State Archives (Kolkata), National Library (Kolkata) and Bangiya Sahitya Parishad (Kolkata). Research trips

(2015, 2018) to the British Library and the Wellcome Library (London, U.K.), along with the Radcliffe Science Library at the University of Oxford (Oxford, U.K.) and the Highgate Literary and Scientific Institution (Highgate, London, U.K.) turned out to be very productive due to accessibility of rare materials unavailable in India.

Questions raised in the course of my research mainly include: Is breastfeeding 'natural'? Why is it necessary to historicise breast- and artificial feeding of infants in colonial Bengal, mainly Calcutta? How are 'tradition', 'modernity', 'science' and 'hygiene' linked with breastfeeding? How does breastfeeding fit into the broader discourse on nutrition? How are various aspects of gender and breastfeeding connected? How was breastfeeding associated with the debates on the age of consent, child marriage and premature maternity? What were the reasons given, in relation to infant feeding, to explain the maternal and infant morbidity and mortality rates at the time? How was infant feeding related to intellection on and processes concerning the medicalisation of childbirth and midwifery? Why was regimentation of breastfeeding and artificial feeding of infants necessary? Why was disciplined weaning of infants important for maternal and infant health? Did breastfeeding or artificial feeding determine if someone was a 'good' versus 'bad' mother? Why was surveillance over 'who' was breastfeeding necessary? Or why were caste, class, and character, only to name a few credentials, relevant when breastfeeding? Could a mother or wet nurse feed milk, diseases as well as values/vices through breast milk? What was the 'ideal' diet of lactating mothers? How were imported baby foods and galactagogues (substances promoting lactation) advertised and did these reveal contemporary worldviews on breastfeeding and artificial feeding of infants? What were the pros and cons of artificial feeding of infants as discussed in English and Bengali print media? In short, rising awareness about what comprised 'modern' maternities and associated 'proper' infant feeding practices was a significant politically charged, 'scientific' mode of interfering with the daily lives of individuals, families and communities. Throughout my book, medical discourses on breastfeeding is situated within the overarching framework of the colonial 'civilising missions' and anti-colonial nation-building.

Outline of Chapters

Following is a brief outline of the five main chapters of this book focused on medicine and the mothering of infants in colonial Bengal, mainly Calcutta. The first chapter is designed to cast a wide net by putting a spotlight on medical and popular handbooks about maternal and infant healthcare in 'tropical' India. It is divided into three sections namely: Milk, Maternities and Manliness; Governing Ideas: *Dais*, Memsahibs and Medicine; and Artificial Foods versus Wet Nursing. It explores, previously underexplored, medical practitioner Frederick Corbyn's *Management and Diseases of Infants* which was one of the earliest medical manuals on memsahibs and childcare in India. Corbyn reinterpreted mainstream ideas about both European and 'native' maternal bodies in the 'tropics' with an extra dose of 'scientific' racialism. This chapter, therefore, problematises, analyses and reinterprets the governing assumption that the tropical environment ruined the nursing capacities of memsahibs whereby Indian wet nurses had to be hired. In the process, it explores army doctor Francis Roberts Hogg's medical advice in detail. It also examines a wide range of representations of the dangerous yet bountiful Indian wet nurse as well as the non-breastfeeding memsahib with faulty lactation in the tropical environment. Finally, it also discusses medical and popular opinions on artificial feeding versus wet nursing of infants in colonial India.

The second chapter situates medical advice on breastfeeding amidst the processes of the medicalisation of childbirth, midwifery and wet nursing. It is divided into two main sections namely: The 'dai question' and Innocence of Maternal Breasts: Divine/Natural/Maternal/Sexual/Economical. The first section explores European and indigenous medical writings on 'scientific' midwifery in colonial Calcutta. The second section questions the 'innocence' of maternal (lactating) breasts. This is compared and contrasted with the elaborate medical lists for the bodily examination of the wet nurse, the economical breast. It also explores gender disparity as a contributing factor in decisions about and/or duration of maternal breastfeeding and/or wet nursing as also discussed by famous 'lady doctor' Haimabati Sen.

The third chapter focuses on a discussion about the concomitant glorification as well as pathologisation and medicalisation of 'Indian mothers' and their mother love in contemporary medical literature in colonial Bengal. It is divided into two sections namely: Customs, Prejudices and Breastfeeding; and Materialities of Modern Motherhood? Clocks, Corsets, and '*Cheleder Khabar*'. The first section provides an analysis of the horrifying customary breastfeeding practice of 'exposure of infants'. This is followed by an examination of the problems associated with the more quotidian breastfeeding practices of prolonged lactation, and 'constantly breastfeeding' whenever the child cried. In the second section, the materialities of 'modern' Indian motherhood in colonial Calcutta – from mechanical clocks to maternal dress and diet – are discussed. It also touches on medicalised discussions about milk-borne diseases associated with the adulterated milk supply amidst the contemporary high infant and maternal morbidity and mortality rates.

The fourth chapter examines the problem of breastfeeding in early motherhood as crucial to the age of consent debates (1890s–1920s) in colonial Bengal. It is divided into three sections namely: 'Premature Maternity' Criticised; 'Premature Maternity' Defended; and 'Mother India' and Childcare. The timeframe of this chapter is delimited by the Age of Consent Act (1891) and the Child Marriage Restraint Act (1929). It contributes towards situating breastfeeding of infants amidst the broader context of intense discussions on the female/maternal body, sexuality, conjugality, early motherhood, nutrition, and high infant and maternal morbidity and mortality in colonial Bengal. It also investigates the *Mother India* controversy and the problems in nursing of infants as discussed in pro-imperialist American journalist, Katherine Mayo's *Mother India* published in 1927.

Finally, the fifth chapter discusses the Health and Child Welfare Exhibition in colonial Calcutta in 1920. Introduction: Exhibition, Knowledge and Power is followed by three main sections namely: From 'Dirty Midwifery' to 'Clean Midwifery'; The *Bhadramahila* Ideal; and a final section Child's Cries to Ticking Clocks. The first section, in particular, interrogates the so-called *bhadra* or 'respectable', often upper caste and middle-class disdain towards the *dai* palpable in the Calcutta Exhibition lectures. The second section critically analyses Bengali instruction offered at the Exhibition about the very making of the 'ideal' *bhadramahila* mother figure. I am interested in the 'women's question' as it related primarily to the Hindu Bengali *bhadramahila* in colonial Calcutta. In the process, it also problematises the contemporary quotidian usage of the very term *bhadramahila*. The third section discusses famous Brahmo and nationalist *daktar* Sundari Mohan Das' works which brought together 'tradition' and 'modernity' as he combined western medicine, Ayurveda and Hinduism in his deification of the breastfeeding 'Indian mother' figure as *Ma Lakkhi* (Hindu goddess of wealth and prosperity) and concomitant pathologisation as *Putana* (Hindu mythological demoness) based on her habit of always breastfeeding whenever the child cried which had to be replaced by the modern clock and regular feeds. Transnational discursive associations are drawn with the global infant welfare movement. This book keeps a keen eye on the fact that the male child/*balak*/*cheley* was mainly addressed in the manuals and periodical essays to advertisements of tinned baby foods, as the only future citizens of the nation. The girl child often remained invisible and implied.

Notes

1 On the sociological concept of 'medicalization', see Ivan Illich, *Medical Nemesis: The Expropriation of Health* (New York: Pantheon Books, first American ed. 1976); Peter Conrad, *Deviance and Medicalization: From Badness to Sickness*. (Philadelphia: Temple University Press, expanded ed. 1992); among others. However, my research builds on and furthers Anna Davin's arguments on medicalised motherhood or 'mothercraft', see Anna Davin, 'Imperialism and Motherhood' *History Workshop*, vol. 5, no. 1, 1978, pp. 9–65; and Supriya Guha's historical analysis of the medicalisation of midwifery and childbirth in colonial Bengal, Supriya Guha, 'A History of the Medicalisation of Childbirth in Bengal in the Late Nineteenth and Twentieth Centuries', Unpublished PhD Thesis, University of Calcutta, 1996.

2 Here, the focus is on the Bengali-Hindu *bhadramahila*/the so-called 'respectable', upper and middle class and caste women usually confined in the seclusion

of *purdah* and homebirths, instead of hospital births, in the 'polluted' and 'dirty' lying-in rooms, the *sutikagriha* or *anturghar*. The *bhadramahila* was gradually addressed as the literate, 'new woman' reader and author, see Partha Chatterjee, 'The Nationalist Resolution of the Women's Question', in Kumkum Sangari and Sudesh Vaid (eds), *Recasting Women. Essays in Colonial History* (New Delhi: Kali for Women, 1989), pp. 233–253; and Meredith Borthwick, *The Changing Role of Women in Bengal, 1849–1905* (Princeton: Princeton University Press, 1984).

3 Nupur Chaudhuri argues that '[t]he term "memsahib" was used originally to show respect for a European married woman in the Bengal Presidency, the first portion denoting "ma'am"; over the years the usage spread throughout the British colonies in Southeast Asia and Africa', Nupur Chaudhuri, 'Memsahibs and Motherhood in Nineteenth-Century Colonial India', *Victorian Studies*, vol. 31, no. 4, 1988, p. 517n3.

4 In Bengal, the Sanskrit term *dhātrī*/'a nurse' refers to both the traditional midwife and wet nurse. It is derived from *dhā* meaning 'to nurse' – Franco Rendich, *Comparative etymological Dictionary of classical Indo-European languages Indo-European – Sanskrit – Greek – Latin*, trans. by Gordon Davis (n.p., 2013), pp. 273–274; also see Guha, 'A History of the Medicalisation of Childbirth in Bengal in the Late Nineteenth and Twentieth Centuries', pp. 114–116 for an interesting discussion on *dais* and terminology. They were hired from lower castes and classes like the 'Dome and the Bagthee caste', among others – Shib Chunder Bose, *The Hindoos as They Are. A Description of the Manners, Customs and Inner Life of Hindoo Society in Bengal* (With a Prefatory Note by The Rev. W. Hastie, B. D. Principal of the General Assembly's Institution; Calcutta: W. Newman & Co., 1881), p. 23, Sujata Mukherjee, 'Medical Education and Emergence of Women Medics in Colonial Bengal', Occasional Paper 37, Institute of Development Studies, Kolkata, August 2012, pp. 17, 27. For a detailed discussion, see chapters 2 and 5 in this book.

5 To gain an understanding of the 'biocultural' and the complex overlaps of biology/culture in a colonial setting like India, useful readings include David B. Morris, *Illness and Culture in the Postmodern Age* (Berkeley: University of California Press, 1998); Molly K. Zuckerman and Debra L. Martin (eds), *New Directions in Biocultural Anthropology* (New Jersey: John Wiley & Sons, 2016); Peter Robb (ed.), *The Concept of Race in South Asia* (Oxford: Oxford University Press, 1995); Meena Radhakrishna, 'Of Apes and Ancestors: Evolutionary Science and Colonial Ethnography', *The Indian Historical Review*, vol. XXXIII, no. 1, 2006, pp.1–23; Ishita Pande, *Medicine, Race and Liberalism in British Bengal Symptoms of Empire* (London: Routledge, 2010); among many others.

6 Judith E. Walsh, *How to Be the Goddess of Your Home. An Anthology of Bengali Domestic Manuals* (New Delhi: Yoda Press, 2005), pp. 2–3.

7 On medicalised motherhood or 'mothercraft', Davin, 'Imperialism and Motherhood'; and Kalpana Ram and Margaret Jolly (eds), *Maternities and Modernities Colonial and Postcolonial Experiences in Asia and the Pacific* (Cambridge: Cambridge University Press, 1998); also on medicalisation and commodification of infant foods see Valerie A. Fildes, *Breasts, Bottles and Babies A History of Infant Feeding* (Edinburgh: Edinburgh University Press, 1986); and Penny Van Esterik, 'The Politics of Breastfeeding: An Advocacy Update', in Carol Counihan and Penny Van Esterik (eds), *Food and Culture a Reader* (New York: Routledge, third ed. 2003), pp. 510–530, among others.

8 The phrase 'clean midwifery' has been quoted from Lt. – Colonel E. E. Waters, I.M.S., Superintendent, Howrah General Hospital cited in 'Chapter II. Opinions of Provinces. I. – Bengal Presidency', in *Improvements of the Conditions*

of Childbirth in India Including a Special Report on the Work of the Victoria Memorial Scholarships Fund during the Past Fifteen Years and Papers Written by Medical Women and Qualified Midwives (Calcutta: Superintendent Government Printing, India, 1918), p. 10. Also, see Margaret I. Balfour and Ruth Young, *The Work of Medical Women in India* (With a foreword by Dame Mary Scharlieb; London: Humphrey Milford Oxford University Press, 1929), p. 140.

9 Maneesha Lal, '"The ignorance of women is the house of illness". Gender, Nationalism, and Health Reform in Colonial North India', in Mary P. Sutphen and Bridie Andrews (eds), *Medicine and Colonial Identity* (London: Routledge, 2003), pp. 14–40; and Geraldine Forbes, *Women in Colonial India. Essays in Politics, Medicine, and Historiography* (New Delhi: Chronicle Books, 2005), pp. 79–100; and Ranjana Saha, 'Milk, Mothering & Meanings: Infant Feeding in Colonial Bengal', *Women's Studies International Forum*, vol. 60, 2017, pp. 97–110

10 See Mary Douglas, *Purity and Danger: An Analysis of the Concepts of Pollution and Taboo* (London: Routledge, ARK ed. 1984, first ed. 1966), especially pp. 37, 124–129. Here Douglas discusses religion and 'germ theory' in relation to 'dirt', and thereafter 'dirt', ritual pollution, body, caste and cooking of food in Hinudism.

11 Georges Canguilhem, *The Normal and the Pathological* (New York: Zone Books, 1991, French ed. 1966), p. 228 in Margaret Lock and Vinh-Kim Nguyen, *An Anthropology of Biomedicine* (Chichester: Wiley-Blackwell, 2010), p. 44.

12 Colin Jones and Roy Porter argue that Michel Foucault was also influenced by Canguilhem's arguments on epistemological 'ruptures' located amidst the backdrop of Fernand Braudel's (of the Annales School) notion of the *longue durée* and Marxist ideas on the human will. Colin Jones and Roy Porter (eds), *Reassessing Foucault Power, Medicine and the Body* (New York: Routledge, 1994), p. 7.

13 Lock and Nguyen, *An Anthropology of Biomedicine*, pp. 37–38, 43–45.

14 Ambalika Guha, *Colonial Modernities Midwifery in Bengal, c. 1860–1947* (London: Routledge, 2018), p. 7.

15 Ibid., pp. 33, 36–39.

16 Michel Foucault, *The History of Sexuality* Volume I: An Introduction Translated From the French by Robert Hurley (New York: Pantheon Books, 1978), pp. 67–69.

17 Ibid., p. 100.

18 Ibid.

19 Ibid., p. 101.

20 Edward W. Said, *Orientalism* (New York: Vintage Books, 1979, reprint of Pantheon Books edition 1978), p. 3. He emphasises that a discourse is not in a 'direct, corresponding relationship with political power in the raw, but rather is produced and exists in an uneven exchange with various kinds of power'. Said stresses on 'the exchange' (of power) between 'power political'/'colonial or imperial establishment', 'power intellectual'/'reigning sciences like comparative linguistics or anatomy', 'power cultural'/'orthodoxies and canons of taste, texts, values', and 'power moral'/'ideas about what "we" do and what "they" cannot do or understand as "we" do'. Ibid., p. 12

21 Ibid., pp. 1–2.

22 Michel Foucault, *Discipline and Punish: The Birth of the Prison.* Translated from the French by Alan Sheridan (New York: Vintage Books, second ed. 1991).

23 Robbie P. Kahn's analysis of 'cyclical' or 'maialogical time' in Robbie P. Kahn, 'Women and Time in Childbirth and During Lactation', in Frieda Johles Forman and Caoran Sowton (eds), *Taking Our Time Feminist Perspectives on Temporality* (New York: Pergamon Press, 1988), pp. 27–29; Fiona Dykes,

Breastfeeding in Hospital Mothers, Midwives and the Production Line (New York: Routledge, 2006), pp. 96–97, 126.
24 Dykes, *Breastfeeding in Hospital*, pp. 80, 85; Alison Bartlett, 'Babydaze: Maternal Time', *Time & Society*, vol. 19, 2010, pp. 122–123
25 Dykes, *Breastfeeding in Hospital*, pp. 170–171. Also, a significant prior study on time, work and family – Tamara K. Hareven, *Family Time and Industrial Time: The Relationship Between the Family and Work in New England Industrial Community* (Cambridge: Cambridge University Press, 1982).
26 Tanika Sarkar, 'Nationalist Iconography: Image of Women in 19th Century Bengali Literature', *Economic & Political Weekly*, vol. 22, no. 47, 1987, p. 2011.
27 Sumit Sarkar, *Writing Social History* (Delhi: Oxford University Press, 1997), p. 191. On clock time, E. P. Thompson, 'Time, Work-Discipline and Industrial Capitalism', *Past and Present*, vol. 38, no. 1, 1967, pp. 56–97. Sumit Sarkar's arguments on the Kaliyuga and print culture need to be read together with his earlier work on the Swadeshi Movement in Bengal. He argues that there were contradictions inherent in the grand narrative of anti-colonial nation-building, primarily about the Swadeshi Movement (against the partitioning of Bengal which called for a boycott of foreign goods and self-reliance). He analyses various kinds of archival and published sources in order to highlight problems associated with idealistic nationalist rhetoric especially the contradictory pulls of moderate/militant and modernist/traditionalist ideas (for instance, Rabindranath Tagore's *Ghare Baire*), *bhadralok* anxieties about class/caste hierarchies, Hindu-Muslim rivalries, and shifts in thinking about gender relations (mainly conjugality) during and after the Movement. See Sumit Sarkar, *The Swadeshi Movement in Bengal 1903–1908* New Edition with a Preface by the author and critical essays by Neeladri Bhattacharya and Dipesh Chakrabarty (Ranikhet: Permanent Black, 2010, first ed. 1973).
28 Sarkar, *Writing Social History*, p. 188.
29 Ibid.
30 Ibid.
31 Ibid.
32 Ibid., p. 190.
33 Ibid., p. 191.
34 Ibid.
35 For examples of clocked feeding in English and Bengali manuals at the time, see Meredith Borthwick, *The Changing Role of Women in Bengal*, pp. 174–175.
36 Davin, 'Imperialism and Motherhood', p. 10.
37 Ibid., p. 13.
38 Ibid., p. 12.
39 Milton Lewis, 'The Problem of Infant Feeding: The Australian Experience From the Mid-Nineteenth Century to the 1920s', *Journal of the History of Medicine and Allied Sciences*, vol. 35, no. 2, 1980, p. 187.
40 See Lal, 'The ignorance of women is the house of illness', pp. 14–40.
41 Lewis, 'The Problem of Infant Feeding', p. 177; Milton Lewis, 'The "health of the race" and infant health in New South Wales: perspectives on medicine and empire', in Roy Macleod and Milton Lewis (eds), *Disease, Medicine and Empire Perspectives on Western Medicine and the Experience of European Expansion* (New York: Routledge, 1988), p. 307.
42 Arthur Newsholme, 'Domestic infection in relation to epidemic diarrhoea', *The Journal of Hygiene*, Camb., vol. 6., no. 2, 1906, pp. 139–148 in Lewis, 'The Problem of Infant Feeding', p. 177.
43 Lewis, 'The Problem of Infant Feeding', pp. 177–178.

44 Lewis, 'The "health of the race" and infant health in New South Wales', p. 301.
45 Ibid., pp. 301, 306.
46 Ibid., p. 308.
47 Ibid.
48 See Daniel R. Headrick, *The Tools of Empire Technology and European Imperialism in the Nineteenth Century* (New York: Oxford University Press, 1981), pp. 11, 205–206, 209.
49 Ibid., p. 209.
50 On racism as racist discrimination and racialism as race theory or so-called 'race science' – see Tzvetan Todorov, *On Human Diversity: Nationalism, Racism, and Exoticism in French Thought* (trans. Catherine Porter, *Convergences: Inventories of the Present*; Cambridge and London: Harvard University Press, 1993) in Ishita Pande, *Medicine, Race and Liberalism in British Bengal Symptoms of Empire* (London: Routledge, 2010), p. 201n103. Pande highlights:

> Tzetvan Todorov adds that when a political end is based on such a knowledge of race, and race theory is put to practice, the racialist joins the racist; it is therefore possible to talk of liberal racism in discussing policies erected on racialist doctrines. Examples abound in colonial Indian history – the denial of positions in the Civil Services to qualified Indians, the existence of separate spaces for natives in public places, the denial of military employment to certain natives based on a 'Martial Races' theory, the refusal to let a qualified native judge preside over a European's trial. See Ibid.

51 David Arnold, *Colonizing the Body State Medicine and Epidemic Disease in Nineteenth-Century India* (Berkeley and Los Angeles, CA: University of California Press, 1993), pp. 9–10; also see Shula Marks, 'What is Colonial about Colonial Medicine? And What has Happened to Imperialism and Health?', *Social History of Medicine*, vol. 10, no. 2, 1997, p. 206.
52 Arnold, *Colonizing the Body*, p. 35.
53 Ibid., p. 10.
54 Ibid., pp. 7–8.
55 Ibid., p. 8.
56 Ibid.
57 Ibid.
58 Ibid., p. 52. Also, on early twentieth-century derecognition of indigenous medical practitioners and revival, see Poonam Bala, *Imperialism a Medicine in Bengal: A Socio-Historical Perspective* (New Delhi: Sage Publications, 1991), especially pp. 80–92.
59 Arnold, *Colonizing the Body*, p. 53.
60 See Pande, *Medicine, Race and Liberalism in British Bengal*, pp. 2–3, 6, 13, 22. My analytical methodology which builds on Pande's Foucauldian approach has been discussed in the following section of this Introduction.
61 Projit Bihari Mukharji, *Nationalizing the Body The Medical Market, Print and Daktari Medicine* (Delhi: Anthem Press, 2012; U.K. and U.S.A. edition 2009), p. 33, 85, 177.
62 Rachel Berger, *Ayurveda Made Modern Political Histories of Indigenous Medicine in North India 1900–1955* (New York: Palgrave MacMillan, 2013), pp. 10–11.
63 Mukharji, *Nationalizing the Body*, p. 82.
64 On '*ledi daktars*' see Mukharji, *Nationalizing the Body*, pp. 108–09. For instance, indigenous medical practitioners like Jodu Nath Mukerje asserted their active agency by his daily medical practice as well as through his medical

treatises. There is a brief dedication to T. E. Charles, EsQ., M.D., Professor of Midwifery and Diseases of Children, at the Medical College, Calcutta included right at the beginning of Mukerje's (Licentiate in Medicine and Surgery or L.M.S. from Calcutta Medical College) book titled *Dhatri Sikkha*. It reads '[t]his little volume is respectfully dedicated as a token of Gratitude and Esteem for his high professional acquirements by His obliged and Obedient pupil the Author'. See Jodu Nath Mukerje, *Dhatri Sikkha: A Guide to the Dhaees or Native Midwives and to the Mothers Written in the Form of a Dialogue in Two Parts* Part 1, (Chinsura: Printed by Greesh Chunder Bhuttacharje, Chitsaprokash Press, third ed. 1875, first ed 1867), n.p. In the Preface, he mentions:

> [I]t is true that native midwives seldom know to read or to write, but if there were in existence a work in their own vernacular giving practical lessons in the art they follow, they would, no doubt, avail themselves of the earliest opportunity of getting at those lessons . . . a book can be adapted to their comprehension by being written in the form of a dialogue, which is the most impressive of all methods of conveying knowledge to simple and unsophisticated minds.

The book was written in two parts, the first part focused on the management of pregnancy, childbirth and proper nursing of the child till two years' old. Here he also added that '[b]esides being of use to native midwives . . . the book may be read by Hindoo-females who will no longer place themselves in the hands of ignorant women in one of the most critical periods of their life'. This excerpt has been cited from Jodu Nath Mukerje, *Dhatri Sikkha*, pp. 1–2. His name is spelt here as in the third edition of his book, *Dhatri Sikkha*. Also, a part of this excerpt has been mentioned in Chapter 2 of this book.

65 Usually the designation *daktar* was a professional, social identity for a 'native' doctor based on local reputation, social background and different levels of training in varied medical traditions mainly western allopathic medicine and homeopathy. Mukharji, *Nationalizing the Body*, pp. 1, 32. Mukharji talks about 'provincializing' of western medicine by *daktars*. His arguments dovetail the wider argument in Dipesh Chakrabarty, *Provincializing Europe Postcolonial Thought and Historical Difference* (Princeton: Princeton University Press, 2000). Also, on this subject, see mainly Deepak Kumar, *Science and the Raj 1857–1905* (Delhi: Oxford University Press, 1995); and Dhruv Raina and S. Irfan Habib, *Domesticating Modern Science: A Social History of Science and Culture in Colonial India* (New Delhi: Tulika Books, 2004).

66 Chatterjee, 'The Nationalist Resolution of the Women's Question'; Jasodhara Bagchi, 'Representing Nationalism: Ideology of Motherhood in Colonial Bengal', *Economic and Political Weekly*, vol. 25, no. 42/43, 1990, p. WS65.

67 Chatterjee, 'The Nationalist Resolution of the Women's Question'. I also build on the argument that the private/public are interrelated spaces from mainly Tanika Sarkar, 'Rhetoric Against Age of Consent: Resisting Colonial Reason and Death of a Child-Wife', *Economic & Political Weekly*, vol. 28, no. 36, 1993, pp. 1869–1878; Mrinalini Sinha, *Mother India* by Katherine Mayo. Edited with an Introduction by Mrinalini Sinha (Ann Arbor, MI: University of Michigan Press, 2000); Satadru Sen, 'The Savage Family: Colonialism and Female Infanticide in Nineteenth-Century India', *Journal of Women's History*, vol. 14, no. 3, 2002, pp. 53–79, among others.

68 Partha Chatterjee, *Our Modernity* (Rotterdam and Dakar: SEPHIS CODESRIA, 1997), p. 14.

69 Ibid.

70 See Pande's analysis of Chatterjee's arguments in Pande, *Medicine, Race and Liberalism in British Bengal*, p. 8. Pande refers to Chatterjee's argument in Partha Chatterjee, *The Nation and Its Fragments: Colonial and Postcolonial Histories* (Delhi: Oxford University Press, 1994), p. 19 in Pande, *Medicine, Race and Liberalism in British Bengal*, p. 8.
71 David Arnold, *The Tropics and the Traveling Gaze India, Landscape, and Science 1800–1856* (Delhi: Permanent Black, 2005), p. 137. Also, see Arnold, *Colonizing the Body*, Biswamoy Pati and Mark Harrison, *The Social History of Health and Medicine in Colonial India* (London: Taylor and Francis, 2011); Peter Robb, *The Concept of Race in South Asia* (Oxford: Oxford University Press, 1995); and Thomas R. Trautmann, *Aryans and British India* (New Delhi: Yoda Press, 2004).
72 Margaret Jolly 'Introduction Colonial and postcolonial plots in histories of maternities and modernities', in Ram and Jolly, *Maternities and modernities*, p. 1.
73 Ibid.
74 Ibid.
75 Ibid., p. 2.
76 Ibid., p. 4.
77 Ibid.
78 Borthwick, *The Changing Role of Women in Bengal*, p. 159.
79 Supriya Guha, '"The Best Swadeshi": Reproductive Health in Bengal, 1840–1940', in Sarah Hodges (ed), *Reproductive Health in India. History, Politics, Controversies* (Hyderabad: Orient Longman, 2006), p. 153.
80 Walsh, *How to Be the Goddess of Your Home*, p. 1.
81 Ibid., pp. 2–3.
82 Ibid., p. 3.
83 Ibid., pp. 2–3; Judith E. Walsh, *Domesticity in colonial India what women learned when men gave them advice* (New York: Rowman and Littlefield Publishers, Inc., 2004), p. 14.
84 Nagendrabala Dasi, *Nari Dharma* (Woman's Dharma), (Calcutta: Published by the author, 1900) in Walsh, *How to Be the Goddess of Your Home*, pp. 135, 150, 159.
85 Walsh, *How to Be the Goddess of Your Home*, p. 9.
86 Dasi, *Nārī Dharma* in Walsh, *How to Be the Goddess of Your Home*, p. 162.
87 See mainly Sumit Sarkar, 'The Women's Question' in Nineteenth Century Bengal', in Kumkum Sangari and Sudesh Vaid (eds), *Women and Culture* (Bombay: Research Centre for Women's Studies, 1994), pp. 103–112; and Chatterjee, 'The Nationalist Resolution of the Women's Question'.
88 Tapti Roy, 'Disciplining the Printed Text: Colonial and Nationalist Surveillance of Bengali Literature', in Partha Chatterjee (ed), *Texts of Power, Emerging Disciplines in Colonial Bengal* (Minneapolis: University of Minnesota Press, 1995), p. 30.
89 *Act XXV of 1867* (reprint Calcutta: Superintendent of Government Printing, 1890) cited in Roy, 'Disciplining the Printed Text', p. 49.
90 Roy, 'Disciplining the Printed Text', p. 49.
91 Ibid.
92 Ibid.
93 Ibid., p. 53.
94 Ibid., p. 54.
95 Ibid.
96 Ibid.

97 On the 'martial races' theory as it was deployed by Lord Roberts, Commander-in-Chief of the Indian army in the 1885–1893, see Indira Chowdhury-Sengupta 'The Effeminate and the Masculine: Nationalism and the Concept of Race in Colonial Bengal', in Peter Robb (ed), *The Concept of Race in South Asia* (New Delhi: Oxford University Press, 1995), p. 288; see also Nirad C. Chaudhuri, 'The martial races of India', *Modern Review*, vol. xlviii, no. 1, 1930, pp. 41–51 and xviii, no. 3, 1930, 295–307 cited in Ibid., p. 288n19; also see Mrinalini Sinha, *Colonial Masculinity. The 'Manly Englishman' and the 'Effeminate Bengali' in the Late Nineteenth Century* (Manchester: Manchester University Press, 1995), mainly p. 27n28, among others.

98 Bernard S. Cohn *Colonialism and Its Forms of Knowledge: The British in India* (Princeton, NJ: Princeton University Press, 1996), p. 4. Also, Bernard S. Cohn 'History and Anthropology: The State of Play', *Comparative Studies in Society and History*, vol. 22, 1980, pp. 198–221, in Frederick Cooper and Ann Laura Stoler, *Tensions of Empire Colonial Cultures in a Bourgeois World* (Berkeley: University of California Press, 1997), p. 15.

99 Cohn, *Colonialism and Its Forms of Knowledge*, p. 4.

100 Ibid., p. 5.

101 Ibid.

102 Ibid.

103 Carol A. Breckenridge and Peter van der Veer, 'Orientalism and the Postcolonial Predicament' in Carol A. Breckenridge and Peter van der Veer (eds), *Orientalism and the Postcolonial Predicament Perspectives on South Asia* (Philadelphia: University of Pennsylvania Press, 1993), p. 12.

104 Anthropology or the 'scientific' study of mankind incorporates ethnography where European travellers, missionaries, scientific explorers and administrators served as ethnographers. Ethnography became moulded in the framework of a universal 'natural science' from the eighteenth century, see Carl Linnaeus (1707–1778, Swedish botanist and zoologist) and his 'Linnaean system of classification' of plants, animals and mankind. See Mary Louise Pratt, *Imperial Eyes Travel Writing and Transculturation* (New York: Routledge, 1992; this edition was published in the Taylor & Francis e-Library, 2003), pp. 24–35.

105 The impulse behind colonial ethnography, anthropometry and the censuses in late nineteenth and twentieth century British India was the need for order. Recording of such details gained enormously from the concomitant development of photography. For further information on the history of colonial anthropology and photography in British India, for example, Christopher Pinney, 'Colonial Anthropology in the Laboratory of Mankind' and John Falconer, 'Photography in Nineteenth Century India', in C. A. Bayly (ed), *The Raj India and the British 1600–1947* (London: Pearson National Portrait Gallery Publications, 1990), pp. 252–263, 278–304, among others.

106 See Susan Bayly, 'Caste and "race" in the colonial ethnography of India' and Crispin Bates, 'Race, caste and tribe in Central India: The early origins of Indian anthropometry', in Peter Robb (ed), *The Concept of Race in South Asia* (New Delhi: Oxford University Press, 1995); pp. 165–218, and 219–259; and Meena Radhakrishna, 'Of Apes and Ancestors: Evolutionary Science and Colonial Ethnography', *The Indian Historical Review*, vol. XXXIII, no. 1, 2006, pp. 1–23; among others.

107 Nicholas Dirks, *Castes of Mind Colonialism and the Making of Modern India* (Princeton: Princeton University Press, 2001), p. 9

108 Ibid., p. 185.

109 Ibid., p. 196.

110 Ibid., p. 3.

111 Ibid., p. 13.
112 Ibid., p. 196.
113 'Brief précis of an article in the Muenchener Medizinische Wochenschrift, dated January 17, 1911, by Walcher, on the subject of artificial changes in the shape of the skull', np. in *Summaries of some essays, etc. relating to census and caste* (Calcutta: The Govt Printing, 1911), Rare Books, WBSA.
114 Radhakrishna, 'Of Apes and Ancestors', p. 10.
115 Ibid., p. 17.
116 Ibid., pp. 2–3, 7–8.
117 Ibid., p. 14.
118 Bates, 'Race, caste and tribe in Central India', pp. 244–245.
119 Herbert Hope Risley, *The People of India* Edited by W. Crooke (Calcutta: Thacker, Spink & Co., second ed. 1915), p. 21.
120 Risley, *The People of India*, p. 22. Edgar Thurston, Superintendent of the Madras Government Museum (1885–1908) was the Superintendent of the Ethnographic Survey of the Madras Presidency. His *Castes and Tribes of Southern India* (7 volumes, 1909) shared Risley's faith in anthropometry. For a discussion on Thurston, see mainly Dirks, *Castes of Mind*, pp. 183–192.
121 Risley, *The People of India*, p. 278.
122 On traditional birthing practices, *dais* and western medicine, see Forbes, *Women in Colonial India*; Guha, 'A History of the Medicalisation of Childbirth in Bengal in the Late Nineteenth and Twentieth Centuries', and Supriya Guha, 'Midwifery in Colonial India The role of traditional birth attendants in colonial India', *Wellcome History*, vol. 28, 2005, pp. 2–3, (Accessed 5 October 2014). www.wellcome.ac.uk/stellent/groups/corporatesite/@msh_publishing_group/documents/web_document/wtx024905.pdf
123 Guha, 'Midwifery in Colonial India', p. 2.
124 Ibid., p. 2.
125 Projit Bihari Mukharji, 'Symptoms of Dis-Ease: New Trends in the Histories of "Indigenous" South Asian Medicines', *History Compass*, vol. 9/12, 2011, p. 887
126 Marks, 'What Is Colonial About Colonial Medicine?, ' pp. 205–219.
127 Pande, *Medicine, Race and Liberalism in British Bengal;* Tanika Sarkar, *Hindu Wife, Hindu Nation Community, Religion and Cultural Nationalism* (Delhi: Permanent Black, 2001), Walsh, *Domesticity in Colonial India*; Forbes, *Women in Colonial India*; Himani Bannerji, 'Fashioning a Self: Educational Proposals for and by Women in Popular Magazines in Colonial Bengal', *Economic and Political Weekly*, vol. 26, no. 43, 1991, pp. WS50–WS62, among others.
128 Pande, *Medicine, Race and Liberalism in British Bengal*, p. 7.
129 Ibid.
130 Ibid., 16.
131 Ibid.
132 Ibid.
133 Gyan Prakash's main argument that continues throughout his book is that indigenised ways of attempting to address the 'colonial difference' mark out subversive and counter-hegemonic notions of subjectification. Prakash does not consider western medicine as a discourse of Othering which maybe disempowered and applied in the process of creating the colonial subject, as illustrated in Pande's arguments in Pande, *Medicine, Race and Liberalism in British Bengal*, p. 6. Also, see Gyan Prakash, *Another Reason: Science in the Making of Modern India* (Princeton: Princeton University Press, 2000).
134 Pande, *Medicine, Race and Liberalism in British Bengal*, pp. 3, 6.

135 Srirupa Prasad, *Cultural Politics of Hygiene in India 1890–1940 Contagions of Feeling* (New York: Palgrave Macmillan, 2015), p. 17.
136 Annada Charan Khastagir, *A Treatise on the Science and Practice of Midwifery With Diseases of Children and Women Manab-Jatna Tattva, Dhatribidya, Nabaprasuto Sishu o Stri Jatir Byadhi - Sangraha* (Calcutta: Author, second ed. 1878, first ed. 1868)
137 Kabiraj Sri Harimohan Dasgupta, *Ayurvediyo Dhatribidya Sangraha. Pratham Khando: A Compilation of Ayurvedic Midwifery* Part 1 (Berhampur: Kabiraj Srinikhilranjan Sengupta Kabibhushan Berhampur Dhanantari Pharmacy, Bengali Year 1324, c.1917).
138 Surendranath Goswami, *Arya Dhatribidya. A Treatise on the Ayurvedic System of Midwifery w*ith Sanskrit text and English translation. Part I (Kumarkhali: Author, 1899)
139 Also, see Saha, 'Milk, "Race" and Nation', p. 155.
140 Guha, *Colonial Modernities*, p. 36.

1

TROPICANA MILK*

The Wellcome Witness Seminar report titled *The Resurgence of Breastfeeding, 1975–2000* (2009), acknowledges that –

> breast-milk was always seen as a good thing. But the fact that it came out of women was the problem. Breastfeeding women weren't supposed to have sex, to be temperamental or red-headed; if they did any of these things their milk wouldn't be good.[1]

It was considered 'better to have the vegetarian, nerveless cow, than a woman who has temper tantrums, is weak, failing, or hasn't eaten well'.[2] This chapter primarily focuses on medical criteria for hiring of wet nurses for European infants in nineteenth and early twentieth century colonial India. Domestic and medical handbooks gradually became popular contemporary genres among British wives of colonial officials who consistently arrived 'to set up "English" style homes in India' from the 1860s onwards following the opening of the Suez Canal and decrease in duration of travel.[3] Medical advice about breastfeeding of European infants in 'tropical' India ranged from the regulation of diet and behaviour to increase the flow of milk in the mother/wet nurse to a detailed bodily examination of the wet nurse and her child for hiring purposes. Colonial medical instruction to memsahib mothers concerning 'ideal' infant feeding was aimed at the management and regeneration of 'racial' and national health and strength in the tropics with imperial and colonial agendas.[4] The main argument is that medical and popular handbooks on maternal and infant healthcare in colonial India, and here I am only focusing on those primarily addressing colonial officials and their families, provided expert knowledge about domesticity and motherhood to tackle anxieties about childrearing in the tropics by creating a specific kind of memsahib mother.[5] I would like to begin with reference to these two excerpts at the start of the chapter that encapsulate the governing assumption that the tropical environment ruined the nursing capacities

DOI: 10.4324/9781003327837-2

of memsahibs which resulted in the hiring of the 'native' Indian wet nurse (*dhai/dai* or *amah*) as 'a virtual milch cow',[6] and/or 'feeding'[7] of infants:

> Whenever a bottle or spoonfed child comes under treatment in England, the medical practitioner is ever anxious for a wet-nurse, and in India a thousand times more so. . . . Wet-nurses are very inconvenient, and goats in many senses a great nuisance, but where there are children there remains no option.[8]
>
> The nursing mother, without being fidgety, should be careful to keep to wholesome and simple food herself; this principle to be followed in the case of the wet-nurse or *dhâi*, and even of the cow, for the sudden change from *bhoosa* to green wheat will affect the cow's milk, and the child's motions through the milk.[9]

Memsahibs weakened by the tropical climate were most often represented as inadequate mothers with 'little milk'.[10] Medical and popular childcare advice literature warned about 'chicanery in the native nurses' who 'generally eat opium' and have the 'extraordinary power of drawing back the suck'.[11] However, despite anxiety, suspicion and contempt about hiring the Indian wet nurse, her breasts were often positively tropicalised in medical handbooks as being blessed with an abundant supply of *natural* and nutritious milk, a tropical bounty at the service of the European families residing in India. This chapter problematises and analyses the representations of the Indian wet nurse as dangerous yet usually bountiful hired as an unavoidable necessity to save the life of European infants as well as the characterisation of the memsahib as deficient mothers in the 'tropics' – both tropicalised and problematic. The first section of this chapter is a case study of one of the earliest medical manuals on maternal and infant care in India, written by surgeon, Frederick Corbyn of the East India Company's Bengal medical establishment.[12] It offered a highly racialised and gendered reinterpretation of the governing assumptions about the nursing of European infants in 'tropical' India. The second section begins with a discussion on 'tropicality' followed by the general climate of medical and popular thought about the nursing of European infants by memsahibs and *dais* in 'tropical' India. In this regard, it explores army doctor Surgeon-Major Francis Roberts Hogg's, previously underexplored, childcare advice in detail. This chapter closes by discussing opinions about artificial foods versus wet nursing of infants and, subsequently, summarises the main conclusions of the chapter.

Milk, Maternities and Manliness

Frederick Corbyn's *Management and Diseases of Infants Under the Influence of the Climate of India* (1828) is one of the earliest medical manuals which addressed (European) 'women' and 'medical men' on guidelines about childcare and infantile diseases in 'tropical' India. It has been largely neglected by prior scholarship on western medical literature concerning the health of memsahibs and their children in the 'tropics'. Corbyn recommended a detailed regimen for maternal and child welfare, including the benefits of disciplined breastfeeding of infants, in 'tropical' India.[13] However, as I argue, his highly racialised and gendered reinterpretation of governing assumptions about the nursing of European infants in the 'tropics' is most significant as a clear indication of his intentions about a broader refashioning of imperial and colonial domesticities and maternities in early nineteenth-century tropical India.[14] 'Race', class and gender figured prominently in his reinterpretation of dominant assumptions about the 'degenerative' effects of the tropical climate on the memsahib mother and her children.[15] He considered the tropics unsuitable for memsahibs' health but he opted for the counterintuitive choice of deploying his medical knowledge and experience as a physician to discard many popular notions about climatic determinism as he used diet as a medical remedy to ensure memsahib's capacity for effective breastfeeding of her children in the 'tropics'.[16]

Pratik Chakrabarti highlights that Corbyn was one of the 'most important scientists in colonial India'.[17] He was born in Manchester in 1792. In 1813, after completion of his medical degree from London, he joined the East India Company's medical establishment in Bengal. He was also the editor of the *Indian Journal of Medical and Physical Science*, and in 1836, he started the periodical *India Review and Journal of Foreign Science and Arts*.[18] Chakrabarti argues that colonial scientists like Corbyn often put forward an 'Orientalist challenge to claims of European superiority' because they were primarily interested in their research alone.[19] As colonialism was a battle for power/knowledge with colonial imperatives, the control of knowledge did not belong to scientists.[20] Building on and moving beyond Chakrabarti's argument here, it is highlighted that Corbyn's plea for government aid for scientific research in India was accompanied by the desire to 'erect the fabric of our rule and future prosperity on a permanent basis'.[21]

Valerie A. Fildes argues that tropical regions posed specific problems for young women who, for example, travelled to India in order to marry and start a family. They 'often married at a particularly young age – the mid and late teens – and were isolated from women of their own acquaintance'.[22] Therefore, they had to manage with little assistance they got from 'native' women or any European, official or soldier's, wives who lived nearby.[23] The 'special problems of young wives in India' were highlighted in 1828 in a book published 'to aid these inexperienced mothers'.[24] It elaborately discussed the problems encountered when hiring *dhyes* or wet nurses in India which were often similar to those experienced in England.[25] This study extends Fildes' arguments further by examining why Corbyn urged even memsahibs with 'little milk' to nurse their own children.[26] Corbyn encouraged memsahibs to breastfeed due to 'medicinal' properties of the 'first milk'.[27] Moreover, instead of agreeing with the governing notion among medical men that 'European ladies in India are not in that climate in which they were born, and where the constitution is braced and strengthened; but in one which, from excessive heat, is unhealthy and debilitating' – Corbyn emphasised that 'I fortunately found it opposed by actual experience, and discovered that ladies of feeble constitution, on nursing, in many instances actually gained strength'.[28] He acknowledged, however, that 'it is true, some instances in which nursing is not admissible; but in ordinary cases, where there is ever so little milk, I would rather give that little', 'subject to the rules I am about to give respecting making good nurses' rather than 'incur the danger arising from native nurses'.[29] About *dhyes*, he boldly claimed that the 'poor and watery milk of a native woman'[30] hardly had any nourishment and the European infant usually cried, screamed and died from nothing but hunger[31]:

> It must be granted, however, that it is the general belief that native women are the best nurses, in comparison with European ladies; but it is but fair to enquire, on what grounds? Is it because they are stronger? – because their food is richer and better; – because they have richer and purer blood flowing in their veins? – because they will partake of the appropriate food, and abide by all necessary instructions as to diet? – because they have more affection and loving feeling towards the child? May we not negative such conclusions, and confidently assert, that the argument is against native nurses? One European will almost overpower, by his innate superior strength, four native men; and may we not assert, that the same proportion of comparative strength belongs to the other sex, begging my fair readers' pardon for making such a simile; but any simile will be acceptable, I trust, in making our argument tenable. As the European is of stronger members than the native, so likewise is the milk of the former stronger and finer than that of the latter. How many poor dear babes are heard screaming and crying, their peevishness being frequently ascribed to sickness or irritability in the bowels, when in all probability it arises solely from hunger, not receiving any substantial nourishment in the poor and watery milk of a native woman. The cause thus being mistaken, castor oil or rhubarb is deemed expedient, which adds to the little sufferer's misfortunes, and tends greatly to increase its screaming: it is then ascribed to some organic affection, calling for calomel and mercurial friction, when the infant, being quite exhausted, falls a victim! So serious are the effects from such causes! so alarming the mistakes from false conclusions! I can only grant, therefore, that in some

> degree, ladies in India have poorer milk, and are considerably more delicate in constitution than those in England: notwithstanding, their milk is comparatively cream to that of any native woman's, and their capacity for nursing is fully four times as great. Ladies must, however, pursue a course different from those in Europe, and make up the deficiency arising from the influence of climate by a peculiar diet. This I now proceed to mention; and if it be rigidly followed, I have no doubt most mothers will become excellent nurses.[32]

In the aforementioned excerpt, 'race' and gender together figured in Corbyn's analysis of the 'danger arising from native nurses'[33] He emphasised the 'biological' superiority of 'whiteness' in his analysis of mothering of European infants in British India. He used the concept of effeminacy, a highly racialised and gendered stereotype of 'femininity-in-masculinity',[34] making sweeping statements about the supposedly weak and frail bodies of 'native' men and, by extension, 'native' women portraying *dais* as physically incapable of effectively nursing European infants.[35] He assigned agency to the breastfeeding memsahib, instead of the *dhye*, to distance the coloniser and colonised as he aimed to reshape imperial and colonial domesticities and motherhood.[36] The present study of Corbyn's arguments about breastfeeding aims to contribute towards a better understanding of 'what was colonial about colonial medicine'.[37]

In the section titled 'Diet for Nurses', Corbyn recommended diet as a medical remedy for scanty lactation in memsahib mothers in tropical India.[38] Corbyn advised that barley soup as a diet was specifically designed for optimum lactation in the memsahib mothers and smooth bowel movement in infants in the tropics.[39] Preferably the soup was to be concocted from 'barley first made into meal', freshly prepared twice a day to avoid 'fermentation after a lapse of a few hours' which then turned acidic, and boiled with constant stirring with a wooden spoon.[40] Besides diet, he advised nursing mothers to pay attention to the period of confinement alongside getting fresh air, adequate sleep, exercise and a steady routine.[41] He also drew attention to class prejudices against wet nurses in Britain, while he advised about the joys of maternal breastfeeding as follows:

> In the higher stations of life in Britain, ladies have deemed the office of nursing derogatory; as in their opinion, it assumes the appearance of the poorer orders of persons. Were it in their power, I have no doubt but they would desire likewise, that their shape, make, and organs, should distinguish them from the inferior class of mankind. . . . Lessening the delicacy of shape, or the elegance of figure, is often urged against nursing; deprivation from balls, routes,

> and parties is a prominent objection: while delicacy of constitution, dread of debility, and general ill health, are among the most plausible arguments. Thus then, the fifth commandment is often broken by children, who are sensible that they have not had tender, nursing mothers; and many, sinking under the indifferent, careless deputy, fall a sacrifice to this separation from maternal affection and care. The mother, likewise, is guilty of the greatest disobedience to the command of God. . . . [T]hose who are desirous of becoming real good nurses, must forego all parties and gay society, for family retirement and domestic serenity, – a hard and a terrible restriction, it must be granted, on the lively, gay, and spirited young lady! But how soon the fascinating prospect of a gay ball, the enchanting hope of a masquerade, the pleasing anticipation of the fancy play, will be found to be vain delusion and empty joy, in comparison with the charms of the playful caresses of a lovely offspring, the enjoyment of health, a fond and affectionate partner, and a peaceful, happy dwelling.[42]

The review of Corbyn's *Management and Diseases of Infants* in *The Lancet*, however, seemed sceptical about the practicality of his strict regimen and thereby commented, 'It is not every lady in India, however, who is so fortunate as to possess these strong temptations to domestic life'.[43]

It is fascinating to note that in mid-nineteenth-century Britain, Queen Victoria expressed similar prejudices against breastfeeding. Julia Baird points out that Queen Victoria despised the 'physical toll' of pregnancy and childbirth which made her 'feel like an animal'. Moreover, she also had an '"insurmountable disgust" for breastfeeding' because she considered it as 'vulgar, and inappropriate for upper-class women', and 'incompatible with performing public duties'. Baird highlights that Queen Victoria did not hesitate to employ wet nurses 'believing it better for the child if a woman who was less refined and "more like an animal" suckled them'.[44] Wet nursing 'infant royal charges' seems like an inhuman practice as Baird points out that '[e]ven wet nurses were advised to breastfeed standing up out of respect'.[45]

Corbyn appears to have been an outlier. His advice about not hiring Indian wet nurses was ignored. Yet his *Management and Diseases of Infants* remains relevant as it opens a window into the subject of anxiety-ridden mothering of European infants in the tropics. It is of particular relevance to note that his medical chauvinistic ideas about childcare by upper- and middle-class European mothers were in contrast to the later medical handbooks on 'family medicine'[46] in the 'tropics' and instead, in alignment with colonial and nationalist medical instruction to *bhadramahila* mothers about their duty to nurse their infants. It is pertinent to note, as also discussed in Chapter 2 of this book, that in 1868, Sub-Assistant Surgeon Ashraf Ali (or Meer Ushruff Ally) from the Agra Medical School was appointed as the teacher of midwifery, diseases of children and women for the Bengali licentiate class at the Calcutta Medical College.[47] He compiled two books based on his lectures and canonical western medical textbooks – *Handbook of Midwifery in Bengalee* (1869) and *Diseases of Children in Bengalee Balchikitsa* (1870), respectively. *Diseases of Children in Bengalee Balchikitsa* focused primarily on breastfeeding along with several do's and don'ts in childcare. It is rather interesting to note that he mentioned 'Dr. Corbyn's Management and Diseases of Infants' among the western medical textbooks consulted in the course of writing this book.[48]

Now, the second section delves into the historical background of the 'tropics' followed by an analysis of the governing assumptions about memsahib mothers and Indian wet nurses in 'tropical' India.

Governing Ideas: *Dais*, Memsahibs and Medicine

David Arnold highlights, 'India was in the tropics, but not necessarily of the tropics'.[49] From the fifteenth and sixteenth centuries onward, European travel and travelogues gradually constructed the 'tropics' both positively and negatively as a 'geographical and perceptual space' and a 'torrid zone' of primitiveness, fecundity, desire, danger and fear.[50] Elaborating about 'tropical' India, Arnold traces the trajectory of the tropicalisation of India – at first, disappointingly identified as the 'poor tropics' lacking tropical 'abundance' and 'fecundity' until it became, from the early nineteenth century onwards, closely associated with the 'tropics' by European travellers in terms of its 'natural violence' and 'extremes' of the 'degree' of disease and climate. He highlights that, between the 1750s and the 1820s, 'scientific tropicality' established the undoubtable 'existence of the tropics' by the 1830s while India was consistently tropicalised and identified as the 'tropics' by the 1840s.[51] Moreover, as specific geographical boundaries did not demarcate most of what is referred to as the 'tropics' – I find it to be closer to Mary Louise Pratt's phrase 'contact zones', or 'social spaces where disparate cultures meet, clash, and grapple with each other, often in highly asymmetrical relations of domination and subordination – like colonialism, slavery, or their aftermaths'.[52] She explores how European travel writing produced the West and 'the rest of the world' for European readership in different stages of European imperialist expansionism.[53] In the process, she deploys Johannes Fabian's phrase the 'denial of coevalness' to describe the processes of 'temporal distancing' between Europe and 'the rest of the world' as a 'textual practice' in such ethnographical accounts.[54]

Eighteenth and early nineteenth century Anglo-Indian medical practitioners often relied on ideas about the impact of climate on health and character as well as comparisons between Europe and Asia going as far back as the Hippocrates' *Airs, Waters, and Places* in 410 B.C.[55] Mark Harrison emphasises, however, that despite the persistence of climatic determinism in various forms, it was superseded by 'human agency' as an explanation of 'filth', 'disease' and 'health' in 'tropical' India especially from the late 1830s onwards with the publication of Bengal Presidency surgeon James Ranald Martin's *Notes on the Medical Topography of Calcutta* (1837) – one of the first detailed medical topographical treatises to have become a medical authority on India and its tropical environment.[56] Early nineteenth-century medical topographical writings, mainly concerned about the male population, were both optimistic and pessimistic about the issue of the adaptability of European constitutions to the 'tropical climate' in British India. Normative understandings of the 'tropics' across the criss-crossing web of empires were underscored by ideas about its climate, corporeality and culture together with 'degenerative', and rarely beneficial, effects on European well-being. The deleterious effects of the 'tropics' on the 'whiteness' of the ruling 'race' were fiercely debated in Europe and its colonies in the nineteenth and twentieth centuries.[57] Philippa Levine argues, '[T]o be British was to embody civilization, to be born to rule, and to be *not* colonized, not enslaved, conditions fundamentally associated with non-whiteness'.[58] Medicine, 'race' and empire, therefore, came to be intimately associated with fears of racial mixing and sexually transmitted diseases as 'racial poison' that would be 'ruinous to Britain's powerful empire' and 'its alleged racial superiority'.[59]

Ann Laura Stoler points out that sterility, prolonged amenorrhea and a host of other health problems, including 'degeneration', were also believed to have resulted from what was considered to be medically hazardous climate, culture, heredity, miscegenation and factors associated with the strain and duration of residence in the colonies.[60] Climatic and medical conditions were often held responsible for the prevalent high infant mortality rates that sealed the fate of the European child.[61] Therefore, household management and childcare advice which instructed European women about hiring wet nurses, breastfeeding practices and suitable alternative milks were meant to bolster their confidence to remain in the tropics. By the early twentieth century, motherhood had become a national, imperial and racial duty globally.[62] In the metropolis and the colony, the ideology of 'scientific motherhood'[63] singled out mothers, whether coloniser or colonised, for the task of childrearing. Motherhood under medical supervision, often popularised as mothercraft, had turned into a disciplined and taught/learnt duty to bolster imperial and national health and vigour.[64] Advice literature paid close attention to European women's household duties, including the maintenance of 'racial purity' in the colonies. '[P]ositive eugenics placed European women of "good stock" as "the fountainhead of racial strength" '.[65]

The general climate of opinion among medical practitioners was that memsahibs were victims of the tropical climate in India and thereby 'native' wet nurses, however problematic, had to be hired to save the life of European infants. As early as in 1836, *A Domestic Guide to Mothers in India*, written by an anonymous physician in Bombay, pointed out:

> I believe it is not generally known how much ladies are incapacitated from becoming good nurses to their babes, during their residence in this country. I agreed at one time with many of my professional brethren, in supposing that ladies, gave themselves airs, and were affected when they said, they could not nurse their children, and that many young mothers laid aside the maternal character, in order to gratify a desire for fashionable visiting; but, after twelve years experience, I have become much more charitable on this point, and have had too many opportunities of witnessing the extent to which a tropical climate undermines, and impairs the energies and power, of an European constitution. Mothers who experience every devotedness for their babes, feel a very natural reluctance to yield them up to native wet-nurses; the mind revolts at the idea of a stranger taking upon herself such a responsible office. All these feelings, however, must give way to imperious necessity; let mothers who are called to subdue these fond heart-yearnings, and to surrender their children in this way to an amah, embrace this consolation, that no infant thrives so well in India as those fed by these women: and more-over it enables the mother to have the child nursed through his teething, a point of immense importance at that critical period.[66]

In nineteenth and early twentieth century colonial India, medical handbooks often forbade memsahibs from breastfeeding as they believed that it emaciated and weakened them in the tropical environment whereby 'native' wet nurses were recommended. As mentioned in *A Domestic Guide to Mothers in India* (1836), teething was also a genuine concern among colonial doctors. With an M.D. degree from Canterbury and on the Bengal medical staff, J. Jackson in his article 'On Midwifery in the East' pointed out that if the European infant survived the threat of tetanus in the initial days, their health might have been endangered particularly during the teething period by the 'native' *dais*, who, on the whole, were 'very good' but 'the irritating effects of their milk' during menstruation were aggravated by the tropical climate[67]:

> European children, for the most part, thrive pretty well for the first few months, until the period of dentition arrives; and then, from the increased irritability induced by the climate, especially in some peculiar constitutions, every tooth has to be watched and free

lancing of the gums to be made. The frequent necessity of employing native nurses, who, on the whole, are very good, and the irritating effects of their milk during the time of the catamenia in the hot weather, has, in several instances within my knowledge, induced an attack of convulsions, which has been more or less continuous for several days, and even weeks, in a mild form, and has established a habit of irritability that has lasted during the whole period of dentition. Convulsions coming on with the first teeth are not unusual; but the first double tooth is a more frequent cause for the attack, and in all such cases, if there be heat of head, and this be allowed for six hours to remain unattended to, or is unrelieved by brisk purgatives, warm bath, or leeching, there will be much cause for apprehension.[68]

Medical opinions varied and therefore, by way of contrast, army doctor Surgeon-Major Francis Roberts Hogg (M.D.) advised that 'menstruation during lactation is objectionable, yet in India often unavoidable, nor does pregnancy during lactation necessarily poison the milk'.[69] He recommended hiring an Indian wet nurse because '[t]hings may prosper for a while until a dirty bottle, a careless nurse, some epidemic effecting human beings, the goats or the cows, else teething troubles, or climatic influences provoke the dreaded diarrhoea'.[70] He emphasised that, by then, medicines were ineffective and it was too late 'to rush off for the first disengaged wet nurse; for the time has gone by for building a constitution to resist disease'.[71]

Like many medical and popular handbooks in colonial India at the time, Hogg also voiced anxieties about '[t]he bewildered mother, a weakly European or Eurasian girl, knowing nothing appertaining to domestic management, may delegate vitally important duties to apathetic natives' – but if 'instructions are not carried out', 'efforts to save little children are completely paralyzed'.[72] Colonial medical practitioners 'universally demonised the wet-nurse'[73] and yet hired them as 'a necessary evil'.[74] Unlike Corbyn's medical views on wet nursing discussed earlier, I find that the Indian wet nurse was usually viewed with a strange mix of appreciation, suspicion and disdain by most colonial physicians.

Here I put a spotlight on previously underexplored Hogg's medical opinions about wet nursing in India, both in the plains and in the hill stations, to highlight that Hogg believed that '[n]otwithstanding all the expense, discomfort, worry, annoyances, extra room, domestic squabbles pleaded in association with wet nursing, the solemn fact cannot be blinked that the child's life trembles in the scales'.[75] He recommended that the

best age for the nurse is between 19 or 30, not too early, when functions are premature and girls ignorant, bewildered, foolish, quite likely to suffocate a baby taken into bed strictly against orders.

> Seduced young women sometimes soon forget the shame, become ungrateful, inclined to flirt . . . Many however are very good and valuable.[76]

The seriousness of hiring a wet nurse is evident from his detailed yet generalised medical checklist – according to Hogg, '[i]nstead of being large, soft, flabby, pendulous, her breasts firm elastic, pear-shaped, should be moderately distended with milk, the skin thin, mottled with veins, the nipple well developed, yet not too large, and free from cracks or fissures'.[77] He advised that the properties of the milk 'opaque, dull white, when standing should throw up plenty of cream; that of a dark woman, richer in sold constituents, and according to Eustace Smith the child should increase 3 to 5 ounces in weight after being nursed'.[78] He advocated that not just the wet nurse and her milk but also her child must be examined thoroughly to confirm 'freedom from sickness, from any eruption, especially about the head', while the 'tongue of the sick child, not altogether free' might require 'a nick underneath with a pair of scissors'. It is relevant to note that, thereafter, Hogg went on to directly mention the European nurse, mainly regulation of her diet and the importance of keeping her away from an 'extortionate' husband, along with her relations and friends.[79]

Hogg alerts us that wet nurses were notoriously rumoured to have run tricks like 'the old trick . . . of imposters drinking largely previous to examination, thus allowing milk temporarily to accumulate, leading to the deceptive idea of abundance in breasts distended for a little while'.[80] It had become normative at the time for most medical handbooks on childcare in India, often based on race/class/caste prejudices, to stress on detailed bodily examinations and medical scrutiny of 'native' wet nurses and their infants at the time of hiring. The wet nurse's barely known socioeconomic background was often directly correlated with her possibly questionable character and disease-ridden body that posed a potential danger to the European infant. Renowned physicians, for example, Sir William Moore, Surgeon-General, Government of Bombay, in the 1870s,[81] and Cuthbert Sprawson, Major in the Indian Medical Service and Professor of Medicine at the Lucknow Medical College,[82] who edited Moore's *Manual of Family Medicine for India*, pointed to an elaborate medical list for the bodily examination of the wet nurse.[83] They, too, advocated that doctors should also be 'warned against the habitual deception of the prospective wet nurse, such as passing off of a borrowed baby as her own, or presenting breasts full of milk by not drawing out the milk for hours before "inspection"'.[84] Hogg regretted, however, that 'it is an unfortunate fact that whilst all the love and interest become transferred to the pale-faced stranger, the poor little black man, making his own arrangements as we say in India, often is ignored'.[85] The 'scientific' scrutiny and commodification of the wet nurse's milk was ideally meant for preserving the health and vigour of the 'white' imperial 'race' in the tropics. Moreover, Hogg was expressing guilt which, as Sen argues, was often voiced by memsahibs 'about the welfare of the amah's own infant'. Memsahibs' opinions varied sometimes leading to guilt-ridden decisions like making separate arrangements for the wet nurse's infant or, on the contrary, fearing that the deceitful *dai* would often hide and prioritise to nurse her own infant, it was considered necessary to take 'the "native" infant' away from the mother.[86] The colonial home was 'a microcosm of the empire'.[87] Bodily examinations and forced separations of mother and child dehumanised the wet nurse into some kind of a 'milch cow' in the service of the British empire, primarily displaying a combination of race, class and gender prejudices.[88] Moreover, in order to complicate the notion of *colonial difference* here, it is important to note that Bengali *daktars*[89] in particular also advocated that the medical criteria for hiring a wet nurse include detailed bodily examinations of mother and child and, if necessary, she should be prepared to be separated from her infant as late as the 1930s.[90]

As also discussed in Chapter 5 of this book, the salient fact is that European and indigenous elite men and women often managed to share power/knowledge as they actively promoted maternal and child welfare measures on a pan-Indian scale.[91] Particularly significant in this regard was the quasi-governmental organisation the National Association for Supplying Female Medical Aid to the Women of India or the Countess of Dufferin's Fund (1885) established as a non-sectarian organisation training women doctors, nurses and nurse-midwives.[92] The Countess of Dufferin's Fund (1885), the Victoria Memorial Scholarships Fund or V.M.S.F. (1903) and, subsequently, The Lady Chelmsford All-India League for Maternity and Child Welfare (1920) and Lady Reading's Baby Weeks programme (1924) were established by vicereines. With government support, these were self-governing in administration and policy, often with funding from philanthropists.[93] Municipal corporations were also pivotal to such power-sharing particularly through the expansion of maternal and childcare services in colonial Calcutta.[94] However unequal such power-sharing and exchange of knowledge was in a colonial setting like India, authors mainly Biswamoy Pati and Mark Harrison, Projit Bihari Mukharji, and Ishita Pande, among others, use a Said-inflected Foucauldian approach to highlight not just the negative but also the positive aspects of western medical discourse which allowed identity formation of the colonised – most often, upper and middle class and/or caste colonised elite – through discoursing about health and hygiene.[95]

In the the service of the empire, the materialities of breastfeeding emerged intimately associated with imperial, colonial and national agendas, scientised and medicalised in medical handbooks as objective and matter of fact suggestions underscored by a civilisational gap between the coloniser and the colonised. Thus, 'dirt' and 'disease' also became loaded terms marking civilisational differences – the employers' concern for 'the cleanliness and health' of the wet nurse whereby she was 'forbidden to go home' was primarily to prevent her breast milk from becoming 'dirty'.[96] Sara Suleri argues in the context of colonial India, the 'economy of the borrowed breast' implied that 'the lactating Indian feeds another's child and loses her own' whereby the 'bond of nurturing between ruler and servant is quite pragmatically a bond of death'.[97] Here I draw parallels with Emily West and R. J. Knight's arguments about the enslaved mothers in the antebellum South – that there was a serious 'manipulation of motherhood' on the part of slaveowners for their own ends, as the black mothers were forced 'to relinquish their own breast-feeding commitments as mothers in order to prioritize the families of their white owners'.[98] This ties up with the fact that, in colonial India, the milk of these 'professional milk mothers' was the 'life force of the Empire' at the cost of the lives of the infants born to them. Despite such harsh realities, however, it is pertinent to note that colonial homes were also uncertain and ambivalent spaces where the *amahs* or the Indian wet nurses also asserted themselves from time to time, often making memsahibs feel helpless, by resorting to tricks or demanding numerous things whereby she was not just objectified but she also sometimes emerged as 'objectified Subjects'.[99]

Furthermore, Hogg recommended benefits of the colder hill stations as a respite from the disease-ridden plains. He lamented that

> [s]cattered about India innumerable instances of ladies, who knowing nothing of the Himalayas, yet contrive in the plains to preserve their little ones through all the perils and dangers of early life, especially those associated with feeding, weaning, and teething.[100]

The Himalayas primarily housed the hill station Simla which was established as the summer capital of the British Raj from 1864, a safe haven for the British.[101] Hogg explained:

> In choosing a native nurse the great hope is not to fall in with one who smokes in excess, or indulges in sedatives or stimulants. At Simla, a very fine child, 2 years of age, had just been weaned after being nursed by the same woman from the commencement, and the following information was kindly given by the proud and happy mother (a strong opponent to the pestilent, pernicious, and in some case, unpardonable system of neglect termed bringing up by hand). The nurse aged 19, of the weaver caste, received 10 rupees a month besides clothes, cooking utensils and *caste money*; never allowed chupaties, green vegetables or potatoes, she would have a cup of tea in the early morning, also for breakfast half a seer of warm milk, half a loaf of bread; for dinner either curry, rice, dhal or kicherie, washed down with water, whilst for tea a whole load of bread and half a seer of warm milk, and the last thing at night perhaps a cup of tea. . . .

> This nurse was one of those from Agra. *The hill women, dirty, comical, savages almost, are very valuable.* A poor little infant rapidly running down hill at Meerut was hurried up to the Himalayas, and thanks to one of these women the tide turned towards recovery.
>
> (emphasis added)[102]

This dovetails contemporary ethnographic representations of aboriginal hill populations, for example the Paharis of Simla, in a typical Rousseaunean manner, most often exemplified 'lineaments of the noble savage' in 'an Edenic tranquility' – Orientalist 'imaginative geography' and colonial agendas were at play in the drawing out of the sharp binaries between the places and the people of the hills versus the dangerous and diseased plains.[103]

It was around this time, when Hogg was writing, in the 1870s, that 'family medicine' began to emerge as a significant research area for the colonial government – although only a handful of medical manuals were exclusively focused on the management of health and diseases of European women and children in 'tropical' India in the nineteenth and early twentieth centuries. Surgeon-Major in the Indian Medical Service (Bombay) Sir William James Moore's very popular *Manual of Family Medicine for India* (1874), mentioned a little earlier, won the prize for being 'the best medical manual' from the colonial government. The 'Indian Medicine Chest' sold with Moore's (1874) Manual contained 67 basic medicines, and equipment like mortar and pestle, syringes, bandages, scales, weights and measuring glasses.[104] As medical manuals on the management of health in the tropical environment were designed primarily by 'male colonial physicians' in alignment with contemporary racialised, gendered, and classed imperialist and colonial agendas – these ran the risk of reducing women to their reproductive health concerns or ignoring her altogether.[105] The demand for medical guides continued undiminished, despite modern modes of transport like railways and motor-cars to nearby dispensaries and pharmacies selling western medicine because medical assistance in some districts was not easily available and people relied on these manuals in their everyday lives.[106]

The following section compares the merits of artificial foods versus wet nursing of European infants as sometimes voiced in domestic and medical manuals, advertisements and personal correspondence in late nineteenth and early twentieth century colonial India.

Artificial Foods Versus Wet Nursing

This section discusses that, by the early twentieth-century colonial India, due to the growing popularity of artificial foods available in the markets,[107] memsahibs were sometimes actively discouraged from hiring wet nurses in the contemporary medical and popular childcare manuals. It highlights that baby food advertisements rarely stated any negative effects of artificial feeding.

Instead, these most often voiced that baby food contents corresponded with mother's breast milk. These also sometimes cited as proof the meticulous medical and personal testimonies promoting artificial foods often together with promotional pamphlets detailing their composition, preparation, feeding bottles, feeding regimen and suitability for infants through their different ages.

In 1876, Hurrish Chunder Gangooly, Assistant Surgeon, Nawadi, in his letter to the editor of the *Indian Medical Gazette* argued that mothers from 'European and Eurasian families at the different railway stations' usually suffered from breasts that were 'dry' or 'do not satisfy baby' whereby the baby of about two months was fed arrowroot, corn flour, tapioca or farinaceous foods leading to various stomach ailments leading to 'excessive mortality from bowel affections amongst the infants, and which is out of all proportion as compared to the families of the well-to-do class of Baboos'. He argued, 'I maintain that the custom which prevails among the well-to-do Baboos, of feeding children up to 2 years of age exclusively on milk, is the only rational one'.[108] As discussed in this book later, this neatly dovetails the fact that 'Indian mothers' – a recurring theme in European and indigenous medical literature in colonial India – were often championed and pathologised due to their tendency for breastfeeding 'too frequently' or 'weaning too late'. The 'ideal' *bhadramahila* mother was often constructed in contrast with the popular 'Bengali stereotype' of the non-breastfeeding memsahibs.[109]

The governing assumption that memsahibs experienced problems with lactation in the 'tropics' whereby they were unable to breastfeed their infants persisted throughout the nineteenth and early twentieth centuries.[110] Many domestic manuals like *The Englishwoman in India* (1864) and *Tropical Trials* (1883) also echoed the doctors and recommended the hiring of Indian wet nurses.[111] Nupur Chaudhuri points out that even though memsahibs often hired wet nurses, they also voiced various reservations about 'native' wet nurses. Memsahibs did not display 'a monolithic perception' or a colonising 'female gaze' instead a 'plurality' of 'white women's perceptions'.[112] These often included, for instance, as Emma Roberts, editor of the *Oriental Observer* highlighted, the notion that they were considered to be the 'most expensive and troublesome appendages to a family. There is no other method in which natives can so rapidly impose upon the European community'.[113] 'Race', class and/or caste and gender prejudices sometimes were explicitly voiced by women writers in the course of the nineteenth century in India as we will go onto discuss in this section.

It is relevant here to point out that 'race' became increasingly visible in both textual and visual representations of defilement of Anglo-Indian bodies and homes during and after the Revolt of 1857. Official rest-houses or the dak bungalows also featured in Mutiny stories. In one of her letters written in Ludhiana, renowned Scottish physician Margaret Ida Balfour (1866–1945), joint-secretary of the Dufferin Fund 1916–1924, and appointed chief medical officer of the Women's Medical Service in 1920,[114] mentioned that the Ludhiana dak bungalow and most Indian houses were haunted by ghosts of Mutiny victims. She argued that a certain lady was visiting who was 'an inspector of schools for Government' and she was staying at the dak bungalow. She had joined them for dinner one evening. Balfour went on to mention the following:

> She enlivened the evening by ghost stories. It seems houses in India are haunted because of the things that happened during the Mutiny. There was a house she stayed at where 14 people defended themselves against the sepoys but they were overpowered and murdered and when the relief party entered the house they found 14 heads in a row on the drawing room mantelpiece that house is very much haunted. I am beginning to hear very queer sounds myself just now.[115]

Many letters and memoirs also attested the loyalty of servants who gave them shelter in the servant quarters. Sen alerts us that colonial accounts of Indian loyalty/disloyalty during the Rebellion were varied. 'A number of non-literary writings feed into the myth of the "ungrateful" and "disloyal" Indian'.[116] However, memsahibs' memoirs and letters together with literary representations also pointed to Indian women's loyalty to the British during the Rebellion – the 'ayahs, dancing girls and the Englishman's Indian concubines and wives – were deployed as part of a larger textual strategy to secure support for the British in the context of the 1857 Rebellion'.[117] The ayah, the most prominent of the 'faithful Indian women' in Mutiny discourse, fitted into the latter category and the memsahib's vital connection with 'native' India.[118]

Alison Blunt analyses 'How the Mutiny came to English homes' (unknown artist, 1857) as a politically charged illustration of an Anglo-Indian home which embodied a 'threat both to imperial domesticity and to imperial rule'.[119] 'With a baby at her breast and a young child playing next to her, the British woman is depicted at the centre of domestic and familial calm that has just been shattered by the invasion of two Indian insurgents'.[120] Her vulnerability is accentuated by the absence of her husband 'whose portrait hangs on the wall behind her' while the box 'England' which is 'on the *chaise longue* suggests that national and imperial power is similarly vulnerable alongside the child'.[121] Yet, as Blunt also points out, the presence of Indian insurgents was the only indication that the home was located in India whereby the Indian rebels are invading a British home and threatening the British Raj.[122] To extend Blunt's arguments, the stark absence of the *dai* (wet nurse) in particular from the Anglo-Indian home seems to promote an 'ideal' of self-sufficient Anglo-Indian motherhood thereby further distancing the coloniser/colonised.

By the late nineteenth century, highly racialised prejudices against wet nursing were sometimes emphatically voiced by women writers like British writer and novelist, Mrs Howard Kingscote or Adeline Georgina Isabel Kingscote (1860–1908) who later in the 1890s started using the pen-name Lucas Cleeve,[123] in her *The English Baby in India and How to Rear It* (1893). She overtly expressed extreme dislike for Indian wet nurses based on ideas about 'race' and disease and also added the element of their potential to impact child character formation[124]:

> I am strongly against an Indian wet-nurse, except where it is absolutely necessary in order to save the child's life. It is almost impossible for any doctor to find out the antecedents or relationship of any low-caste woman in India. They marry and intermarry till they do not themselves know what relation they are to each other; they lie so readily and so craftily that the sharpest of detectives find it difficult to cope with them, and where the mother cannot herself nurse the child it is more important not only that the wet-nurse be strong and healthy herself, but that she should come of a strong and healthy stock, and this is a thing about which you could never have a certainty; and the diseases that pervade India are so terrible and so loathsome that the English child should have no closer contact with such a race than is necessary. Then I have the old-fashioned idea that through the milk is impressed, in a certain degree, the character and disposition of the nurse, and there is nothing in the Indian disposition that one would covet for one's child. Therefore we hope that the reader will, if possible, avoid an Indian wet-nurse, and advise her friends to do so. If the mother cannot nurse, let her have a cow or Swiss milk for her child, but never a wet-nurse in India.[125]

It was sometimes feared that along with breast milk, the nurse's virtues and vices were also transferred into the child. Nupur Chaudhuri argues that similar fears about the wet nurse's breast milk contaminating the child's character also had parallels in nineteenth-century Britain 'where wet nurses were generally country women or unwed mothers in impoverished circumstances'.[126] Adriana S. Benzaquén goes further back to early eighteenth-century Britain when medical treatises like *The Nurse's Guide* by 'an Eminent Physician' published in London in 1729 aimed at reshaping the roles of wet nurses, mothers and doctors:

> Every Mother that is in perfect Health ought to nurse her own Children herself, because she will be sure to take more care of them than

> a Nurse . . . only she could give him the 'best Milk' and with it 'the most Virtuous Sentiments'.[127]

It is pertinent to note that this became mixed with the element of caste in Bengali childcare advice, for instance, Kabiraj Srijukta Girijabhushan Ray Sengupta's article titled '*Sishupalan*' or 'Child-Rearing', advised against hiring a wet nurse as alongside her milk, her nature and qualities were transferred into the child. Instead, if mother's milk was available, it was the most suitable for the child and there would have been no need to hire a low caste wet nurse.[128]

There were, however, differences of opinion, for example, Flora Annie Steel and Grace Gardiner's very popular household management manual *The Complete Indian Housekeeper & Cook* (1921, first ed. 1888), which went into multiple editions, contradicted such baseless fears and emphatically urged memsahibs to be grateful instead. They pointed out that Anglo-Indians, even missionaries, due to race prejudice feared 'lest the milk of a native woman should contaminate an English child's character' while that of the beasts 'is held to have no such power'[129]:

> The horror of native wet-nurses universally expressed, even by missionary ladies, in the answers received from their correspondents, have impressed the authors so deeply that they feel bound to call special attention to it. No good purpose would be served by quoting the actual expressions used, but it must surely rouse surprise and regret that even those who profess to love the souls of men and women should find the bodies in which these souls are housed more repulsive than those of a cow or donkey or a goat? The milk of all these, it is true – to the shame of humanity be it said – is free from a certain specific contagion; but it is a contagion from which, alas! the West is no more immune than the East. Therefore the objection cannot be on this ground. What remains, therefore, but race prejudice to account for the fatuity of fearing lest the milk of a native woman should contaminate an English child's character, when that of the beasts which perish is held to have no such power? The position is frankly untenable. Therefore if the Western woman is unable to fulfil her first duty to her child, let her thank Heaven for the gift of any one able to do that duty for her.[130]

Steel and Gardiner's concerns about 'race prejudice' when it came to wet nursing of European infants, however, should not overshadow their broader conviction that any 'Indian household' had to be governed like the 'Indian Empire'.[131] In the colonial home, the memsahib belonged to 'the master race' often only in the presence of the 'native' who hailed her as 'memsahib' or literally, 'madam boss'.[132]

In colonial India, wet nursing was also prevalent across class boundaries. Éadaoin Agnew discusses that even for a public figure like Vicereine Lady Lytton, being 'the perfect colonial wife' to perform her 'imperial duties' at the Delhi Durbar meant neglecting 'her maternal duties'.[133] As it was not possible for prominent figures like Lady Lytton to breastfeed baby Victor 'in the appropriate manner while travelling' and in order to 'fulfil her duties' at the Durbar, she borrowed the nurse of Lytton's Private Secretary's wife until she managed to employ someone to take care of her son. Her racialised prejudices are starkly visible in her comment that due to the short notice, she had to hire a 'dirty little brown wet nurse'.[134] Chaudhuri also emphasises that there were differences between the metropolis and the colony as well – the contemporary practice of hiring wet nurses, usually low-caste and/or class Hindus or Muslims,[135] meant that whereas by the 'mid-nineteenth century the use of wet nurses by the middle class in Britain was rapidly declining because of concern about the consequences of intimate associations with lower-class women' – memsahibs faced a dilemma about 'how to imitate the shifting practice of their social class in Britain and yet reconcile the conflict of perceived need for wet nurses with racist contempt for indigenous women'.[136]

By the turn of the century, consumerism was on the rise and many imported baby food advertisements began targeting both memsahib and Indian mothers, sometimes by even incorporating 'codes of local culture'[137] in English and regional vernacular newspapers and periodicals in India. Instructions about and merits and demerits of baby foods available in the market were often seen in both domestic and medical manuals and periodicals at the time, including the popular Steel and Gardiner's *The Complete Indian Housekeeper*. Besides also promoting maternal breastfeeding,[138] Steel and Gardiner pointed out that, at the time, artificial foods were brought to 'great perfection' through 'scientific research' and consequently, wet nurses were rarely being employed – 'opinion is very strong against it, only to save life or in the case of very delicate children is it recommended'.[139] In an elaborate endnote to their chapter on this subject in *The Complete Indian Housekeeper*, they tried to dispel useless racist prejudices against the *dai* – discussed already on the previous page. They also highlighted that while a 'good ayah', under the memsahib's supervision, of course, would have been ideal, especially for 'tiny babies', British mothers in India preferred an Anglo-Indian or Eurasian nurse who was accustomed with the practice of bringing children up by hand.[140] Steel and Gardiner also mentioned several baby foods like Paget's Milk Food, which did not require boiling and thereby ideal for travels and emergencies, while the 'great attraction of Allenbury Foods is the system of progressive feeding':

> No.1 is for the first three months, and can be given alternately with the breast, in the event of a deficiency of milk, without risk. No.

> 2 is No. 1 with the addition of some preparation of farinaceous food, whilst No. 3 is malted farinaceous, needing the addition of cow's milk to prepare it for use. All these foods are in dry powder hermetically sealed, and will keep indefinitely and in any climate'.[141]

They also added that to supplement the 'malted condition of Allenbury's Food', 'orange or grape juice, fresh bananas and raw meat juice occasionally' were recommended.[142] They also pointed to Mellin's Food and echoed contemporary advertisements of Mellin's Food, which claimed that it supplied 'any deficiency of breast milk', or it was an ideal 'substitute containing substances which represent the components of mother's milk'.[143]

Rima D. Apple, in the context of America, argues that on the basis of 'scientific' infant formulas like Mellin's Food alongside meticulous comparative analyses of human and cow's milk, there was a rationale in place for increasingly bringing childcare within the purview of medicine.[144] In colonial India, breastfeeding was also often considered 'unscientific' because of the very nature of breast milk as 'nervous'/'chemical'/'glandular' and the quantity of milk flow being undetermined. Preferences for artificial infant feeding were often rationalised based on drawing correlations between quantity and quality of food, proportion of various ingredients and their nutritive values, and duration of feeding dependent on age of the infant, and so on.[145] As Apple argues, '[O]nce their research had disclosed the variable nature of breast milk, some physicians promoted artificial feeding with a food compounded of known ingredients in preference to the uncertainty of maternal nursing'.[146] Thus, unlike that in Britain, New Zealand and colonial India, which mainly promoted medicalised clocked breastfeeding as discussed in detail in Chapter 5 of this book, '[m]others' changing perceptions coupled with developments in medical practice, the growth of infant-food manufacture, and scientific research' ultimately resulted in American mothers predominantly opting for 'bottle feeding their infants under medical supervision'.[147] It is relevant to note, as Apple also highlights, that popular artificial infant foods, primarily Mellin's Food, also came with instruction booklets which contained testimonials from mothers in the United States.[148] An in-depth study of such a booklet for India, *The Care of Infants in India* (1895 edition) which went through several editions, reveals the way in which the promotional booklet targeted memsahibs and Indian ladies of 'high caste and better educated classes' as the 'ideal' consumers of this product:

> *Every mother has sooner or later forced upon her notice the question of the selection of an artificial food for her baby.* It may be that during the earlier periods of maternity she can supply her child with food, but a time comes when a substitute for mother's milk must be found. In India the tendency and ability of mothers to suckle their babies seems to be decreasing, and it therefore, in many cases, becomes

> necessary for mothers to employ some artificial substitute for breast milk . . . very often young mothers in India are ignorant of those simple truths which should guide them in the feeding of their little ones. Those blind rule-of-thumb practices, which are only too frequently followed by the ayah in feeding young children, cost thousands of infants' lives annually. . . . *The advice given is mainly intended for Anglo-Indian mothers, but it is hoped that this little work will receive the attention, not only of such, but also that of the native ladies of high caste and better educated classes.*
>
> (emphasis added)[149]

I would argue here that mention of 'the native ladies of high caste and better educated classes' should not stand out as an anomaly. Although my focus here in this chapter is on memsahibs and English language advertisements of imported baby foods, I would like to point out that Indian mothers were also gradually under the radar of such food companies. For example, the very interesting and detailed Mellin's 1922 calendar captioned in both English and Bengali and illustrated with a young Lord Krishna playing the flute next to an ornamented cow surrounded by her calves on the ground signifying that the Mellin's Food products like Mellin's Lacto were prepared from 'rich cow's milk' and protected by what seems to be the protective hood of the Ananta Nag snake above (Figure 1.1).[150] This is reminiscent of Adi Sesha Nag or Ananta, often a hooded 'couch to Vishnu' and the 'sacred eternal creature on whom the world rests'.[151] Ananta Nag also protected the passage of infant Krishna across the Yamuna implying protection and good health guaranteed by the product. By way of contrast to the protective role of the snake in the Mellin's calendar, as Rudyard Kipling's father, artist and museum curator John Lockwood Kipling, mentions, Krishna, 'India's cerulean Apollo', appears in 'modern bazaar pictures' standing on the 'head of the great black snake'.[152] In this regard, it is relevant to mention Madhuri Sharma's take on the advertisement of Gripe Water in the 1930s, which uses the theme of *kaliyamardan* – the defeat of the snake-king, Kaliya by Krishna, a triumph of good over evil or illness.[153] These advertisements reveal that imported baby food and drug advertisements were often Hinduised in colonial India.

'Part II Fac-Simile Letters of Parents and Photographs of Anglo-Indian Infants *Reared upon Mellin's Food*' appended in this same edition of the book *The Care of Infants in India* (1895 edition) provides a treasure trove of letters from various parts of India with testimonies of how delicate babies could become 'healthy' babies raised, in many cases exclusively, on Mellin's Food. For example, one letter stated 'Ethel Florence Griffiths has been fed entirely on Mellin's Food and is remarkably rosy and healthy for a Calcutta child'.[154] At the time, the generalised biocultural stereotype was of the so-called pale or sickly children of Calcutta versus the rosy cheeks of those who had recently

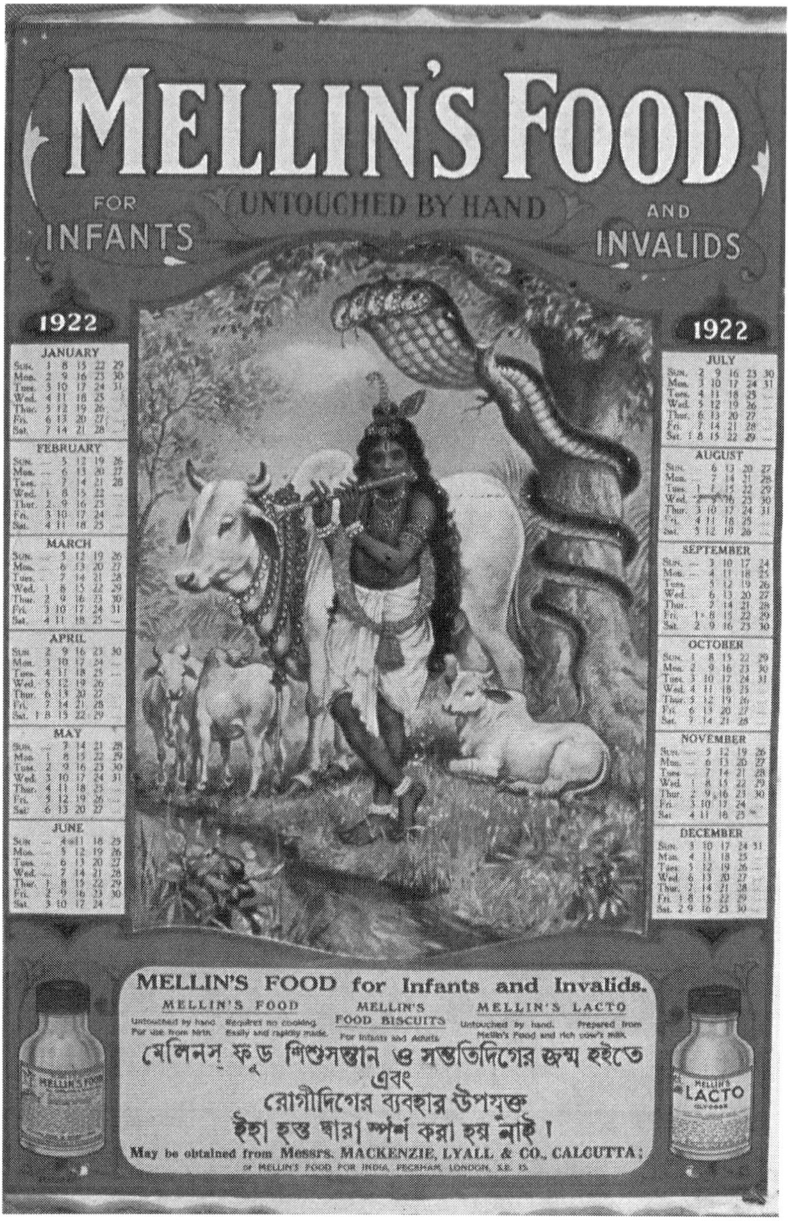

Figure 1.1 'Mellin's Food: Untouched by Hand for Infants and Invalids' which shows Lord Krishna playing a flute, 1922 Mounted Calendar Series.

Source: Film Lobby Cards, Calendars and Other Advertisements from the Collection of Parimal Ray, CSSSC Hitesranjan Sanyal Archives [with permission from the CSSSC Hiteshranjan Sanyal Archives].

visited the colder climates of Britain or the hill stations. As Elizabeth Buettner points out, these were a part of the repertoire of 'colonial common sense' in colonial India.[155] In Part III, 'Directions for the Preparation of Mellin's Food' written in languages like 'Guzerati, Marathi, Telegu, Persian, Sindhi, Urdu',[156] is interspersed with few letters from parents in England with success stories of the baby food. Even the Empress of Germany's testimonial to using Mellin's Food with best results was also translated into English and several other vernacular languages, included at the end of the book.

Testimonies, based on personal experiences of mothers and medical experts in India or Britain, appeared in imported baby food advertisements in colonial India. For example, a full-page advertisement of Glaxo, baby food and galactagogue (material promoting lactation) in *The Statesman and Friend of India* during the First World War led with the caption 'The Future of the Empire lies in the arms of every Nursing Mother',[157] in order to primarily authenticate the product for both British and Indian mothers as its ideal consumers. Personal testimonies of parents also appeared in advertisements for Mellin's Food, for instance, in *The Statesman and Friend of India* at the time: 'Mellin's has suited *her* admirably in the trying Indian Climate. So the mother of this happy little one year old *girl* writes from "The Croft", Lahore'. (emphasis added)[158] The advertisement highlighted that 'when prepared as directed, it provides the proper substitute for mother's milk in the tropics'.[159] Unlike most baby food advertisements which focused on the boy child, Mellin's Food adverts like this particular one featured a 'happy little one year old girl' and claimed that Mellin's Food, was 'the proper substitute for mother's milk in the *tropics*' (emphasis added). Not only Mellin's Food, as Mridula Ramanna argues, in early twentieth-century Bombay newspaper advertisements, for instance, 'Allenbury's product was declared to be particularly suited to tropical climates'.[160] In the late nineteenth and early twentieth century Calcutta popular newspapers and periodicals like *The Statesman*, *Amrita Bazar Patrika* and the *Calcutta Journal of Medicine*, among many others, baby foods like Nestle's Milo Malted Food, and Mellin's Food were often advertised as – 'UNTOUCHED BY HAND'.[161] Srirupa Prasad argues that typically labelled 'completely untouched by hand'[162] was a trademark of modern, mechanised imported baby foods which emphasised the English or British origins of the commodities as 'a guarantee of the genuineness, purity, and superiority of those products'.[163] It was meant to reassure consumers about the quality of the product as free from any 'tropical' contagion. Infant formula, 'science' and modernity together created a 'discourse on "vitalism"' – the way in which imported baby food advertisements combined an ideal of the 'purity' of one place to the lack of the same in another, namely the 'hot climate of India'.[164] Prasad also adds, 'untouched' had several layers of meaning –[165] as Utsa Ray elaborates in the context of Bengali middle-class society – 'meanings were interwoven' and 'the rhetoric of science' could coexist with 'an overt cultural rhetoric about purity', implying primarily class/caste taboos.[166] There was a growth in the new vocabulary of consumerism, health and vitality in the Indian market primarily due to the entry of imported products such as Robinson's Barley, Cadbury's Cocoa, Nestlé's Swiss Milk Chocolate, and Ovaltine, only to name a few.[167]

Moreover, 'Mellin lacto food and biscuits were recommended for infants and invalids'.[168] Similarly, Nestle Milo Malted Food was also described as food for the 'infants, children, and invalids'.[169] Physician at the King's College Hospital, London, Burney Yeo, in 1889, commented on the possible logic behind

> this very important connection between invalids and infants-namely, that they are commonly dependent on others for the provision or selection of their food, and it is for this reason, I presume, that we are invited to consider their food wants together.[170]

Nestle Milo Malted Food also claimed to help grow 'strong bones', 'sound flesh' and 'ensure vigorous and healthy growth'. It is a food whose merits just could not be doubted as apparently it was 'The Latest & the Best being recommended by all home doctors'[171] Nestle Milo Malted Food was certainly making mother's milk optional by promoting their 'Newest and Most Scientific Food'.[172] Like most baby food advertisements claiming to be an equivalent of breast milk at the time, Nestle's Milo also made the claim that its contents corresponded with mother's milk.[173] It was supposed to have been prepared by the 'Choicest Milk' and 'Finest Wheat Flour' that have been 'prepared in such proportions as to correspond to the amount of fat, sugar, proteids and salts of mother's milk'.[174] Deborah Valenze points out that nutritional analysis of milk by Henri Lebert for the Nestlé company actually weighed against mother's breast milk and its capacity to properly nourish infants with the requisite nutrients and quantity. H. Lebert's *A Treatise on Milk and Henri Nestlé's Milk Food* published in 1881 claimed that Nestlé baby food was an ideal replacement for wet nursing, breastfeeding by mother and the problem of adulterated animal milk while it resolved a host of problems associated with infant and adult nutrition.[175]

Yacoob's Food promoted as 'A challenge to Mellins or Nestles Food' (Figures 1.2 and 1.3), was advertised as 'a Swadeshi[176] preparation' – 'Unlike the foreign preparations this is purely a vegetable, or herbal preparation'. It was appended at the end of Munshi Mohamed Yacoob's ('Unani Doctor'/'Hakim and Special Magistrate', Ellore, Kistna district, Madras) book titled *The Cry of the Child & the Calf* (1908). Yacoob's Food was supposed to be 'sweeter than Nectar' and intended 'especially for babes to grow round and healthy'. '*Babies relish this food more than the natural milk of mother's*, as this would check vomitting and purging so common to babies' (emphasis added), while it was also for 'young and old, males and females' as a substitute for the harmful

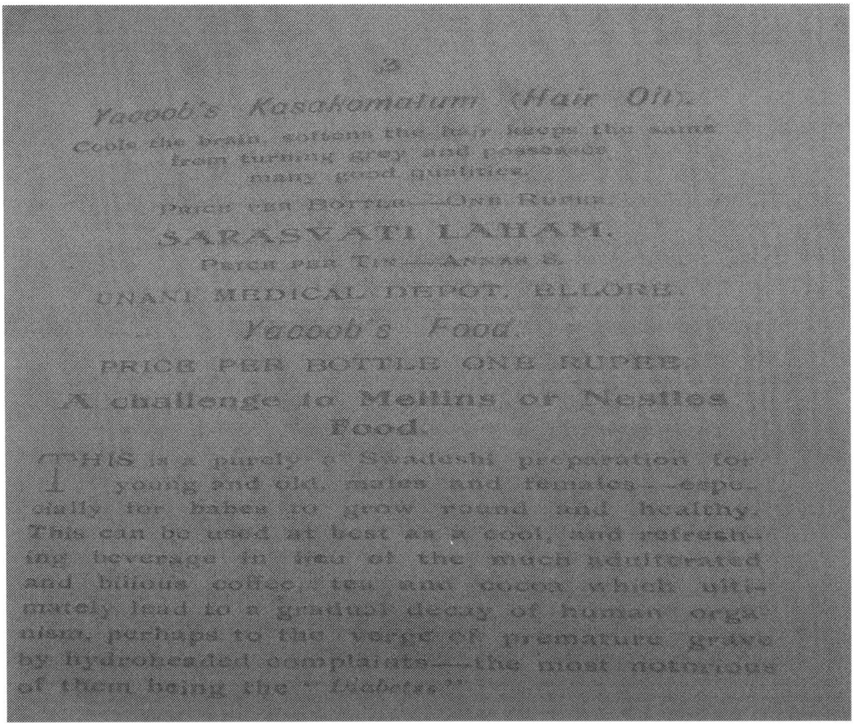

3

Yacoob's Kasakomalum (Hair Oil).

Cools the brain, softens the hair keeps the same from turning grey and possesses many good qualities.

PRICE PER BOTTLE—ONE RUPEE.

SARASVATI LAHAM.

PRICE PER TIN—ANNAS 8.

UNANI MEDICAL DEPOT. ELLORE.

Yacoob's Food.

PRICE PER BOTTLE ONE RUPEE.

A challenge to Mellins or Nestles Food.

THIS is a purely a Swadeshi preparation for young and old, males and females—especially for babes to grow round and healthy. This can be used at best as a cool, and refreshing beverage in lieu of the much adulterated and bilious coffee, tea and cocoa which ultimately lead to a gradual decay of human organism, perhaps to the verge of premature grave by hydroheaded complaints—the most notorious of them being the "*Diabetes.*"

Figure 1.2 Advertisement of Yacoob's Food (and Other Items).

Source: Munshi Mohamed Yacoob, *The Cry of The Child & The Calf*, p. 3 [with permission from the British Library].

'coffee, tea and cocoa'. Unlike such 'Narcotics and similar shabby preparations rife all over India', Yacoob's Food 'acts on the digestive organs more mildly yet magically' as it 'aids digestion', 'braces the nervous system', 'sharpens the facial angle of the brain' and is the 'favourite beverage' for 'debilitated brain workers' and 'diabetic patients'. It also 'purifies the blood', and it is a 'sure anticeptic and antespasmodie'. It is relevant to note that it was also marketed as a 'sure cure for Spermatoriea'[177] together with 'heart and lung affections if systematically used by adults'. He emphasised, 'This preparation has after all been brought to the notice of the public after much experience and experiment to suit the Indian and European constitutions alike'.[178] In his book, however, he blamed animal milk for 'beastly qualities and habits among the degenerated races of India'. He argued that children imbibed the so-called low and mean views of the wet nurses while those fed on animal milk became beastly men, and a cannibal. He believed that nectar or milk of 'godly mothers' will have a bracing effect upon the baby growing to manhood. He promoted mother's breast milk instead of

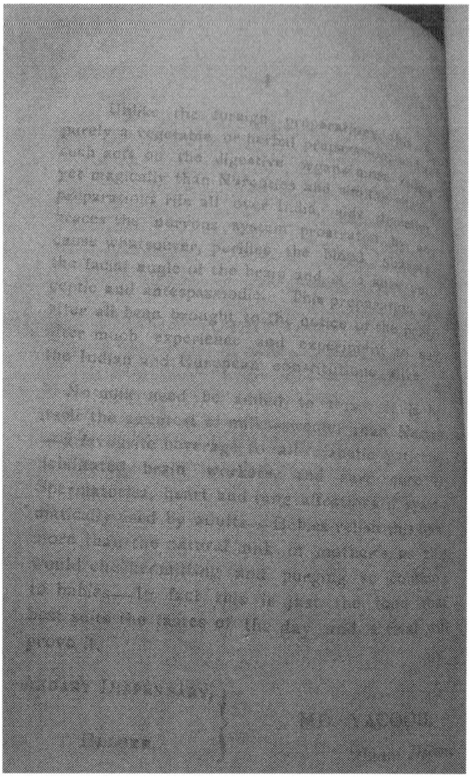

Figure 1.3 Second Page of Advertisement of Yacoob's Food.

Source: Munshi Mohamed Yacoob, *The Cry of the Child & the Calf*, p. 4 [with permission from the British Library].

animal milk for babies also to support the cause of the 'Society for the prevention of cruelty to animals' by prioritising the health of the calf. Yacoob also made an interesting case about how to make a 'good Aryan' and realise the 'cry of the Indians for self-Government or Swaraj' through naturalising and sacralising maternal breastfeeding while discarding wet nursing, animal (mainly cow) milk and even artificial milk.[179]

On the other hand, 'British Empire' and the 'British Government' were specifically mentioned in advertisements of Lactagol, a popular galactagogue (materials promoting lactation) at the time advertised in both Britain and colonial India, mainly Calcutta. Yet medical practitioners like famous nationalist and Brahmo, Calcutta *daktar* Sundari Mohan Das who deified Indian mothers as '*Ma Lakkhi*'[180] due to their tendency to always breastfeed their baby, as the opposite of the non-breastfeeding memsahib, a popular 'Bengali stereotype',[181] also promoted the use of the imported galactagogue, Lactagol.[182] Sarasi Lal

Sirkar (M.A.), Civil Surgeon, Chittagong Hill Tracts, also recommended several measures, including the use of Lactagol to promote lactation; however, these were presented as suggestions by European medical practitioners in his article published in the *Indian Medical Record* in 1917, as follows:

> The fact should be clearly borne in mind that the initial secretion of milk in the mother's breast reside in the child and not the mother, i.e., to say, the secretion of milk is controlled chiefly by the sucking of the child. . . . For example, in the Lancet 1913 ii 911, Cameron states that a device which he has often found very effective, when the milk supply of the mother for the newborn child to be growing less is to put back to the breast the child of a year old, which had been weaned only a short time before. . . . If . . . rapid loss of weight . . . more food is required for the child. This is best supplied by giving the milk drawn off by the breast pump after the infant has finished sucking. If this is insufficient, nothing remains but to give artificial food. . . . There is so much prevailance of the diseases of children as infantile diarrhoea, infantile liver, with very high infant mortality, because the mothers of children either do not look properly to their own health or comfort, or under the circumstances prevailing in their family, they are not in a position to do this properly. However the mothers can often improve their health greatly if they pay some attention to this for the sake of their children. H. R. Riddle in Med. Press and Circular 1913 ii, 643 records a series of cases showing the beneficial effects of Lactagol in increasing the amount of milk secreted and in raising its fat content.[183]

Lactagol was, in fact, advertised as a prerequisite for creating a 'normal mother' in Britain and her Empire.[184] Similarly, in colonial Calcutta, particularly during the First World War, a Lactagol advertisement caption read: 'Lactagol for Nursing and Prospective Mothers 100,000 Babies Sacrificed'.[185] This advertisement cited a 'British Government Report' stating that the 'deaths amongst children under three months of age either wholly or partially fed on artificial foods are fifteen times as great as they are among an equal number of infants fed on breast milk'. It went onto point out that '[w]ith this terrible indictment of artificial feeding before her, can any fond mother condemn her baby to the bottle without having first tried every possible means to feed *him* herself?' (emphasis added). It used the help of 'science' as 'the aid of suffering humanity' stating that 'the discovery of Lactagol has provided the means of enabling every *normal mother* to breastfeed her baby' (emphasis added). Why? It claimed boldly that

> Lactagol when taken by the Nursing Mother, *increases remarkably*, the flow of milk, at the same time *enriching* its quality so that it

> fully satisfies baby's growing needs. *It strengthens the mother, and baby through the mother, building up a foundation of robust health and increasing the powers of resistance to disease.*
>
> (emphasis added)[186]

Thus, Lactagol was supposed to improve mother's milk together with creating a strong and robust (male) baby.[187] Lactagol here was advertised as being manufactured by its 'Sole Manufacturers E. T. Pearson & Co. Ltd. London' and sold by 'Agents for India J. Murray & Co. Bombay, Calcutta and Madras'. It was marketed as a *natural* yet medical remedy unlike 'artificial feeding', curbing high infant mortality and it was explicitly stated in the advertisement that it was being used widely across maternity hospitals in Britain.[188] Another Calcutta Lactagol advertisement around this time commented:

> Physicians everywhere will tell you the way LACTAGOL *increases and enriches* mother's milk is as helpful to mother as it is to baby. Baby is saved the danger of disease from artificial foods and mother the distressing pains, fatigue and overstrain of the nursing period.
>
> (emphasis added)[189]

Some Lactagol adverts were also catering to the needs of European (or Europeanised) families as suggested with an illustration of a suited father, mother in a western dress and their baby (addressed as a male child).[190]

It is pertinent to note that despite the availability of baby foods in the market, as Sen argues, advice about hiring wet nurses continued to be visible well into the early twentieth century.[191] Like most medical manuals by male physicians and domestic advice by memsahibs in tropical India, Delhi-based physician, Kate Platt's *The Home and Health in India* published in 1923, also expressed mixed feelings about the wet nurse but ultimately recommended the hiring of 'native' wet nurses as 'the best solution'.[192] About the Indian wet nurse, Platt emphasised on a full bodily examination by a doctor and a thorough background check alongside the need to discipline her and keep her under constant supervision:

> When the mother's milk fails to appear, the best substitute is that of a wet nurse, provided that it is possible to obtain one who is satisfactory in health and disposition. Doubtless the prejudice which exists against native foster-mothers is not without foundation, but with a delicate or premature child and difficulty in obtaining fresh cow's milk or other artificial substitutes, a wet nurse is the best solution of the difficulty. *No wet nurse should be employed without a thorough examination by a doctor, and a careful enquiry into her antecedents and personal habits. Indian foster-mothers are usually*

> *devoted to their charges, but they need continual supervision. It is difficult to introduce order and regularity in their care for the child.*
> (emphasis added)[193]

As also discussed in the following chapter, the demonisation of the *dai* ('native' midwife and wet nurse) and the rhetoric of their constant supervision and infantilisation need to be located amidst the broader context of the 'psychological force of colonialism'.[194] In a colonial setting, the aspirations and acts of resistance of indigenous populations were often represented as juvenile tantrums of ' "unruly" children' thereby erasing the serious nature of their resistance.[195]

As evidence of the practice of wet nursing and yet in stark contrast to the meticulous medical advice about how to hire an Indian wet nurse for the nursing European infants – Balfour lamented:

> Rather an odd thing happened the other day. After breakfast an old man was discovered sitting in front of the house. He was nearly blind & had a little boy with him. In the little boy's arms there was a bundle about the size & shape of a small coconut, which turned out to be a baby. They said they had brought the baby to give to us. It was evidently not theirs as they were very low caste & it was apparently high caste. Probably the old man had been given a rupee or so to get rid of it & of course it was a girl rather than kill it brought it here. It was 8 days old & very little for its age. Miss Greenfield was away & no one also felt inclined to adopt it so they were told to bring it back in the evening to see her. Now comes what I consider the dreadful part of the story. Miss G. did take it but gave it out to one of the Christian woman to nurse, a woman of the worst character & who has a dreadful disease brought on by her bad living (sic). She will in all probability communicate to the poor little child. Both Miss Popon & I spoke to Miss G. as soon as we heard of it & remonstrated with her but she only said it was not certain the child would get the disease. Her last 2 babies have died of it though the present one seems so far healthy. If Miss G. had tried everywhere to get a proper wet nurse & failed & if she had tried honestly to bring it up on the bottle & the child were really dying for want of suitable food it might be a question whether it would be kinder to let it die or give it to that woman but as it is I consider it simple wickedness on Miss Gs. part. She made not the slightest effort to find anyone else. Went straight for this woman & gave the child to her. I would like to ask her if she would have done the same by a child of her own. But I don't suppose it is any good saying more than I have. She knows the consequences herself as well as any one. You know Miss Andrews did the same by that child she has taken home with her and it has got

> the disease. Though at present only slightly. It is astonishing what thoroughly bad things good people can do.[196]

In this letter, it seems Balfour expressed her horror about the racism and indifference of the hospital staff hiring a Christian woman, of 'the worst character' and with 'a dreadful disease', in this particular case to nurse an abandoned, 'high caste' Indian girl child, instead of opting to search for a suitable wet nurse or available artificial foods.[197] It is relevant to note here that, in India, the birth of a girl child was not always welcome and she sometimes faced death.[198]

In conclusion, this chapter primarily examined the elaborate medical criteria for hiring of Indian wet nurses to nurse European infants in 'tropical' India. As Sen argues, the colonial home was 'a microcosm of the empire'.[199] Wet nursing had to be medically crafted in order to tackle various kinds of 'tropical' contagion. The materialities of breast milk, therefore, emerged as political and biocultural tools in nation and empire building. These were intimately associated with 'scientific' and matter of fact suggestions for maternal and child welfare considered appropriate in a colonial setting. Colonial and indigenous medical advice about wet nursing stereotyping the Indian wet nurse 'ideal' and advocating detailed bodily examinations of the wet nurse and her child involved the contradictory processes of both acknowledging and dismissing her capacity to mother effectively, unless under constant supervision. Rare archival materials from medical manuals and periodical essays to advertisements, promotional pamphlets and personal correspondence offered novel entry points into the subject together with opening up pathways for a reinterpretation of the dominant historiographical worldviews. Extant scholarship on the subject of wet nursing in the tropical environment of India stressed on ambivalences within the colonial nursery and yet when it came to discussing European (predominantly male) physicians' and memsahibs' advice mainly in medical and domestic manuals about the medical criteria for hiring of an Indian wet nurse – they believed it to be predominantly within the ambit of *colonial difference*. While this remains true to a large extent, I highlight, mainly in Chapters 2 and 5 of this book, that both European and indigenous medical practitioners often coopted and applied problematic medicalised distinctions between the pathological and the normal when hiring a *dai*, whether the traditional untrained Indian midwife or a wet nurse. After all, 'it is in discourse that power and knowledge are joined together'.[200]

Notes

* A revised version of this chapter has been submitted to the *Gender & History* journal which is currently under final round of review. I am grateful for the invaluable anonymous reviews. I am particularly indebted to Professor Siobhan Lambert-Hurley for her insightful suggestions.

1 Gabrielle Palmer cited in S. M. Crowther, L. A. Reynolds and E. M. Tansey (eds), *The Resurgence of Breastfeeding, 1975–2000.* Wellcome Witnesses to Twentieth Century Medicine, Volume 35. (London: Wellcome Trust Centre for the History of Medicine at UCL, 2009), p. 26. Here Palmer refers to Valerie Fildes, 'Infant feeding practices and infant mortality in England, 1900–19', *Continuity and Change* vol. 13, 1998, pp. 251–80.

2 Ibid., p. 26. Palmer mentions about the phrase 'it is better to have the vegetarian, nerveless cow' - 'Miss Chloe Fisher has often used this quotation from Dr Eric Pritchard, an early twentieth-century British paediatrician. [Pritchard (1907)]', 'Note on draft transcript, 3 September 2007.' On Eric Pritchard, see Eric Pritchard, *Infant Education* (London: Marylebone Health Society, 1907).

3 Indrani Sen, 'Memsahibs and Health in Colonial Medical Writings, c.1840 to c.1930', *South Asia Research*, vol. 30, no. 3, 2010, p. 256.

4 In alignment with the main arguments in Anna Davin, 'Imperialism and Motherhood', *History Workshop*, vol. 5, no. 1, 1978, pp. 9–65., Sen, 'Memsahibs and Health in Colonial Medical Writings', and Ranjana Saha, 'Milk, "Race" and Nation: Medical Advice on Breastfeeding in Colonial Bengal', *South Asia Research*, vol. 37, no. 2, 2017, pp. 147–165.

5 Nupur Chaudhuri, 'Memsahibs and Motherhood in Nineteenth-Century Colonial India', *Victorian Studies*, vol. 31, no. 4, 1988, p. 517n3. There was also a wide range of childcare advice for Indian mothers, for example, Siobhan Lambert-Hurley, *Muslim Women, Reform and Princely Patronage Nawab Sultan Jahan Begum of Bhopal* (New York: Routledge: 2007), pp. 124–143.

6 Sen, 'Memsahibs and Health in Colonial Medical Writings, p. 253.

7 Hand-feeding was often referred to as 'feeding' of infants. See, for instance, Frederick Corbyn, *Management and Diseases of Infants Under the Influence of the Climate of India Being Instructions to Mothers and Parents in Situations Where Medical Aid Is Not to Be Obtained and a Guide to Medical Men, Inexperienced in the Nursery and the Treatment of Tropical Infantile Disease* (Illustrated By Coloured Plates; Calcutta: Thacker and Co., 1828), p. 32; Jacqueline H. Wolf, 'Low Breastfeeding Rates and Public Health in the United States', *American Journal of Public Health*, vol. 93, no. 12, 2003, p. 2001, among others.

8 Francis Roberts Hogg, 'Notes on Infantile Diseases of India', *Indian Medical Gazette*, vol 11, no. 10, 1876, p. 260.

9 Flora Annie Steel and Grace Gardiner, *The Complete Indian Housekeeper & Cook Giving the Duties of Mistress and Servants The General Management of the House and Practical Recipes For Cooking in All its Branches* (London: William Heinemann, 1909, 1888), p. 170. *Bhoosa* is chaff, Ibid., p. 105.

10 Corbyn, *Management and Diseases of Infants*, p. 12.

11 Ibid., pp. 10–11. The problems of hiring *dais* including 'drawing back the suck' are mentioned in 'F. Corbyn, *Management and Diseases of Infants, under the Influence of the Climate of India . . .*, (Calcutta, 1828)' cited in *Lancet*, vol. 16, 1828, p. 760 in Valerie Fildes, *Wet Nursing: A History From Antiquity to the Present* (Oxford: Basil Blackwell, 1988), pp. 204–205; and also 'F. Corbyn, *Management and Diseases of Infants, Under the Influence of the Climate of India . . .* (Calcutta, 1828) cited in *Lancet*, 16 (1828): 760. See Valerie Fildes, "The Demise of the Wet Nurse c. 1800–c. 1914," in *Wet Nursing: A History from Antiquity to the Present* (London/New York, 1988), pp. 204–205' cited in Swapna M. Banerjee, 'Blurring Boundaries, distant companions: non-kin female caregivers for children in colonial India (nineteenth and twentieth centuries)', *Paedagogica Historica*, vol. 46, no. 6, 2010, p. 780. However, both authors did not touch on Corbyn's racist and gendered arguments about the *dais* which has

been discussed here in this chapter in detail. Also, on *dais* and opium, see Charu Gupta, *The Gender of Caste. Representing Dalits in Print* (Ranikhet: Permanent Black, 2016), p. 36.

12 Saha, 'Milk, "Race" and Nation', p. 148.
13 Corbyn, *Management and Diseases of Infants*, pp. 30–33.
14 Saha, Milk, 'Race' and Nation', pp. 149–151.
15 For instance, see Corbyn's recommendations about Bengal climate for infants during dentition, Corbyn, *Management and Diseases of Infants*, pp. 420–422.
16 Saha, 'Milk, "Race" and Nation, p. 149.
17 Pratik Chakrabarti, *Western Science in Modern India Metropolitan Methods, Colonial Practices* (Delhi: Permanent Black, 2004), p. 35.
18 Ibid., pp. 35–36.
19 Ibid., pp. 47, 90; Saha, 'Milk, Mothering & Meanings: Infant Feeding in Colonial Bengal', *Women's Studies International Forum*, vol. 60, 2017, pp. 100–101.
20 Ibid., p. 90.
21 Frederick Corbyn, 'Preface', in F. Corbyn (ed), *The India Review and Journal of Foreign Science and the Arts*, vol. I, 1837, p. iv. http://dli.serc.iisc.ernet.in/scripts/FullindexDefault.htm?path1=/data2/upload/0048/5968&first=1&last=745&barcode=4990010194444 (consulted on 10 November, 2015). Also, see Saha, 'Milk, Mothering & Meanings, p. 100; Saha, 'Milk, "Race" and Nation', pp. 150–151.
22 Fildes, *Wet Nursing*, p. 204. Also, on Corbyn's book as intended to give advice to young European mothers on childrearing in order to guide them and to curb the problem of infant mortality, see Corbyn, *Management and Diseases of Infants*, pp. v–vi.
23 Ibid.
24 Ibid.
25 Ibid.
26 Corbyn, *Management and Diseases of Infants*, p. 12.
27 Ibid., p. 11; also on the use of castor oil as a purgative for infants, see Ibid., pp. 22–23; also see Saha, 'Milk, "Race" and Nation', p. 150.
28 Corbyn, *Management and Diseases of Infants*, p. 14.
29 Ibid., p. 12
30 Ibid., p. 15.
31 Ibid.
32 Ibid., pp. 14–15. Also, Corbyn, *Management and Diseases of Infants*, pp. 14–15 cited in Saha, 'Milk, Mothering & Meanings', p. 101.
33 Corbyn, *Management and Diseases of Infants*, p. 12.
34 Revathi Krishnaswamy, *Effeminism: The Economy of Colonial Desire* (Ann Arbor, MI: University of Michigan Press, 1998), p. 9.
35 See Saha, 'Milk, "Race" and Nation', p. 151. On 'native effeminacy' and the 'white race' as the 'male of the species', see Anne McClintock, *Imperial Leather Race, Gender and Sexuality in the Colonial Contest* (New York, Routledge, 1995), p. 55; on the fluid definitions of effeminacy changing over time, Michèle Cohen, *Fashioning Masculinity: National Identity and Language in the Eighteenth Century* (New York: Routledge, 1996), p. 7; on the 'martial race' theory, Mrinalini Sinha, *Colonial Masculinity The 'Manly Englishman' and the 'Effeminate Bengali' in the Late Nineteenth Century* (Manchester: Manchester University Press, 1995), pp. 8, 27–8, 70–94. This study also aligns with Mark Harrison's arguments on the 'fluid' perceptions of 'race' as a 'socio-cultural' and 'physical' category, and the '"racial turn" in Anglo-Indian culture' by the 1820s following the Burma War, and climatic determinism accompanied by

human agency as an explanation of 'filth', disease and health in India from the 1830s onwards, see Mark Harrison, 'Differences of Degree: Representations of India in British Medical Topography, 1820-c.1870', in Nicolaas A. Rupke (ed), *Medical Geography in Historical Perspective* (London: Wellcome Trust Centre for the History of Medicine at UCL, 2000), pp. 51–69. On 'native' agency and germ theory in the late nineteenth century, see David Arnold, *Colonizing the Body State Medicine and Epidemic Disease in Nineteenth-Century India* (Berkeley: University of California Press, 1993), pp. 89, 210.

36 Saha, 'Milk, "Race" and Nation', p. 151.

37 Shula Marks, 'What is Colonial About Colonial Medicine? And What Has Happened to Imperialism and Health?', *Presidential Address, Social History of Medicine*, vol. 10, no. 2, 1997, pp. 205–19.

38 See Corbyn, *Management and Diseases of Infants*, pp. 15–18

39 Ibid., p. 16.

40 Ibid.

41 Ibid., pp. 16–18; also see Saha, 'Milk, "Race" and Nation', p. 150.

42 Corbyn, *Management and Diseases of Infants*, 9–10.

43 Review of *Management and Diseases of Infants Under the Influence of The Climate of India Being Instructions to Mothers and Parents in Situations Where Medical Aid Is Not to Be Obtained and a Guide to Medical Men, Inexperienced in the Nursery and the Treatment of Tropical Infantile Disease.* Illustrated By Coloured Plates. *By* Frederick Corbyn, Esq., Surgeon on the Bengal Establishment; and Author of a Treatise on the late Epidemic Cholera and Taraii Fever, M.R.C.S.L. Calcutta, Thacker and Co. Royal 8 vo. Pp. 463.1828; *The Lancet* MDCCCXXVIII-IX In Two Volumes Volume II, ed. Thomas Wakley, 1829, p. 762.

44 Julia Baird, *Victoria The Queen: An Intimate Biography of the Woman Who Ruled an Empire* (New York: Random House, 2016), pp. 219–220. Furthermore, Baird points out that whereas she bore one child after another, her own mother possibly benefitted from the contraceptive effects of having breastfed Victoria for six months. At the time, aristocratic women preferred to hire wet nurses often due to the fashion of wearing corsets which ruined their ability to produce milk. Ibid., p. 12–13.

45 Ibid., p. 186.

46 See Sen, 'Memsahibs and Health in Colonial Medical Writings', pp. 256–258.

47 WBSA, General Department, Education Branch, Proceedings 8–11, 12–13, 18–22, February 1868 cited in Ambalika Guha, *Colonial Modernities Midwifery in Bengal, c. 1860–1947* (London: Routledge, 2018), pp. 70–71.

48 Meer Ushruff Ally, *Handbook of Midwifery in Bengalee* (Calcutta: Das and Sons, 1869); and *Diseases of Children in Bengalee Balchikitsa* (Calcutta: Das and Sons, 1870). For details, see Ally, *Diseases of Children in Bengalee*, p. 1 (of Preface, pp. 1–2).

49 David Arnold, *The Tropics and the Traveling Gaze India, Landscape, and Science 1800–1856* (Delhi: Permanent Black, 2005), p. 114.

50 Arnold, *Colonizing the Body*, p. 29; and *The Tropics and the Traveling Gaze*, p. 111.

51 Arnold, *The Tropics and the Traveling Gaze*, pp. 112–113, 132–133, 142; also useful, David Arnold, *The Problem of Nature Environment, Culture and European Expansion* (Oxford: Blackwell Publishers Ltd., 1996); and Saha, 'Milk, "Race", and Nation', p. 149.

52 Mary Louise Pratt, *Imperial Eyes. Travel Writing and Transculturation* (New York: Routledge, 1992, 2008 second edition), p. 7.

53 Ibid., p. 4.
54 Johannes Fabian, *Time and the Other: How Anthropology Makes Its Object* (New York: Columbia University Press, 1983), p. 35 cited in Pratt, *Imperial Eyes*, p. 63. On identity formation of the colonised, see 'autoethnography', Pratt, *Imperial Eyes*, p. 9.
55 Harrison, 'Differences of Degree', p. 59.
56 Ibid., pp. 55–62, 66–67; Arnold, *Tropics and the Travelling Gaze*, pp. 140–141.
57 See Mark Harrison, *Climates and Constitutions Health, Race, Environment and British Imperialism in India, 1600–1850* (Oxford: Oxford University Press, 1999).
58 Philippa Levine, *Prostitution, Race and Politics Policing Venereal Disease in the British Empire* (New York and London: Routledge, 2003), p. 4.
59 Ibid., pp. 4, 5, 9. Also, see for example, Erica Wald, *Vice in the Barracks Medicine, the Military and the Making of Colonial India, 1780–1868* (New York: Palgrave Macmillan, 2014).
60 Ann Laura Stoler, 'Making Empire Respectable: The Politics of Race and Sexual Morality in 20th-Century Colonial Cultures', *American Ethnologist*, vol. 16, no. 4, 1989, p. 649; also see Saha, 'Milk, "Race" and Nation, p. 149.
61 Ch. Grall, *Hygiene Coloniale Appliquee* (Paris: Bailliere 1908), p. 65; and Grenfell A. Price, *White Settlers in the Tropics* (New York: American Geographical Society, 1939), p. 204 cited in Stoler, 'Making Empire Respectable', p. 650.
62 Davin, 'Imperialism and Motherhood', p. 13, among others cited in Stoler, 'Making Empire respectable', p. 649.
63 Rima D. Apple, *Perfect Motherhood Science and Childrearing in America* (New Brunswick: Rutgers University Press, 2006); and Rima D. Apple, *Mothers and Medicine: A Social History of Infant Feeding, 1890–1950* (Madison, WI: The University of Wisconsin Press, 1987), Part III Scientific Motherhood, pp. 95–132.
64 On 'mothercraft', midwifery, and child welfare exhibitions in a colonial Indian context, see for example, Saha, 'Motherhood on display'.
65 Hugh Ridley, *Images of Imperial Rule* (New York: Croom & Helm, 1983), p. 91; and Davin, 'Imperialism and Motherhood', p. 12 cited in Stoler, 'Making Empire Respectable', p. 644.
66 *A Domestic Guide to Mothers in India Containing Particular Instructions on the Management of Themselves and Their Children*, By a Medical Practitioner of Several Years' Experience in India (Bombay: American Mission Press, 1836), pp. 57–58.
67 J. Jackson, M.D., 'On Midwifery in the East' (Communicated by Dr. Metcalfe Babington), *Transactions of the Obstetrical Society of London* II, 1860, p. 41.
68 Ibid. On 'dirt' and 'disease' see Mary Douglas, *Purity and Danger an Analysis of the Concepts of Pollution and Taboo* (London: Routledge, ARK ed. 1984, first ed. 1966); and Swati Chattopadhyay, *Representing Calcutta Modernity, Nationalism and the Colonial Uncanny* (London: Routledge, 2005); among others; also on 'dirt, disease, child marriage and 'Indian pathologies', see Ishita Pande, *Medicine, Race and Liberalism in British Bengal. Symptoms of Empire* (New York: Routledge, 2010), pp. 151–176
69 Francis R. Hogg, *Practical Remarks Chiefly Concerning the Health and Ailments of European Families in India, with Special Reference to Maternal Management and Domestic Economy* (Benares: Medical Hall Press, 1877), pp. 23. Also, on menstruating mothers and various other issues connected to diarrhoea and the need for wet nurses particularly in India, see Francis R. Hogg, 'Notes on Infantile

Diseases of India', *Indian Medical Gazette*, vol. 12, no. 7, 1877, p. 181. On the trajectory of Hogg's career, see for example, 'Address of John Marshall, F.R.S. President At the Annual Meeting, March 1st, 1883' in *Medico-Chirurgical Transactions* Published by The Royal Medical Chirurgical Society of London Second Series Volume The Forty-Eighth, (London: Longmans, Green, Reader, and Dyer, Paternoster Row, 1883) pp. 2–3.

70 Hogg, *Practical Remarks Chiefly Concerning the Health and Ailments of European Families in India*, p. 22.

71 Ibid.

72 Hogg, 'Notes on Infantile Diseases of India', p. 181.

73 Indrani Sen, *Gendered Transactions: The White Woman in Colonial India, c. 1820–1930* (Manchester: Manchester University Press, 2017), p. 163.

74 Ibid.

75 Hogg, *Practical remarks chiefly concerning the health and ailments of European families in India*, p. 22.

76 Ibid., p. 22.

77 Ibid, p. 23.

78 Ibid.

79 Ibid.

80 Ibid.

81 Sen, 'Memsahibs and Health', p. 271n4.

82 Ibid., p. 271n5.

83 Cuthbert Allan Sprawson, Moore's *Manual of Family Medicine and Hygiene for India* Eighth edition, re-written by the editor. Foreword by Charles Pardey Lukis. (London: J.&A. Churchill, 1916), p. 492 in Sen, 'Memsahibs and Health', p. 269. Also, about bodily examination and regulation of diet of the 'native' wet nurse, see W. J. Moore, *A Manual of Family Medicine for India* (London: J. & A. Churchill, 1874), mainly pp. 487–489.

84 Ibid., p. 493 in Sen, 'Memsahibs and Health', p. 268.

85 Hogg, *Practical remarks chiefly concerning the health and ailments of European families in India*, p. 24.

86 See detailed discussion in Sen, *Gendered Transactions*, pp. 134–135; on the nature of the memsahib-wet-nurse interactions, see mainly p. 132.

87 Indrani Sen, 'Colonial Domesticities, Contentious Interactions: Ayahs, Wet-Nurses and Memsahibs in Colonial India', *Indian Journal of Gender Studies*, vol. 16 no. 3, 2009, pp. 299, 324. It is relevant to note that unlike ayahs, wet nurses were hired for a much shorter duration in the colonial home. Ibid., p. 317.

88 Sen, 'Memsahibs and Health', p. 269.

89 On Bengali *daktars*, see Projit Bihari Mukharji, *Nationalizing the Body The Medical Market, Print and Daktari Medicine* (Delhi: Anthem Press, 2012; U.K. and U.S.A. edition 2009).

90 For example, see discussion in Chapter 2 in this book, pp. 93–4.

91 For a detailed discussion on this subject, see Saha, 'Motherhood on display'.

92 Cecelia Van Hollen, *Birth on the Threshold Childbirth and Modernity in South India* (Berkeley, CA: University of California Press, 2003), p. 42. On organisational structure and main objectives of the Dufferin Fund – see Harriot Dufferin, 'The National Association for Supplying Female Medical Aid to the Women of India', *Asiatic Quarterly Review*, vol. 1, 1886, pp. 260–261 in Maneesha Lal, 'The Politics of Gender and Medicine in Colonial India: The Countess of Dufferin's Fund, 1885–1888', *Bulletin of the History of Medicine*, vol. 68, no. 1, 1994, p. 35.; also see The Countess of Dufferin's Fund, *Fifty Years' Retrospect*

India 1885–1935 (London: The Women's Printing Society Ltd., 1935), p. 5, File: Countess of Dufferin's Fund, PP/MIB//C/4, Wellcome Library.

93 Van Hollen, *Birth on the Threshold*, pp. 42–43.

94 Guha, *Colonial Modernities*, p. 126. As also discussed elsewhere in this book, Ambalika Guha mentions that in Calcutta as early as in 1908 maternal and child welfare services were begun by the Corporation and from 1915 trained 'corporation midwives' provided domiciliary midwifery services, Guha, *Colonial Modernities*, pp. 127–128; municipal maternal and infant welfare work in Delhi had already commenced in 1915 and the first infant welfare centre opened in May 1918. DSA, New Delhi; Chief Commissioner Series, File 5(56) 1929, Review on Maternity and Child Welfare work at Delhi for the year 1928.

95 Biswamoy Pati and Mark Harrison, 'Introduction Health, Medicine and Empire: Perspectives on Colonial India', in Biswamoy Pati and Mark Harrison (eds), *Health, Medicine and Empire Perspectives on Colonial India* (New Delhi: Orient Longman, 2001), p. 1; Projit Bihari Mukharji, *Nationalizing the Body The Medical Market, Print and Daktari Medicine* (Delhi: Anthem Press, 2012), p. 11; and Ishita Pande, *Medicine, Race and Liberalism in British Bengal Symptoms of Empire* (London: Routledge, 2010), p. 7.

96 Ann Laura Stoler, *Carnal Knowledge and Imperial power Race and the Intimate in Colonial Rule* (With a New Preface; Berkeley: University of California Press, 2002, 2010), p. 197.

97 Sara Suleri, *The Rhetoric of English India* (Chicago: University of Chicago Press, 1992), p. 81.

98 Emily West and R. J. Knight, 'Mothers' Milk: Slavery, Wet-Nursing, and Black and White Women in the Antebellum South', *The Journal of Southern History* vol. 83, no. 1, 2017, p. 47. West and Knight also complicate their argument by pointing out that white women also sometimes nursed enslaved infants for various reasons. Ibid., 37. On exploitation of enslaved bodies, see Jennifer L. Morgan, *Laboring Women: Reproduction and Gender in New World Slavery* (Philadelphia: University of Pennsylvania Press, 2004), 27–36 cited in Ibid., p. 40.

99 Sharon Jacob, *Reading Mary Alongside Indian Surrogate Mothers Violent Love, Oppressive Liberation, and Infancy Narratives* (New York, Palgrave Macmillan, 2015), p. 13; Jacob primarily builds on Indrani Sen's argument from Sen, 'Colonial Domesticities, Contentious Interactions', p. 318.

100 Hogg, 'Notes on Infantile Diseases of India', p. 181.

101 Dane Kennedy, *The Magic Mountains Hill Stations and the British Raj* (Berkeley, University of California Press, 1996), p. 14.

102 See Hogg, *Practical remarks chiefly concerning the health and ailments of European families in India*, p. 24. In the excerpt, caste money possibly meant money for reinstatement of caste following pollution of suckling an infant outside their caste – for example, this has been mentioned in a different context in Edwin T. Atkinson, *Statistical Descriptive and Historical Account of the North-Western Provinces of India* Volume III Meerut Division Part II (Allahabad: North Western Provinces Government Press, 1876), p. 51. Sen also highlights that even Muslim wet nurses were believed to have imbibed 'caste prejudices' from the Hindus mostly 'daily 'pollution' from the touch of European infants' whereby they were blamed for extracting extra compensatory money for purchasing their reinstatement to caste'. See Emma Roberts, *Scenes and Characteristics of Hindoostan*, Volume II (London: W. H. Allen, 1835), p. 121 in Indrani Sen, *Gendered Transactions The white woman in colonial India, c. 1820–1930* (Manchester: Manchester University Press, 2017), p. 133. Sometimes they might have belonged to higher castes whereby they made domestic management difficult for memsahibs, see Julia Maitland, *Letters from Madras, During*

the Years 1836–39, by a Lady (London: John Murray, 1846, first ed. 1843), p. 52 in Sen, *Gendered Transactions*, p. 133. On the tropical climate and the benefits of the British hill stations for children, see primarily Elizabeth Buettner, *Empire Families Britons and Late Imperial India* (New York: Oxford University Press, 2004), pp. 29–33, particularly p. 30n7, among others.

103 Kennedy, *The Magic Mountains*, pp. 64–65, 87.

104 Sen, 'Memsahibs and Health', p. 271n8.

105 Ibid., p. 256.

106 Ibid., p. 255.

107 Patent and farinaceous foods were being imported in bulk into British India by the early twentieth century. 'Milk foods for infants and invalids are wanted, imports increasing from a value of Rs. 22,52,757 in 1925–26 to Rs. 32,9,376 in 1928–29; the trade is almost entirely in British hands'. Furthermore, 'Sales of condensed and preserved milk are rapidly increasing imports in 1928–29 being valued at Rs. 89,02,713, compared with Rs. 62,03,787 in 1925–26. The U.K. and the Netherlands were the main suppliers, however, Australia, Italy, Denmark, and Norway also competed in this market. W. H. Wilson, *Markets of Empire* (London: Effingham Wilson, 1930), pp. 104–105. It is interesting to note as K. Stanford wrote, that in general, 'no lady ever demeaned herself to visit the bazaar and buy her own food. She left that entirely to her native cook'. See J.K. Stanford, *Ladies in the Sun: The Memsahib's India, 1790–1860* (London: The Gallery Press, 1962), p. 69 in Cecelia Leong-Salobir, *Food Culture in Colonial Asia A taste of empire* (London: Routledge, 2011), p. 65.

108 Hurrish Chunder Gangooly (L. M. S. Assistant Surgeon, Nawadi), '"Infant's Food To The Editor of the "Indian Medical Gazette"', *Indian Medical Gazette*, vol. XI, no. 6, 4th May 1876, June 1876, p. 164; also see Saha, 'Milk, mothering & meanings', p. 104. Around the same time, see Hogg's advice on the benefits of prolonged lactation in preventing diarrhoea – F. R. Hogg, 'Notes on Infantile Diseases of India', *Indian Medical Gazette*, vol 11, no. 10, 1876, p. 260. Hogg also mentioned the problem of 'hill diarrheoa', see Ibid., pp. 260–261.

109 Meredith Borthwick, *The Changing Role of Women in Bengal, 1849–1905* (Princeton: Princeton University Press, 1984), pp. 171–172.

110 Sen, *Gendered Transactions*, p. 162.

111 Chaudhuri, 'Memsahibs and Motherhood in Nineteenth-Century Colonial India', p. 529.

112 Indrani Sen, *Memsahibs' Writings. Colonial Writing on Indian Women* (New Delhi: Orient Longman, 2008), p. xxv.

113 Emma Roberts, *Scenes and Characteristics of Hindostan with Sketches of Anglo-Indian Society*, Volume I (London: W. H. Allen, 1837), p. 336 in Nupur Chaudhuri, 'Memsahibs and Motherhood in Nineteenth-Century Colonial India', *Victorian Studies*, vol. 31, no. 4, 1988, p. 529.

114 'Obituary Dr. Margaret Balfour', *The Times*, 3 December, 1945 in Samiksha Sehrawat, Colonial Medical Care in North India *Colonial Medical Care in North India Gender, State and Society c. 1840–1920* (New Delhi: Oxford University Press, 2013), p. 184.

115 Letter from Balfour to Jamie, Ludhiana, dated December 19, 1893, File PP/MIB/B/3 Letters 1893, Wellcome Library.

116 Indrani Sen, 'Discourses of "gendered loyalty" Indian women in nineteenth-century "mutiny" fiction', in Biswamoy Pati (ed), *The Great Rebellion of 1857 in India Exploring transgressions, contests and diversities* (London: Routledge, 2010), p. 119.

117 Ibid., p. 126

118 Ibid., p. 119.
119 Alison Blunt, 'Embodying war: British women and domestic defilement in the Indian 'Mutiny', 1857–8', *Journal of Historical Geography*, vol. 26, no. 3, 2000, pp. 403, 407.
120 Ibid., p. 407.
121 Ibid.
122 Ibid.
123 For details see T. J. Carty, *A Dictionary of Literary Pseudonyms in the English Language* (New York: Routledge, 2014, published in 2000 in the U.K. by Mansell Publishing), p. 553. Also, 'Mrs Adeline Kingscote, née Wolff ("Lucas Cleeve") (1860–1908)', available at www.headington.org.uk/history/famous_people/kingscote.htm (consulted on 18 August, 2017).
124 See Mrs. H. Kingscote, *The English Baby in India and How to Rear It* (London: J. & A. Churchill, 1893), p. 110 cited in Saha, 'Milk, 'Race' and Nation', p. 150.
125 Kingscote, *The English Baby in India and How to Rear It*, pp. 109–110.
126 Chaudhuri, 'Memsahibs and Motherhood', p. 529.
127 *The Nurse's Guide* by 'an Eminent Physician' (London: Printed for John Brotherton; and Lawton Gilliver, 1729), pp. 21–22, 25 cited in Adriana S. Benzaquén, 'The Doctor and the Child', in Anja Müller (ed), *Fashioning Childhood Fashioning Childhood in the Eighteenth Century Age and Identity* (Aldershot: Ashgate, 2006), p. 15.
128 Kabiraj Srijukta Girijabhushan Ray Sengupta, 'Sishu-Palan' ('Child-Rearing'), *Janmabhumi*, Ashar or Monsoon season, Bengali Year 1317 or c.e. 1910 in Pradip Basu (ed), *Samayiki Purano Samayik Patrer Prabondho Sankalan, Ditiyo Khanda: Griha and Paribar* (Kolkata: Ananda Publishers Private Limited, 2009), p. 715. Title Translation: *Journal on Current Topics Collection of Old Essays from Periodicals* Second Volume: Home and Family.
129 Flora Annie Steel and Grace Gardiner, *The Complete Indian Housekeeper & Cook* (London: n.p., revised ed. 1921, first ed. 1888), p. 176 in Chaudhuri, 'Memsahibs and Motherhood in Nineteenth-Century Colonial India', p. 529. On beastly qualities from animal milk and the transfer of 'low and mean views' from wet nurse to the child, see Munshi Mohamed Yacoob, *The cry of the Child & the Calf*. (Ellore: 1908), p. 10.
130 Steel and Gardiner, *The Complete Indian Housekeeper*, p. 176, also see Indrani Sen, *Memsahibs' Writings Colonial Writing on Indian Women* (New Delhi: Orient Longman, 2008), pp. 71–72; and Flora Annie Steel and Grace Gardiner, *The Complete Indian Housekeeper & Cook* (London: Heinemann, 1904, rev. ed.), p. 176 cited in Narin Hassan, 'Feeding Empire: Wet Nursing and Colonial Domesticity in India', in Poonam Bala (ed), *Medicine and Colonial Engagements in India and Sub-Saharan Africa* (Newcastle Upon Tyne, Cambridge Scholars Publishing, 2018), p. 79.
131 Steel and Gardiner, *The Complete Indian Housekeeper*, p. 9.
132 Rosemary Marangoly George, *The Politics of the Home Postcolonial Relations and Twentieth-Century Fiction* (Berkeley: University of California Press, 1999), p. 50.
133 Éadaoin Agnew, *Imperial Women Writers in Victorian India Representing Colonial Life, 1850–1910* (Cham: Palgrave Macmillan, An Imprint of Springer Nature, 2017), p. 86. For a detailed discussion about the representations of British authority at this 'Imperial Assemblage', see Bernard S. Cohn, 'Representing Authority in Victorian India' In Eric Hobsbawm and Terence O. Ranger, *The Invention of Tradition* (Cambridge: Cambridge University Press, 1983), pp. 165–210.

134 Edith Bulwer Villiers Lytton, *India, 1876–1880* (London: privately printed at the Chiswick Press, 1899), p. 43 cited in Agnew, *Imperial Women Writers in Victorian India Representing Colonial Life*, p. 86.
135 Chaudhuri, 'Memsahibs and Motherhood in Nineteenth-Century Colonial India', p. 529. On imperial constructions of religious identities and caste prejudices, see for example, Sen, 'Colonial Domesticities, Contentious Interactions', pp. 303–304.
136 Chaudhuri, 'Memsahibs and Motherhood in Nineteenth-Century Colonial India', p. 529. It is also relevant to note the class factor here as many working-class mothers would often send their babies for nursing during the day, for example, see Alfred Greenwood, 'Some Conditions under which infants are nursed away from home', *The Hospital*, vol 44, no. 1133, 1908, 171–174. Renowned physician and medical officer for Kent Alfred Greenwood (MD) focused on the region of Blackburn, Lancashire, England in this article.
137 Madhuri Sharma, 'Creating a consumer Exploring medical advertisements in colonial India', in Biswamoy Pati and Mark Harrison (eds), *The Social History of Health and Medicine in Colonial India* (London: Routledge, 2009), pp. 215.
138 See discussion in Buettner, *Empire Families*, p. 44.
139 Steel and Gardiner, *The Complete Indian Housekeeper*, p. 166.
140 Ibid.
141 Ibid., p. 168.
142 Ibid.
143 Ibid.
144 Rima D. Apple, *Mothers and Medicine*, p. 4. For a discussion on infant feeding in Canada, especially for references to Mellin's food, see Tasnim Nathoo and Aleck Ostry, *The One Best Way? Breastfeeding History, Politics, and Policy in Canada* (Waterloo, Ontario: Wilfrid Laurier University Press, 2009), pp. 32–33, 68; on modern motherhood in Mexico, see for example, Nichole Sanders, 'Mothering Mexico: The Historiography of Mothers and Motherhood in 20th-Century Mexico', *History Compass*, vol. 7, no. 6, 2009, pp. 1542–1553, among others.
145 Saha, 'Milk, mothering & meanings', p. 108; also see G. Sankaran., 'Physiological bases of infant nutrition. *Indian Journal of Pediatrics*, vol. VIII, no. 29, 1941, pp. 1–20.
146 Apple, *Mothers and Medicine*, p. 4.
147 Ibid., p. 5. Here I have built my argument based on Linda Bryder, 'Breastfeeding and Health Professionals in Britain, New Zealand and the United States, 1900–1970', *Medical History* vol. 49, no. 2, pp. 179–196.
148 Apple, *Mothers and Medicine*, p. 11.
149 G. Mellin, *The Care of Infants in India A Work for Mothers and Nurses Upon the Feeding and Rearing of Infants* (London: G. Gill & Sons, second ed. 1895), 10, 12.
150 For a detailed analysis of the different properties of breast milk, animal milk, and various imported baby foods including Mellin's Food Rames Chandra Ray, 'Rogi O Sishudiger Khadya', *Chikitsa-Prokash*, vol. III, No. 9, Bengali Year 1317, pp. 248–55.
151 John Lockwood Kipling, *Beast and Man in India A Popular Sketch of Indian Animals in their Relations with the People* (London, Macmillan, 1891), p. 338.
152 Ibid., p. 339.
153 Madhuri Sharma, 'Creating a consumer Exploring medical advertisements in colonial India', in Biswamoy Pati and Mark Harrison (eds), *The Social History of Health and Medicine in Colonial India* (London: Routledge, 2009), p. 217.

154 Florrie Griffiths, Letter from 6 Hare Street, Calcutta, Dated January 31, 1892 in Mellin, *The Care of Infants in India*, n.p. The photograph with the letter was captioned Miss Griffiths 8 Months old.
155 Buettner, *Empire Families*, p. 46.
156 *The Care of Infants in India*, n.p.
157 Glaxo Advertisement 'The Future of the Empire lies in the arms of every Nursing Mother', *The Statesman and Friend of India*, Calcutta, 17 March, 1918, p. 20, Nehru Memorial Museum and Library, New Delhi (NMML). On gendered aspects of the advertisement, see discussion in Chapter 3 of this book.
158 Mellin's Food 'Untouched By Hand' Advertisement, *The Statesman and Friend* of India, January 17, 1918, Calcutta, p. 8, NMML.
159 Ibid.
160 Mridula Ramanna, *Health Care in Bombay Presidency 1896–1930* (Delhi: Primus, 2012), p. 122.
161 Also, see Saha, 'Milk, mothering & meanings', p. 105.
162 Srirupa Prasad, *Cultural Politics of Hygiene in India 1890–1940 Contagions of Feeling* (New York: Palgrave Macmillan, 2015), p. 108.
163 Ibid.
164 Ibid.
165 Utsa Ray, 'Constructing a "Pure" Body: The Discourse of Nutrition in Colonial Bengal', Institute of Development Studies Occasional Paper 40, 2012, p. 15 in Prasad, *Cultural Politics of Hygiene in India 1890–1940*, p. 32. On implications of 'purity' and caste, see also, 'untouched' in the context of general food items like bread, see Utsa Ray, *Culinary Culture in Colonial India A Cosmopolitan Platter and the Middle-Class* (Cambridge: Cambridge University Press, 2015), pp. 161, 175.
166 Ray, *Culinary Culture in Colonial India*, p. 161. She alerts us, however, that crisis situations like that of the Bengal famine of 1943 had revealed the materiality of fluidity of caste barriers in reality, despite their mention in books, Ibid., p. 191.
167 Ibid.
168 Ramanna, *Health Care in Bombay Presidency*, p. 122. However, she points out that Mahatma Gandhi did not approve of Mellin's food because he felt 'it is a sin to use any foreign products in India' and 'polluting even when they do not contain animal fat or alcohol'. *Collected Works of Mahatma Gandhi* Volume 11 (New Delhi: Publications Division, 1999), 18 February 1912, pp. 237–238 cited in Ibid., p. 122.
169 For example, see Nestle Milo Malted Food advertisement in *Calcutta Journal of Medicine*, vol. XXIV, no. 7, 1905, n.p., https://archive.org/details/calcuttajournal16unkngoog/mode/2up?view=theater; also, see *Calcutta Journal of Medicine*, vol. XXV, no. 10, October, 1906, n.p. (this advert mentions a gold medal received at the 'Capetown Exhibition' and 'Certificate of Merit by the Institute of Hygiene, London'), https://archive.org/details/calcuttajournal09unkngoog/page/n47/mode/2up?view=theater (Date Accessed: 02.02.14).
170 Burney Yeo, 'A Discussion on Foods for Invalids and Infants' In the Section of Pharmacology and Therapeutics at the Annual Meeting of the British Medical Association, held in Leeds, August, 1889, *British Medical Journal*, vol. 2, no. 1510, 1889, p. 1261.
171 Advertisement of Nestle Milo Malted Food, *Calcutta Journal of Medicine*, vol. XXVI, no. 12, 1907, n.p., https://archive.org/details/calcuttajournal11unkngoog/page/n3/mode/2up?view=theater (Date Accessed: 02.02.14).
172 Advertisement of Nestle Milo Food. *Calcutta Journal of Medicine*, vol. XXIV, no. 7, 1905, n.p. Also see Saha, 'Milk, mothering & meanings, p. 105.

173 Ibid.
174 Ibid.
175 See Henri Lebert, *A Treatise on Milk and Henri Nestlé's Milk Food, for the Earliest Period of Infancy and in Later Years* (Vevey, 1881), 13–15, 21 cited in Deborah Valenze, *Milk A Local and Global History* (New Haven: Yale University Press, 2011), p. 175; and see Henri Lebert, *A Treatise on Milk and Henri Nestlé's Milk Food, for the Earliest Period of Infancy and in Later Years* (Vevey, Switzerland: Published by Henri Nestlé, 1881), pp. 10–20.
176 On 'Swadeshi', see mainly Sumit Sarkar, *The Swadeshi Movement in Bengal 1903–1908* New Edition with a Preface by the author and critical essays by Neeladri Bhattacharya and Dipesh Chakrabarty (Ranikhet: Permanent Black, 2010, first ed. 1973).
177 Spermatorrhea, or a constellation of symptoms often associated with involuntary loss of semen due to nocturnal emissions, premature ejaculations, and even impotence, among others, became a 'disease entity' that caused panic in British medicine, see Robert Darby, 'Pathologizing Male Sexuality: Lallemand, Spermatorrhea, and the Rise of Circumcision', *Journal of the History of Medicine and Allied Sciences*, vol. 60, no. 3, 2005, pp. 283–319. In case of colonial India, see discussion in Douglas E. Haynes, 'Vernacular Capitalism, Advertising, And the Bazaar in Early Twentieth-Century Western India', in Ajay Gandhi, Barbara Harris-White, Douglas E. Hayne, and Sebastian Schwecke (eds), *Rethinking Markets in Modern India Embedded Exchange and Contested Jurisdiction* (Cambridge, Cambridge University Press, 2020), pp. 128, 130; also Ishita Pande, 'Time for Sex: The Education of Desire and the Conduct of Childhood in Global/Hindu Sexology', in Veronika Fuechtner, Douglas E. Haynes, and Ryan M. Jones (eds), *A Global History of Sexual Science, 1880–1960* (California: University of California Press, 2018), p. 290.
178 See Yacoob's Food advertisement in Munshi Mohamed Yacoob, *The Cry of the Child & the Calf*, pp. 3–4; also Saha, 'Milk, mothering & meanings', p. 107.
179 For a detailed discussion, see Yacoob, *The Cry of The Child & The Calf*, pp. 1–28, see mainly pp. 14, 16–17.
180 Sundari Mohan Das, *Saral Dhatri-Sikkha o Kumar-Tantra* (Calcutta: Oriental Enterprises Syndicate, third ed. 1922). Title Translation: Simple Education in Midwifery and Doctrines of Childrearing., p. 102; Sundari Mohan Das, *Sishu Mangal Pratham Shikkha* (Calcutta: Shri Premananda Das and Shri Jogananda Das, 1927), p. 43; also Saha, 'Milk, "Race" and Nation', p. 156. For a detailed discussion on Das' childcare manuals, see Chapter 5.
181 Borthwick, *The Changing Role of Women in Bengal*, p. 171.
182 See Das, *Sishu Mangal*, p. 44; Saha, 'Milk, "Race" and Nation', p. 156.
183 Sarasi Lal Sirkar, M.A., Civil Surgeon, Chittagong Hill Tracts; 'Some Observations on Infant Feeding', *Indian Medical Record*, vol. XXXVII, 1917, pp. 3–4.
184 Advertisement of Lactagol. *Journal of the Royal Sanitary Institute*, vol. XLI, no. 3.1921, p. iii https://archive.org/details/n3royalsocietyof41roya/page/n5/mode/2up?view=theater (Date Accessed: 02. 02. 14).
185 Advertisement of Lactagol. *The Statesman and Friend of India*, Calcutta, January 20 1918, p. 19, NMML.
186 Ibid.
187 Ibid.
188 Ibid.
189 Advertisement of Lactagol. *The Statesman and Friend of India*, Calcutta, June 17 1917, p. 14, NMML.
190 Ibid.
191 Sen, *Gendered Transactions*, p. 134.

192 Ibid.
193 Kate Platt, *The Home and Health in India and the Tropical Colonies* (London: Baillière, Tindall and Cox, 1923), pp. 83–84.
194 Ashis Nandy, *The Intimate Enemy: Loss and Recovery of Self under Colonialism* (Delhi: Oxford University Press, 1983) in Van Hollen, *Birth on the Threshold*, p. 50; also see Nandy, *The Intimate Enemy*, pp. 11–15 cited in Maneesha Lal, 'The Politics of Gender and Medicine in Colonial India: The Countess of Dufferin' Fund, 1885–1888', *Bulletin of the History of Medicine*, vol 68, no. 1, 1994, pp. 29–66, p. 46.
195 Rosemary Marangoly George, *The Politics of the Home Postcolonial Relations and Twentieth-Century Fiction* (Berkeley: University of California Press, 1999), p. 50.
196 Margaret Ida Balfour, undated letter no place, File: PP/MIB/B/30 Partial and Undated Letters C. 1890s–1930s; Wellcome Library, London, U.K. It is most likely at Ludhiana as Balfour has mentioned Miss Greenfield or Miss G. in her other letters from Ludhiana.
197 For a positive testimony of an artificial food, Mellin's Food, saving an abandoned baby girl Sophy Fateyl in Agra – see Sophia Bland, Letter from 1 Westfield Terrace, Ballatern, Dated August 22, 1894 in Mellin, *The Care of Infants in India*, n.p.
198 See discussion on female infanticide in Chapter 3 of this book.
199 Sen, 'Colonial Domesticities, Contentious Interactions', pp. 299, 324.
200 Michel Foucault, *The History of Sexuality* Volume I: An Introduction Translated from the French by Robert Hurley (New York: Pantheon Books, 1978), p. 100.

2

DAIS, MIDWIFERY AND WET NURSING

This chapter emphasises that both British and Bengali medical practitioners promoted 'clean' or 'scientific' midwifery and voiced the urgent need to either replace or medically train the 'ignorant' and 'dirty' *dais*. They discursively drew intimate biocultural connections between midwifery, confinement, childbirth, lactation and nursing of infants in colonial Bengal, mainly Calcutta. The dark and insanitary lying-in room of the *bhadramahila*, which represented the 'physical embodiment of the impurity associated with childbirth',[1] together with the unfavourable traditional midwifery practices, was held responsible for the prevalent high maternal and infant morbidity and mortality rates in colonial Bengal.[2] Derived from the word *dhā* meaning 'to nurse' – *dhatri/dhai/dai* refer to both the traditional midwife and wet nurse.[3] The chapter begins with a discussion about why the traditional hereditary untrained midwife or *dai* was often considered a major obstacle to European and indigenous male and female doctors as well as the medically trained midwives' efforts at providing antenatal and postnatal care across colonial India. It touches on the debates about 'clean midwifery'[4] versus 'dirty midwifery'[5] as entry points into the processes of the modernisation and 'medicalisation'[6] of maternal and child healthcare in colonial Calcutta.[7] The second section mainly explores the job role, selection, and supervision of the wet nurse as outlined in Bengali midwifery manuals. It begins by questioning the 'innocence' of maternal (lactating) breasts and explores why and how the mother's breasts were desexualised and sacralised.[8] Furthermore, it examines the fact that maternal breasts, lactation and breast milk were usually supposed to be following the laws of Nature, God-given and *natural*. Yet Bengali childcare manuals paid attention to the mother's background, morality and behaviour as essential to the medical criteria for effective lactation. In the process, the conceptualisation of the 'innocent' maternal breasts is compared and contrasted with the medical checklists for the detailed bodily examination of the wet nurse's body for hiring purposes.

DOI: 10.4324/9781003327837-3

The 'dai question'[9]

> 'The indigenous dai cannot be trained adequately in modern methods. . . . Education of the masses is what appears really the stumbling-block, so that they will ask for the services of something superior and less dangerous than the indigenous women'.[10]

By the late nineteenth century, the traditional, hereditary *dai* (midwife) was conceptualised as 'dirty', 'meddlesome' and 'dangerous' who was usually blamed for the very high maternal and infant mortality figures in colonial India.[11]

> Opinion among European doctors was divided: some thought harnessing the *dai* the only realistic way to extend at least a modicum of European influence into the birthing chamber; others thought the *dai* so uneducated and entrenched in her ways ('ignorant' and 'prejudiced' were the terms normally used) that attempts to introduce her to western medicine were a waste of time.[12]

To begin with, in 1864, sanitary commissions were set up in the presidencies and later, from 1866 to 1867, in the provinces.[13] By the late 1860s, midwifery training schemes were also introduced, although haphazardly, by missionary doctors and medical practitioners across colonial India.[14] In 1871, the Inspector-General of Hospitals, Indian Medical Department, pointed out:

> The instruction of dhaies in the Medical College and General Hospitals was sanctioned as early as 9th December 1869, and a stipend of Rs 6 per mensem assigned to 6 women at each institution. The surgeon to the General Hospital reported (29th April 1870) that the midwifery practice there was very limited, and not sufficient to serve purposes of practical instruction. Dr. Chevers reported . . . after having endeavoured by every means in his power to obtain students of this class, he was entirely unsuccessful. It was suggested by one of the native gentlemen with whom he had communicated on the subject, that the stipend was too low. Accordingly, Rs 9 per mensem were sanctioned (financial resolution No 1376, dated 22nd June 1870,) for eight dhaies to be instructed at the Medical College only up to the close of the year. The movement was unsuccessful, but since then it promises better.[15]

He further added, under the heading 'Lying-in Patients, Women, and Children up to the Age of Seven' – the number of patients treated in obstetric physician, Dr. T. E. Charles' ward 'was 747, against 662 in 1869, 774 in

1868, and 802 in the preceding year'.[16] 'There were 56 deaths, or 74.96 per mille, against 84.59 in 1869, and 76.2 in 1868'.[17] 'The number of confinements was 139, against 142, 173, 134, and 174 in the four preceding years'.[18] To corroborate his argument further, he included the annual returns of out and in-patients at the Medical College Hospital, Calcutta, for the year ending December 31, 1870 while also listing diseases of women treated namely: diseases of the uterus, diseases of the breast, and milk fever, among others.[19] Moreover, in 1870, the total number of confinements in the lying-in wards was listed as follows: Europeans (9), Indo-Europeans (45) and Natives (85), respectively.[20]

On February 24, 1873, a Government of Bengal Resolution expressed that midwifery training was intended to 'spread a knowledge of the advantage of European over native obstetrics even in simple cases'.[21] Sujata Mukherjee points out that, in Bengal, a vast majority of the members of the Calcutta Medical College (CMC) Council opposed the idea that women should get any medical training. Instead, they believed that 'women would better serve as nurses or midwives'.[22] There was resentment towards the entry of women in the medical profession as midwifery was less threatening. This was also evident from Surgeon-General Campbell Brown's statement that 'I am not an advocate for establishing female medical schools for the general teaching of the medical art. In my opinion, teaching should be confined to midwifery, and the common diseases of women and children'.[23] It is of particular interest to note that he also recommended 'stuffed models of mother and child, life-size' for midwifery training to 'aid generally in theoretical teaching' and 'in preparing novices to understand practical cases'.[24] These recommendations were probably also meant to compensate for the lack of hands-on experience in midwifery training due to low levels of hospital childbirths at the time.[25]

In the course of the nineteenth century in Calcutta, a 'new scientized *bhadralok* class'[26] had also evolved providing enormous support for the reform of traditional birthing practices. As early as in 1840, indigenous medical practitioner Madhusudan Gupta argued that traditional beliefs and practices about confinement and childbirth needed to be altered because confinement took place in a 'damp dark room very ill ventilated, with one small door only, and no window or opening in the nature of a chimney'. The doors were usually closed due to 'ritual impurity'[27] associated with childbirth which, in turn, implied:

> [C]hildren too suffer, by being kept in the same smoky room, the treatment of the mother has bad effects upon her milk, and this also disorders the child . . . I do not see in the town of Calcutta any children who are of perfect health.[28]

Madhusudan Gupta was the first to draw attention to the need for midwifery training.[29] However, Ambalika Guha argues that when questioned about the usefulness of a scheme to establish a lying-in hospital by the Fever Hospital and Municipal Improvement Committee in 1838, Gupta was against the building of the lying-in hospital as he believed that due to the prevalent prejudices, the lying-in hospital would only be used by lower classes as well as Muslim and Christian women. Instead, he made the modest proposal of creating a lying-in ward with 20 beds to be attached with the Fever Hospital and proposed the establishment of a 'school of midwifery'. The lying-in hospital was established in the Calcutta Medical College in 1840 and midwifery also came to be included in the medical curriculum from 1841.[30] The Bengali class started in 1851, which was further split into the apothecary section and the vernacular licentiate class in 1864 intended to provide medical care in the countryside.[31] In 1867, the Bengali licentiate class voiced their desire to be educated in theoretical and practical midwifery and diseases of women and children. In 1868, Sub-Assistant Surgeon Ashraf Ali (or Meer Ushruff Ally) from the Agra Medical School was appointed as the teacher of midwifery, diseases of children and women for the Bengali licentiate class at the Calcutta Medical College, a position made permanent in 1868.[32]

Sub-Assistant Surgeon Meer Ushruff Ally compiled two books based on his lectures and canonical western medical textbooks – *Handbook of Midwifery in Bengalee* and *Diseases of Children in Bengalee* – respectively. Written in simple Bengali (with an English Preface) for the Bengali licentiate class as well as lay persons, *Handbook of Midwifery in Bengalee* provided a detailed discussion on how to manage, and problems likely to be encountered in, antenatal and postnatal maternal care including various ailments like milk fever,[33] while *Diseases of Children in Bengalee* began with a brief chapter on 'Hygiene and Physical Education of Young Children'[34] focused primarily on breastfeeding along with several dos and don'ts in care of the newborn followed by an elaborate discussion of various infantile diseases. It is rather interesting to note that he mentioned 'Dr. Corbyn's Management and Diseases of Infants' among the canonical western medical textbooks consulted in the course of writing his *Diseases of Children in Bengalee*.[35] As discussed in the previous chapter, one of the earliest medical manuals on maternal and infant care in 'tropical' India, Surgeon Frederick Corbyn's book, made a few highly racist and gendered remarks. He questioned 'the general belief that native women are the best nurses' and boldly claimed that the 'poor and watery milk of a native woman'[36] which hardly had any nourishment was unsuitable for the European infant.[37]

In the Preface of his *Handbook of Midwifery in Bengalee*, Ally had also highly praised homeopathic and allopathic practitioner Annada Charan Khastagir's *A Treatise on the Science and Practice of Midwifery With Diseases of Children and Women*.[38] It is pertinent to note here that there were similarly titled vernacularised adaptations like Shri Kshirodaprasad Chattopadhyay's (L.M.S.) *Dhatribidya Subikhyato Daktar W. S. Playfair Sahiber: A Treatise on the Science and Practice of Midwifery*[39] based on famous obstetrician William Smoult Playfair's *A Treatise on the Science and Practice of Midwifery* (Volumes I and II).[40] In nineteenth and the early twentieth century Calcutta, Bengali midwifery manuals, encompassing detailed advice on maternal and infant care, also gradually became very popular giving instructions in simple language and addressed to Bengali mothers, medical students and midwives. Medicine also emerged as a cultural practice as 'the break between medical and popular ideas was not always sharp'.[41] Meredith Borthwick argues that Brahmo reformer Shib Chunder Deb, an administrator and 'not a doctor', published his childcare manual titled *The Infant Treatment* First Part in 1857 which was possibly the first among the series of Bengali maternal and infant care manuals created generally on 'English prototypes'.[42] 'His experience of having lost two sons because of the ignorance of midwives, inadequate conditions for birth, and the lack of after-care was a contributing motive'.[43] He specifically adapted Scottish physician and phrenologist, Andrew Combe's *Treatise on the Physiological and Moral Management of Infancy* to the 'wants of Hindoo Society' in Calcutta.[44] In the first of the series of essays published in the Brahmo women's magazine *Bamabodhini Patrika* about reorganisation of the lying-in room, Shib Chunder Deb's influence is perceptible.[45] *Bamabodhini Patrika* was started to educate the *bhadramahila* in health science through 'home tutoring'.[46] Along these lines, one of the earliest and very popular Bengali midwifery manuals like famous Jodu Nath Mukerje's *Dhatri Sikkha* mentioned that '[b]esides being of use to native midwives . . . the book may be read by Hindoo-females who will no longer place themselves in the hands of ignorant women in one of the most critical periods of their life'.[47]

From being 'ignorant', 'dirty' and feared as 'a sorceress' to having a 'hereditary claim on the family of her patient' – I aim to highlight the contradictions inherent in the dichotomous representations of 'dirty'/'clean' midwifery in European and Bengali medical print media on midwifery, encompassing maternal and infant care. Lieutenant Colonel E. E. Waters (I.M.S), Superintendent of the Howrah General Hospital, elaborately discussed the difficulties associated with the 'dai question' being 'the religious and social prejudices of the patients and patients' family, and the vested interest of the dai class itself'. He emphasised that '[t]he indigenous dai is of a low caste, usually Chamar or something equally ignoble', who often held a 'hereditary claim on the family of her patient, in that she or her mother, and possibly her grandmother, have attended successive generations'.[48] He also highlighted:

> I have made many attempts to induce dais to come for training. The older ones won't come, the younger ones usually attend irregularly. Their husbands get jealous, their children want them, some one must cook the family meals, and so on. What advantage are they to gain by coming? An Eden-trained dai makes about Rs. 50 to Rs.

> 100 per mensem in Calcutta. An untrained dai makes about Rs. 25 to Rs. 50 per mensem, with presents of food, saris, and other gifts. This she does easily without any continued attendance at a hospital or restriction of any sort.[49]

Waters alerted that despite the fact that the 'ignorant untrained dai is still extensively employed there is a growing demand for Eden Hospital trained nurses. This is especially noticeable in the educated classes of Calcutta and gets less marked as one leaves the metropolis behind'.[50]

In fact, from the 1870s onwards, midwifery training also attracted the *bhadramahila* as few Brahmo and Hindu women enrolled for the midwifery course offered by the Calcutta Medical College (CMC).[51] Mukherjee emphasises that the Eden Hospital midwifery programme was ultimately difficult requiring a basic knowledge of English and regular attendance thereby ruling out the enrolment of the traditional *dais*.[52] Mukherjee also points out that midwifery candidates had to undergo elaborate training including courses in the 'Sick Nursing Certificate' programme alongside others in anatomy, signs and symptoms of pregnancy and natural labour, breastfeeding and management of newborn infants, etc.[53] In her memoir, famous 'lady doctor' at the Hooghly Lady Dufferin Women's Hospital, Chinsurah, Haimabati Sen's vivid description of her experience of the death of her newborn during childbirth and how she coped also mentioned renowned trained midwife Hemangini Das (Mrs. Sundari Mohan Das), who had passed the Midwife course at Eden Hospital in 1880 and often worked together with her husband, Dr. Sundari Mohan Das (M.B.) as follows[54]:

> They held me down and placed the chloroform cup on my mouth. I struggled a little and then lost consciousness. I had never seen anyone in this situation with my own eyes. This was the first occurrence of an event which I then found so unnatural. I had not totally lost consciousness. I could feel Mrs. Das pulling at something. She could only partially pull it out. I was dimly aware of all that was happening. Sundari Babu pulled out that thing. It seemed the child moved its feet several times when he had come half way out but I have no knowledge of what happened after. . . . When I woke up, I found my husband seated near me. He looked sad . . . he got up and showed me the dead child. I had never seen such a beautiful child in my life. He broke down as he brought the child to me . . . My husband asked, 'Can you stay alone?' I said, 'Why?' He said, 'I have to go and dispose of this thing.' I said, 'You may go.' . . . The doctor and his wife started coming both in the morning and the evening. At the time I did not understand what was happening. They took great care of me and did not charge any fees. . . . I could not understand why such a storm had passed over my life,

> why I had lost my child. My heart was seared with grief for that child. I became mad in my obsession with the one thought: why didn't I die? I developed some symptoms of insanity. . . . Sometimes I feared the police would come and arrest me; at other times I feared that people would hold me down and apply chloroform. . . . My husband moved house. He rented a room on the ground floor in Thakamani Ghosh's house. Another family of tenants also lived there; this Gobinda Majumdar was a very fine person. He had a large number of children including a newborn baby. I spent all my time with those children and breast-fed the baby. I had an excessive quantity of milk in my breast which I had previously squeezed out. Now Robin drank my milk. His mother did not have enough milk in her breasts but he became quite chubby on mine. Naren and Mini had their meals with me. I dressed their hair and they also slept beside me. They came to their 'Aunt' for everything.[55]

As midwifery training was usually about teaching *dais* and trained midwives about simple deliveries, cleanliness and when to call a doctor in case of abnormal labour – critical cases still had to be attended by doctors. Progressive colonial and indigenous opinion, therefore, supported training of female doctors in India. Kumari Jayawardena points out that initially there was also considerable hostility towards the entry of women medical students into universities in Victorian Britain in the 1870s. Women students who were rejected by Edinburgh University, such as Sophia Jex-Blake, Edith Pechey and others, opened the London School of Medicine for Women in 1874 while, in 1876, the British Parliament removed restrictions on the entry of women as medical students into Universities in Britain.[56] It was with the passage of the Russell Gurney Enabling Act and 'the 1877 decision of the King's and Queen's College of Physicians of Ireland to examine women and thus potentially admit them to the Medical Register' which 'seemed to end the battle for women's entry into medicine'.[57] Maneesha Lal highlights that colonial India provided a platform for social mobility and a justification for extending the permissible roles, in the face of restrictions in England, particularly for educated middle-class English women.[58] In India, female medical students gained entry to Madras Medical College in 1875, followed by Grant Medical College in Bombay and Calcutta Medical College in 1883. Mary Scharlieb, private medical practitioner and eugenicist, recalled the resentment against female medical students from her experiences in Madras in 1875 – 'Dr. Branfoot expressed himself as to the folly of educating women to be doctors'. She pointed out that '[h]e told us that the Government had sent us to him, and he could not prevent us from walking round the wards, but that he was firmly determined that he would not teach us'.[59]

As already mentioned briefly in Chapter 1 of this book, in 1885, the Countess of Dufferin's Fund was set up as a non-sectarian medical service which trained women doctors, midwives and nurses.[60] The vicereines of India took the following maternal and child welfare initiatives: the Countess of Dufferin's Fund or Dufferin Fund by Lady Dufferin (1885), the Victoria Memorial Scholarships Fund or V.M.S.F. by Lady Curzon (1903), The Lady Chelmsford All-India League for Maternity and Child Welfare by Lady Chelmsford (1920) and Lady Reading's Baby Weeks programme (1924). These funds received governmental support but these were independent in administration and dependent on funds raised by philanthropists.[61] The quasi-governmental organisational structure 'demonstrates that ultimately the government did not consider maternal health to be an issue of the state, and without full government support it was difficult for these funds to survive'.[62] As Samiksha Sehrawat argues, by the early twentieth century in colonial India, the state left medical care of Indian women to the Dufferin Fund, Association of Medical Women in India (AMWI, 1907), and the Women's Medical Service (1913) which functioned as 'saviours of Indian womanhood'.[63] At the same time, it is pertinent to note that both European and indigenous elite men and women often shared power/knowledge, for example, by promoting maternal and child welfare ideas and initiatives, particularly through these quasi-governmental organisations on a pan-Indian scale.[64]

In particular, in case of the medicalisation of childbirth through midwifery training by the aforementioned Victoria Memorial Scholarships Fund (V.M.S.F) – for European and indigenous, male and female medical practitioners alike, the main concern was whether the *dai* could be medically trained and if it was possible to replace traditional 'dirty midwifery' with 'clean midwifery'. The Countess of Dufferin's Fund headed the V.M.S.F. However, unlike the V.M.S.F., the Countess of Dufferin's Fund aimed to train 'a new cadre of midwives who were not hereditary dais'.[65] Even though midwifery training was initially intended for women from better educated classes as by the Dufferin Fund, Supriya Guha points out that ritual pollution and caste structure were complex and problematic issues when it came to childbirth with traditional low caste *dais* and their assistants as '*narkata*' or 'cord-cutters' whereby the V.M.S.F. specifically targeted them for midwifery training.[66] It was founded in 1903, closely following in the footsteps of the first Midwives Act in England in 1902 to check unlicensed midwifery.[67] As also mentioned in the Introduction of this book, it bore the imprint of the Director of the Ethnographic Survey of India, Herbert Hope Risley's '*idées fixes*' about the 'immutability of caste-related practices' which reveals 'political sensitivity' to the question of customary childbirth practices.[68] In colonial India, the establishment of the V.M.S.F. was meant to restrict untrained *dais* from practising their trade and thereby creating 'trained midwives' out of them.[69]

Midwifery training was integral to maternal and infant welfare as evident from the arguments put forward by Y. Sen, Women's Medical Service, Raj Dufferin Hospital in Bettiah. She pointed out that maternal and infant welfare measures like education of the mother would ensure that the girl child is brought up 'in such a way from her infancy that she grows up to be *an ideal woman as well as an ideal mother*' (emphasis added).[70] Sen emphasised that

> we must have strong healthy mothers and strong healthy babies. . . . If we want to see India great, we must take care of our mothers and babies.[71]

Moreover, she believed that midwifery training would eliminate the danger from the unhygienic birthing practices of the untrained traditional *dais* or 'dirty midwifery'[72] responsible for deadly diseases like tetanus. This may be located amidst the widely prevalent so-called *bhadra* or 'respectable', usually upper caste and/or middle-class contempt towards the *dai*, often '*Chamarni*, *Dosad* or *Hari* women'[73] visible in early twentieth-century Bengali midwifery advice. 'Dirty' was most often symbolised by the main figure of 'the Chamar *dai*'.[74] The 'vilification of the Chamar *dai*' as 'barbaric', 'non-scientific', and 'inherently dirty' and 'evil' – 'all combined the logic of caste with a modern civic discourse'.[75] Midwifery training attempted

> to dislodge the Chamar *dai* from her hereditary occupation and increasingly came to construct her as unintelligent, ignorant, dirty, filthy and debased, burdened with the inability to learn new methods. Systems of surveillance thus came to appear around Dalit female reproductive technologies.[76]

Sen had also highlighted that often the real problem was that 'the hereditary dais (indigenous) are looked upon as women gifted with abnormal powers, and the public while having great faith in them are afraid of them' because 'they believe that these women when offended can harm them in various ways, being a kind of sorceress'.[77] As Charu Gupta argues, by the late nineteenth century, the Chamar *dai* was often constructed and vilified as 'barbaric, as extremely dangerous for women, as the killer of children, as a witch'.[78]

Margaret Ida Balfour and Ruth Young's *The Work of Medical Women in India* (1929) added:

> As long as the patients did not demand a higher standard of skill in their attendants at childbirth, there was no inducement for the *dais* to seek it. All were alike in the matter of training though some might be more skilful as a result of natural gifts or experience. Had the patients appreciated the need for another kind of midwife, and been willing to pay for her, the *dais* would have been forced to come for training through fear of losing their clients, even if they did not do so from pure love of knowledge.[79]

Balfour and Young believed that at the pan-Indian level, the response to the training of *dais* was 'rather meagre'. Some centres showed 'good and successful work' while others admitted 'failure and actually gave up'.[80] They highlighted that women in the villages were usually without trained midwives which made them dependent on *dais*. Due to their lack of interest alongside financial and time constraints, *dais* would not travel to the nearest town for lessons.[81] Balfour and Young also drew attention to the main causes behind maternal mortality in India to have been most often related to 'bad attendance at the time of childbirth' and the 'lack of any legislation requiring registration and supervision of midwives', followed by 'lack of medical aid and of women's hospitals', 'lack of antenatal centres, both for treatment and research'; and 'the existence of certain serious and fatal diseases connected with pregnancy, such as anaemia and osteomalacia'.[82] However, they believed that trained midwives significantly reduced maternal mortality associated with childbirth in India as evident from their rough estimate of maternal mortality rates mainly in Bombay, Calcutta and Madras (Table 2.1)[83]:

Based on research conducted in 1930s Calcutta (areas under Health Officer of the Calcutta Corporation excluding Howrah and Garden Reach), Professor of Maternity and Child Welfare at the All-India Institute of Hygiene and Public Health in Calcutta, M. I. Neal Edwards' (MD, W.M.S.) *Report of an Enquiry Into the Causes of Maternal Mortality in Calcutta* estimated that maternal deaths[84] in Calcutta related to childbearing was 5.85% when attended by trained midwives and 27.82% by untrained *dais* (Table 2.2).[85] Ambalika Guha referring to the same report highlighted the '"growing popularity of institutional delivery" in the city'.[86] The Calcutta Municipal

Table 2.1 Maternal Mortality Rates in Childbirth in India

Source of Information	*Cases*	*Maternal Deaths*	*Rate per 1000 births*
Bombay Corporation Health Officer's Report, 1924	21,838	365	16.7
Calcutta Corporation Health Officer's Report, 1924	17,219	320	18.0
Madras Corporation Midwives, 1924	7,027	33	4.7
Bombay Corporation Midwives, 1924	1,850	9	4.8
Calcutta Corporation Midwives, 1924	4,380	9	2.0
Delhi Municipal Midwives, 1925–1926	306	nil	
Simla Municipal Midwives, 1925–1926	600	4	6.5
Bengal Enquiry, 1919–1925	3,844	47	12.2

Source: Margaret Ida Balfour and Ruth Young, *The Work of Medical Women in India*, p. 189 [with permission from the British Library].

Attendant at Delivery

Attendant.	Deaths due directly to childbearing		Deaths due to associated diseases.		Total.
Trained—					
Midwives	41	5·85%	11	5·91%	52
Private Doctors	15	2·14%	6	3·23%	21
Hospitals	268	38·23%	42	22·58%	310
Maternity Homes	22	3·14%	10	5·38%	32
Untrained—					
Relatives	44	6·28%	16	8·60%	60
Dais	195	27·82%	65	34·95%	260
Irrelevant cases (undelivered, threatened abortions)	113	16·12%	35	18·81%	148
Unknown	3	0·42%	1	0·54%	4
	701		186		887

Table 2.2 Maternal Deaths and Attendants at Delivery

Source: M. I. Neal Edwards, *Report of an Enquiry into the Causes of Maternal Mortality in Calcutta*, Table 15, p. 32 [with permission from the British Library].

Corporation's role was pivotal to the expansion of domiciliary midwifery services, health visitors and a chain of maternity homes.[87] Furthermore, Neal Edwards emphasised that, out of a total of 887 maternal deaths, the report stated that 80% of the women observed purdah – Muslim women usually followed 'strict purdah' while Hindus were usually confined to the house thereby living without fresh air and exercise.[88] 'Purdah as Pathology'[89] implied that Muslim women were often perceived as 'the most disadvantaged'.[90] Moreover, as Samiksha Sehrawat argues, rhetoric about the 'backwardness' of Indian women in purdah, usually identified as a 'passive' and 'undifferentiated' 'aggregate', went hand in hand with the supposed benevolence of the Raj and superiority of western medicine trying to meet Indian women's medical needs and 'rescue' them from Indian patriarchy.[91] Supriya Guha emphasises that colonial civilising missions and modern reproductive health facilities might have inaugurated the 'modern family' by disrupting 'traditional household structures' but purdah hospitals promoted 'the idea of a highly prized fundamental modesty among Bengali women of the *bhadra* classes, while displaying their commitment to a scientific and rational way of life'.[92] Neal Edwards also calculated, besides maternal deaths, the accompanying foetal and infant deaths which were as follows: 46% of infants were alive at birth and 28% stillborn. 'The total foetal mortality including abortions, ectopics and undelivered case was 50 per cent'. However, 'it was reported that 55 per cent of the infants born alive had died by time the mothers' deaths were followed up. This gives a combined foetal and neonatal mortality of 65.77 per cent'.[93] She added that there was also a shortage of available maternity beds alongside the fact that maternity wards usually lacked facilities for accommodating infant care, unlike infant welfare centres (Table 2.3).

Official vernacularised manuals like the 38-page booklet *Bharater desi daider jonno dhatrisikkha* (Midwifery Education for the Indian Indigenous Midwives) by the famous Margaret Ida Balfour, as also mentioned in Chapter 1 of this book, she was joint-secretary to the Dufferin Fund (1916–1924) and appointed chief medical officer of the Women's Medical Service in 1920,[94] aimed to spread awareness about a range of issues particularly related to midwifery and postpartum maternal and infant care. In Chapters 5 and 6 titled

Institutional Midwifery, Calcutta, 1935

Name of Institution.	Antenatal clinic.	No. of Obstetric Beds.				No. of Midwives.		Total deliveries.
		Antenatal.	Maternity.	Others available.	Total.	Trained.	Pupil.	
Hospitals.								
Eden	Yes	No separate ward.	36	26	62	10	54	2,294
Dufferin	Yes	Ditto	30	..	30	4	14	884
Chittaranjan Seva Sadan	No	Ditto	54	..	54	21	46	1,946
Chittaranjan	No	Ditto	15	6	21	7	26	408
Campbell	Yes	Ditto	22	..	22	2	..	667
Carmichael Medical College	No	Ditto	46	28	74	3	..	1,652
Marwari Hospital	No	Ditto	13	8	21	4	..	183
Sambhu Nath Pandit	No	Ditto	12	6	18	6	..	178
Calcutta Medical School Hospital	Yes	Ditto	30	10	40	4	6	236
Corporation Maternity Homes.								
1. Baldeodas	No	No	35	No	35	5	9	2,591
2. Kidderpore	No	No	24	No	24	4	..	931
3. Chetla	No	No	40	No	40	3	..	657
4. Manicktola	No	No	20	6 (septic).	26	3	..	298
Ramkrishna Mission Shishumangal Pratisthan.	Yes	2	13	5	20	3	12	448
		2	390	95	487	79	167	13,273

Table 2.3 Institutional Midwifery in Calcutta in 1935

Source: M. I. Neal Edwards, *Report of an Enquiry into the Causes of Maternal Mortality in Calcutta*, p. 33 [with permission from the British Library].

'*Matake Jotno Karan*' (Taking Care of the Mother) and '*Sishur Rakkhanabekkhon*' (Infant Care), Balfour insisted that the midwife was supposed to attend to both the mother and the child on every visit. She argued that the infant must be put to the breast as soon as possible after birth. Colostrum was recommended in order to cleanse the bowels. She pointed out that milk is eventually produced by the mother usually from the third day. She advised that breastfeeding should occur at regular intervals of two and a half hours then feeding would occur eight times in a day. Also, one feed at night was necessary. She instructed that every time the child cried, disciplined feeding routine should not be broken. Instead the midwife should explain to the mother that she needed to pay attention to any pain or discomfort the child might be facing instead of feeding every time she heard the infant crying. Advice was also to be given on how to sterilise and humanise cow's milk (often by adding water and a little bit of sugar) and to-dos related to bottle feeding and cleaning instructions before and after feeding.[95]

Ruth Young, renowned medical practitioner in northern India and later Director of the Maternity and Child Welfare Bureau, wrote *Antenatal Work in India* which was 'a small handbook which could be used by midwives as well as health visitors and even by sub-assistant surgeons'.[96] Young explained that antenatal work involved educating the mother and also influencing the 'expectant father' – who 'was more easy to influence than the expectant mother'[97] in some cases, and the 'training of dais'. She emphasised:

> [T]he health visitor must be careful not to correct the dai in front of the patient, or make any remarks considered as implying that the dai had done something wrong. On the contrary, the dai's prestige should be increased and the attitude should be that of treating the dai as a 'colleague'.[98]

During an antenatal examination, the *dai* was meant to learn by watching the doctor or health visitor about how to inquire about a case as well as how to wash hands and prepare a patient. She explained:

> In classes for dais, it is often difficult to secure that the dais examine normal cases before delivery and learn the presentations and positions on living persons. Without this, it is almost impossible to convince the dais that external examination can tell us all we want to know in normal cases. Antenatal work gives us just this opportunity and we should not be slow to avail ourselves of it. The benefit both to the mothers and dais is great.[99]

'An antenatal clinic is a special session at a child welfare centre or in connection with child welfare scheme' where mothers and toddlers are examined, and often mothers were advised about 'mother-craft'.[100] She also advised that cards for filling in the 'history of confinement' and 'details of the

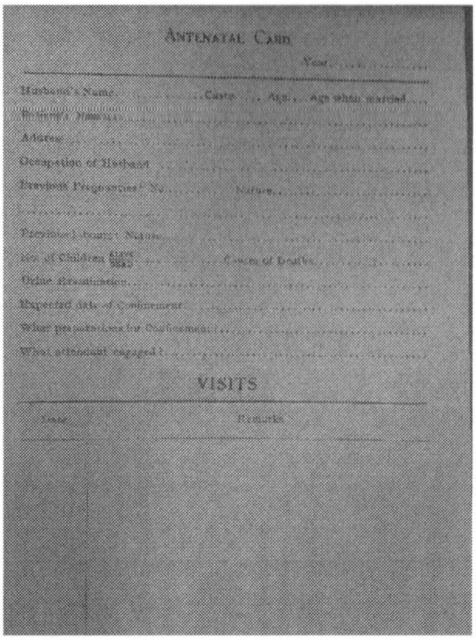

Antenatal Card

Year

Husband's Name ... Caste ... Age ... Age when married ...

Address

Occupation of Husband

Previous Pregnancies: No. ... Nature ...

No. of Children ... Causes of Deaths ...

Expected date of Confinement

What attendant engaged?

VISITS

Date	Remarks

Figure 2.1 Patient Card (Front).

Source: Ruth Young, *Antenatal Work in India*, p. 105 [with permission from National Library, Kolkata].

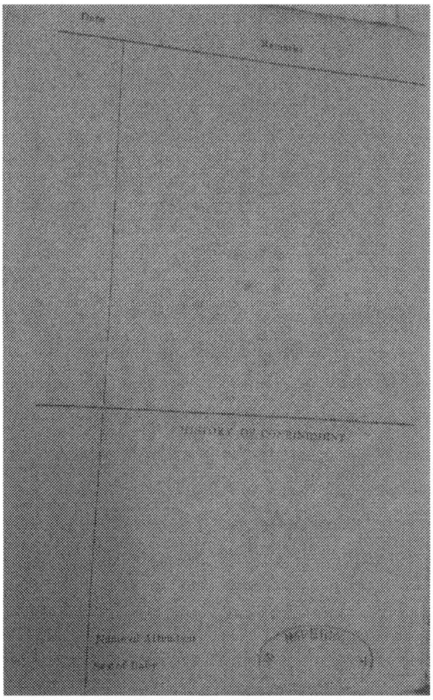

Date	Remarks

Figure 2.2 Patient Card (Back).

Source: Ruth Young, *Antenatal Work in India*, p. 106 [with permission from National Library, Kolkata.

examination' of the patient must be ready.[101] 'The same cards may be used, but red ink can be used for clinic visits and blue for home ones'.[102]

Thus, in late nineteenth and early twentieth century colonial Bengal, *dais*, like the traditional Burmese female midwives or *wan zwe* ('pulling the womb' in Burmese), were usually stereotyped as dangerous, barbarous and unchanging in their ways and thereby blamed for the prevalent high maternal and infant mortality rates.[103] The demonisation of the 'native' untrained midwives as 'purveyors of death'[104] alongside the 'infantalization'[105] of 'ignorant' indigenous mothers like children need to be contextualised amidst the wider processes of infantilisation of entire indigenous populations as the 'psychological force of colonialism'.[106] Both European and Bengali medical practitioners discursively drew intimate biocultural connections between midwifery, confinement, childbirth and nursing of infants in colonial Bengal, mainly Calcutta. These, therefore, also provided discursive 'elite nationalist maps for female agency'[107] meant to discipline, replace or reconfigure beliefs and practices of 'dirty midwifery', ritual pollution associated with childbirth, and Indian mother love. It is pertinent to note, however, as Lang argues:

> The low estimation in which the *dai* was held was partly an issue of caste, and partly a comment on her perceived level of competence . . . By no means were all *dais* as incompetent as the stereotype suggests . . . when they could point to a record of successful deliveries.[108]

Innocence of Maternal Breasts: Divine/Natural/Maternal/ Sexual/Economical

> Wet-nursing- If for any reason the child can not be fed by its mother, the best substitute is 'wet-nursing' i.e. nursing with the breast milk of another woman.[109]

This section focuses on the medical criteria outlined by Bengali *daktars* for the selection and supervision of the *dai* or wet nurse. It begins by exploring the notion that motherhood along with maternal breasts, lactation and breast milk were usually supposed to be following the laws of Nature, God-given and *natural*. Yet, in maternal and infant welfare manuals, the 'ideal' mother was often deified while scrutinising her morality, temperament and behaviour, all essentials in medical advice for effective maternal breastfeeding. The 'innocence' and divinity inherent in representations of maternal lactating breasts, however, contrast with the elaborate medical lists for the selection and supervision of the wet nurse, the economical breast.

In Renaissance paintings about divine maternity, the nursing Madonna was 'the prototype of female divinity' – the maternal act of smiling at her baby in her arms and pressing her breast with two fingers in order to aid the flow of milk.[110] Marilyn Yalom argues that next to the blood of Jesus Christ, the Virgin Mary's milk was supposed to be one of the holiest fluids capable of producing miracles whereby numerous vials of Mary's milk were placed in churches.[111] Moreover, Yalom emphasises that dramatic changes in breast lore have taken place across the centuries, for example, the nursing Madonna appeared in the fourteenth century to the erotic bosom of the sixteenth century and the political breast of the eighteenth century.[112] By the early nineteenth century, the nursing and the sexualised breasts that had been separate during the Renaissance were reunited into a 'multipurpose bosom'.[113] With 'erotic overtones', however, the maternal breast was frequently 'called upon to serve various national interests',[114] to 'inspire political rather than sexual feelings'.[115]

The 'glorification of the maternal breast'[116] also depended on the fact that 'breasts were divided into two categories: the 'corrupted' or 'polluting' breast, linked to wet nursing; and the maternal breast, linked to familial and social regeneration'.[117] In Europe, the wet nurse controversy involved, for instance, the famous Swedish physician and botanist Carolus Linnaeus (1707–1778) as he argued, in his Latin treatise *Nutrix Noverca* (which approximately translates as 'Unnatural Mother'), that wet nursing 'violated the laws of nature and endangered the life of both mother and child'.[118] He is remembered, however, not as 'a wet-nursing abolitionist' but as a zoological taxonomist who coined the term 'mammalia' or mammals from the Latin 'mammae' or 'milk-secreting organs' to distinguish suckling animals from all other creatures.[119] Singling out the mammae dovetailed eighteenth-century politics favouring maternal breastfeeding and an exclusively domestic role for women.[120] For Linnaeus, like many Enlightenment thinkers, breastfeeding was 'a matter of maternal instinct', believed to be 'inborn in animals, including humankind'.[121]

Valerie A. Fildes argues that the eighteenth century was the most significant period for the emergence of new ideas about wet nursing and maternal breastfeeding as medicine and science advanced.[122] This 'century of the Enlightenment was, above all, concerned with Nature and the pursuance of the natural method in areas such as infant feeding'.[123] In the medical world, as 'new ideas about man and Nature' were pursued daily, '[w]omen were advised to imitate the brute beasts in the way in which they fed and cared for their babies'.[124] Medical handbooks for mothers advocated simplicity and non-interference while it forbade the use of 'strange' and 'inferior' women to nurse babies since it was considered as '*highly unnatural*' (emphasis added).[125] One of the most influential published works in England was William Cadogan's (1711–1797) *An Essay Upon Nursing and the Management of Children* published in 1748.[126] The London Foundling Hospital adopted Cadogan's work as 'the tenet of care for their infant foundlings'[127] He criticised wet nursing and recommended 'every father to have his child nursed under his own eye, to make use of his own reason and sense in superintending and directing the management of it'.[128] He advised 'every mother that can . . . to suckle it. If she be a healthy woman, it will confirm her health; if weakly, in most cases it will restore her'.[129] Fildes highlights that from letters and other sources of upper class families in Britain and France, there is proof that many tried to use Cadogan and particularly Rousseau's childrearing advice in bringing up their children.[130] It is impossible to gauge, however, the extent to which such authors influenced childcare as we do not have any clarity about the numbers that read their books or followed the guidelines they contained.[131] However, as Fildes emphasises, it may be certainly argued that these two authors were highly influential in the popular movement towards maternal breastfeeding, particularly in upper and middle-class society in Britain, Europe and North America from the mid-eighteenth century onwards.[132]

Enlightenment *philosophe*, Jean-Jacques Rousseau (1712–1778), was enormously influential in his campaign against wet nursing popularised (primarily through negative publicity as his book was banned as blasphemous) through his educational treatise *Émile* published in 1762. He argued that maternal breastfeeding was a natural means to regenerate family and society.[133] Rousseau believed that 'the earliest education is most important and it undoubtedly is woman's work. If the author of nature had meant to assign it to men he would have given them milk to feed the child'.[134] He urged authors to address their treatises to women as they watch over their children more closely and are more affectionate towards them than men together with their highly influential role in educating their children and for the proper functioning of the family as a whole.[135] About breastfeeding, he went on to argue:

> The woman who nurses another's child in place of her own is a bad mother; how can she be a good nurse? She may become one in time; use will overcome nature, but the child may perish a hundred times before his nurse has developed a mother's affection for him. . . . But when mothers deign to nurse their own children, then will be a reform in morals; *natural feeling* will revive in every heart; there will be no lack of citizens for the state, this first step by itself will restore mutual affection.
>
> (emphasis added)[136]

Mary Seidmen Trouille argues that even though Rousseau's educational treatise was addressed to aristocratic women,[137] the 'implied reader of *Emile* is generally male and its point of view distinctly masculine'.[138] As Yalom also highlights, the 'sexist worldview' inherent in '[t]he Rousseauist idea that woman was by nature a giving, loving, self-sacrificing, contingent creature' was crucial to the new cult of idealising motherhood that became normative across Europe and America for the next two centuries.[139] Yalom finds consolation in the fact that today we have learned from anthropological and medical research that breast feeding is not instinctive but a learned activity like any other social behaviour.[140]

Similarly, Ruth Perry points out that, by the mid-eighteenth century in Europe, '[m]aternal feeling, as the medical establishment increasingly made clear, was biologically determined; women who lacked it were abnormal'.[141] However, motherhood was also coercive when it became '[n]atural but learned'[142] – as taught by many, mainly medical men. Biological and *natural* motherhood was supposed to be the outcome of intelligible bodily processes.[143] Mother's breasts underwent deliberate 'desexualization',[144] in combination with the 'sentimental trope' of motherhood which represented a 'productive view of heterosexual relations'.[145] Breasts also became the 'site of the struggle' as the maternal and sexualised bodies were counterposed often leading to the victorious emergence of 'a mother-self at the service of the family and the state'.[146] It 'represented in both physiological and psychological terms' what 'would seem to be a paradox – the asexual mother, a contradiction in terms'. Feminists continue to debate over the categories 'sexual' and 'maternal' and whether their attributes are 'mutually exclusive' or not.[147]

In the context of colonial Bengal, divinity and purity associated with maternal breasts and the mother-child bond is compromised if one pays attention to the less openly discussed viewpoint, as Nripendra Kumar Bose and Aradhana Debi highlight, that a nursing mother can give up sexual intercourse with her husband between the third and up to the ninth month following delivery of a child possibly because the 'lactating mother has some form of sexual equivalent in the sucking of the baby'.[148] However, as Tanika Sarkar argues, the female/maternal body was largely imagined in nationalist iconography through the deployment of the cult of the 'Mother Goddess' and as a 'race of mothers – "*mayerjati*" ' embodying a 'domesticated gentle feminity' and '*Shakti*' or strength with 'innocent', 'full breasts' responsible for raising 'patriotic' sons who would regenerate and reclaim their 'sacralised and feminised' 'mother's breasts'/'motherland'/'*Bharatmata*' or 'Mother India'.[149] Sarkar emphasises that nationalist iconography in nineteenth-century Bengali literature connected, what Partha Chatterjee has demarcated as separate inner/spiritual versus the outer/materialist domains, especially through the powerful imagery of '*mayerjati*'. She argues that for Bengalis especially, who were habituated with worship of various female cults, 'emotional resonances connected with an enslaved mother figure tended to be particularly powerful' whereby '[d]uring the Salt movement, for example, the alienation of salt-making rights from Indians was expressed through a representation of the salt earth, as the full breasts of the mother to which none other than the child may have access'.[150]

In ancient India, full breasts, breast milk and breastfeeding were iconic prerequisites in the imaginings of motherhood with the mother as *naturally* a nurturing figure which, in turn, underscores the significance of reproductive functions in the very definition of womanhood. Rahul Peter Das argues that teleological connections were often implied between the female body, mother love, effective lactation and breastfeeding. As 'motherly feelings' or 'love for the child' was supposed to determine successful lactation and breastfeeding, 'one can only speculate on what distress this notion must have caused women having difficulty in breastfeeding'.[151] He points out that, in canonical medical texts like the *Susruta Samhita*, the governing assumption was that a woman could have milk shooting from her breasts at the thought of pregnancy or of a child.[152] He emphasises that a woman's body and breasts were perceived in myriad ways – milk could be periodically present in a woman's breasts at certain times like pregnancy and after childbirth (and may or may not be present in her body otherwise), or she could have been perceived to have been 'always pregnant or else breastfeeding' or 'always has milk in her breasts' or in her body as one of 'the constituents of the body'.[153] It could also be that women, other than pregnant women or mothers, were not considered worthy of discussion at all whereby we mainly come across references to women as 'always pregnant or else breast-feeding'.[154]

Kaviraj Kunja Lal Bhishagratna, a resident of Calcutta, translated the *Susruta Samhita* into English in three volumes. In the second volume, there was an analogy between breast milk and semen. He argued that breast milk is 'secreted, and flows out at the touch, sight or thought of the child in the same manner as the semen is dislodged and emitted at the sight, touch or recollection etc. of a beloved woman'.[155] Both semen and breast milk are delineated as 'the product of the essence of digested food, this essence being converted into milk in women'.[156] Thereafter, there is a brief discussion about the selection of a wet nurse 'from among the matrons of its own caste (Varna) and possessed of the following necessary qualifications'[157]

> [S]he should be of middle stature, neither too old nor too young (middle-aged), of sound health, of good character (not irascible or easily excitable), not fickle, ungreedy, neither too thin nor too corpulent, with lips unprotruded, and with healthy and pure milk in her breasts which should neither be too much pendulent nor drawn up.[158]

Moreover, it had to be ensured that 'her skin is healthy and unmarked by any moles or stains, she being free from any sort of crime (such as gambling, day-sleep, debauchery, etc.). She should be of an affectionate heart, and with all her children living'.[159] She should also have been 'of respectable parentage and consequently possessed of many good qualities, with an exuberance of milk in her breasts'.[160] There were also incantations for breastfeeding and several dietary remedies listed to increase the flow of milk as follows:

> The face of the child should be turned towards the north, while the nurse should look to the east at the time. Then, after first having a small quantity of the milk pressed out and the breast washed and consecrated with the following Mantras (incantations) the child should be made to suck her right breast. . . . 'O, thou beautiful damsel, may the four oceans of the earth contribute to the secretion of milk in thy breasts for the purpose of improving the bodily strength of the child. O, thou with a beautiful face, may the child, reared on your milk, attain a long life, like the gods made immortal with drinks of ambrosia'.
>
> The loss or suppression of the milk in the breasts of a woman is usually due to anger, grief, and the absence of natural affection for her child, etc. For the purpose of establishing a flow in her breast, her equanimity should be first restored, and diets consisting of Śáli-rice, barley, wheat, Shashtika, meat-soup, wine (Surá), Souviraka, sesamum-paste, garlic, fish, *Kas'eruka*, *S'ringátaka*, lotus-stalk, *Vidári-kanda*, *Madhůka* flower, *S'atávari*, Naliká, *Alávu*, and *Kála-S'áka*, etc. should be prescribed. . . . A child should not be allowed to take the breast of a hungry, aggrieved, fatigued, too thin, too corpulent, fevered, or a pregnant woman, nor of one in whom the assimilated food is followed by an acid reaction, or of one who is fond of incongenial and unhealthy dietary, or whose fundamental principles are vitiated.[161]

Also, around this time, Kabiraj Sri Harimohan Dasgupta aimed to propagate in simple Bengali the 'enormous progress' made by Ayurveda, especially in midwifery, which was written in the difficult Sanskrit language. He translated into Bengali the canonical Indian medical compendiums like *Susruta Samhita*, *Caraka Samhita* and others. Pratik Chakrabarti points out that Ayurveda was central to the emergence of a 'Hindu "national" identity' through the 'restoration of Indian epistemologies to their supposedly glorious past'.[162] Ayurveda was promoted through the vernacularisation of Sanskrit Ayurvedic texts as simple guidelines for quotidian life. About breastfeeding, Dasgupta cited elaborately from the *Susruta Samhita*, recommending honey and ghee/clarified butter to the infant for the first three or four days prior to breast milk secretion. He also cited ways of discerning 'pure' and 'polluted' milk primarily based on behaviour, diet and disease, various factors needing to be taken into consideration for the onset of lactation, like sight and touch of the baby, and different prerequisites (including caste criterion) for hiring a wet nurse.[163]

Sukumari Bhattacharji points out that, in ancient India, after completion of Hindu rituals following childbirth to drive away evil spirits, 'the father touches the infant's mouth with gold and other auspicious articles and feeds him with clarified butter and honey *before* handing him to the mother. Only then is the baby put to the breast'.[164] Fildes also mentions incantations from the *Susruta Samhita* for the initiation of breastfeeding.[165] She discusses several ancient Indian ceremonies and practices associated with childbirth and infant feeding from the *Susruta Samhita* and *Caraka Samhita*. She highlights that the *Susruta Samhita* insisted on initiating infant feeding with honey and ghee or clarified butter until breast milk was produced on the fourth day. It is of particular relevance to note that such practices of giving honey and other substance to a newborn were not so alien in Europe as analogous practices were found in, for instance, Galenic humoral medicine (Galen – 130–200 A.D.) which was very popular until the eighteenth century. Galen recommended honey or honey mixed with goat's milk for its purgative properties for the first three days followed by putting the baby to the mother's breast after the colostrum or 'first milk' was either 'sucked out by a stripling or expressed by hand' because it was believed to have been 'too thick and unsuitable for a neonate'. She adds that different perspectives about breastfeeding coexisted at any time; however, it is possible to argue that putting the child to the breast right after childbirth through realisation of the benefits of colostrum for the infant and also a decrease in maternal morbidity and mortality from milk fever occurred alongside prioritising the effects of breastfeeding on both the mother and infant, instead of only focusing on infant health, in the course of the eighteenth century and thereafter.[166]

In this context, it is pertinent to mention that Bengali *daktars* like Gangaprasad Mukhopadhyay (B.A., M.B.) combined simple Bengali and western medicine in their advice manuals for educating mothers about when to commence breastfeeding. Supriya Guha argues that Mukhopadhyay aimed to correct 'old wives' tales' as he pointed out that 'women were told to put the infant to the breast too soon after birth' but 'medical opinion' advised waiting for three to four days.[167] By way of contrast, it is argued here that Mukhopadhyay had a more nuanced medical argument as he also pointed out that the popular belief that there was no milk in the breasts right after childbirth was not always correct. He correlated the number of pregnancies and the nature of lactation to argue that if earlier the child had been put to the breast right after childbirth it led to the secretion of a milk-like substance for two or three weeks prior to the following childbirth. In such cases, within 12 hours following childbirth, the breasts hurt, and within 24 hours, milk was secreted and the child could be easily breastfed. He advised that it was necessary to begin breastfeeding after delivery if she has been pregnant for one or two times already. In case of the first or second pregnancy, he argued that breast milk was not produced until the third or the fourth day. On the other hand, medical practitioners like the famous Calcutta *daktar* Sundari Mohan Das emphasised on the benefits of colostrum and putting child to breast right after childbirth.[168] Mukhopadhyay also went against the popular belief that if the child was not put to the breast immediately after childbirth then forming that habit later was difficult. Instead of '*dugdhaheen stanakarshan*' or empty breastfeeding, he recommended training the child with a feeding bottle or the wick of a lamp rather than an empty breast which irritated both the mother and her baby.[169]

Bharati Ray argues that 'proper' childrearing advice was usually given to middle-class mothers to teach them 'good' mothering. Mothers particularly from an aristocratic background, however, 'do not seem to have been burdened by it, however patriotic they might have been. A convention in affluent homes was that newborn children were nursed not by mothers, but by professional wet-nurses'.[170] Meredith Borthwick emphasises that the dominant 'Bengali stereotype of English women' characterised them as ignoring their maternal duty to breastfeed their own children. Yet, in Bengal, 'wet-nursing was not simply a caricatured form of Anglicization, but was an established practice among the wealthy'.[171] Swapna M. Banerjee also confirms that wet nursing was a common practice among well-to-do Bengalis.[172] She also points out that the profession of wet nurse was not a separate category in the censuses of India as they were 'subsumed under female domestic workers'.[173] These 'non-kin caregivers for children are still "distant companions" hidden in the secret history of domesticity'.[174] Banerjee highlights that one of the earliest Bengali feminists, Sarala Devi Chaudhurani, Rabindranath Tagore's niece, actually began her autobiography by mentioning that '[i]nstead of receiving their mother's milk babies were nursed and looked after by wet nurses. Soon after they were born babies left their mothers and were entrusted to the care of a suckling midwife and a supervising maid'.[175] In her description:

> A convention of affluent homes those days was also rigorously followed in the Tagore home at Jorasanko – the newborn children were nursed not by their mothers but by professional wet nurses. Immediately after birth, the infant was separated from the mother and handed over into the custody of a wet nurse and maidservant. The child thereafter had little or no connection with the mother. Neither did I. . . . Mothers were aloof, inaccessible queens. Maidservants' arms replaced mothers' arms, and we were no exceptions. We had no conception of what a mother's love could be, for no mother ever kissed us.[176]

As you might recall from the previous section, famous Bengali 'lady doctor' at the Hooghly Lady Dufferin Women's Hospital (Chinsurah), Haimabati Sen, also reflected about the practice of wet nursing, together with her experience of gender disparity in maternal breastfeeding, in her memoir[177]:

> In the expectation that my mother would give birth to a son, everybody entertained her with ritual celebrations and shower parties.

> After all these were over and after a full ten months of gestation and three days of labor pains, I was born. When it was clear she had given birth to a girl, my mother took to her sick bed in sorrow and disappointment. . . . But my father was so pleased that he ordered celebratory music for an entire month. There was also a festival of lights. The entire house was illuminated with wreaths of lamps. He told everyone, 'No one must describe my child as a girl.' . . . She spent her days in tearful sorrow and I was given over to an untouchable woman of the hadi caste. She used to feed her daughter (older than me by one month) at one breast, and me at the other. In time my mother also softened towards me and occasionally she too would breast-feed me. But how long did I have this privilege? I had to be weaned at the age of seven months, because my mother became pregnant again. It was then my Punti-ma [the hadi woman] who continued to bring me up. . . . When I was about one and a half, my mother got the male child she had so desired. The wife of my father's youngest brother had given birth to a male child a few months before that. Now that my mother had a new baby in her arms, I no longer went near her. When I felt like being breast-fed, I went to Punti-ma. The rest of the time I spent in the outer quarters of the house.[178]

Besides the affective worlds of the *dai* and her charges sketched in Bengali memoirs, detailed intellection on hiring of wet nurses were also available widely across Bengali domestic and medical manuals and periodical essays – for example, Kumudini Bose's[179] (M.A.) essay series 'Sishu Palan' (or childrearing) spread across several issues of *Ayurved* in 1919. Bose discussed an elaborate criteria for selection of a wet nurse (preferably educated and religious, from *uccha-bangsho*/good lineage, and with good health, disposition and character as she pointed out that mother or wet nurse's traits were passed on through breast milk) along with milk charts comparing nutritive values of mother's milk with cow, goat and buffalo milk respectively.[180] She admitted, however, that hiring a wet nurse with good lineage was most unlikely whereby she recommended relatives as wet nurses if possible, or feeding animal milk instead.[181] She also provided detailed up-to-date statistical data on infant mortality together with medicalised regular breastfeeding guidelines.[182] In fact, the job role, selection and supervision of the *dugdhabati dhatri*[183] were meticulously medicalised and authenticated with references to canonical medical texts and incorporated in the very definition of *bhadra* or 'respectable' mothering in the course of the nineteenth century.[184] Various detailed medical criteria for selection of wet nurses were provided by European and indigenous medical practitioners alike. *Daktars*' advice on wet nursing will be discussed in order to highlight the medicalised objectification and commodification of the wet nurse's body and breast milk.

To begin with, William Smoult Playfair's (1836–1903), M.D., F.R.C.P.,[185] *A Treatise on the Science and Practice of Midwifery* referenced by contemporary midwifery books across Britain and colonial Bengal, and also vernacularised by Shri Khirodaprasad Chattopadhyay's *Dhatribidya* (2 volumes) published in 1886, mentioned the following medical checklist for hiring a wet nurse:

> *Selection of a Wet Nurse.* In selecting a wet nurse we should endeavor to choose a strong, healthy woman, who should not be over 30, or 35 years of age at the outside, since the quality of the milk deteriorates in women who are more advanced in life. For a similar reason a very young woman of 16 or 17 should be rejected. . . . The breasts should be pear-shaped, rather firm, as indicating an abundance of gland-tissue, and with the superficial veins well marked. Large, flabby breasts owe much of their size to an undue deposit of fat, and are generally unfavorable. The nipple should be prominent, not too large, and free from cracks and erosions, which, if existing, might lead to subsequent difficulties in nursing. On pressing the breast the milk should flow from it easily in a number of small jets, and some of it should be preserved for examination. It should be of a bluish-white color, and when placed under the microscope, the field should be covered with an abundance of milk corpuscles, and the large granular corpuscles of the colostrum should have entirely disappeared. If the latter be observed in any quantity in a woman who has been confined five or six weeks, the inference is that the milk is inferior in quality. It is not often that the practitioner has an opportunity of inquiring into the moral qualities of the nurse, although much valuable information might be derived from a knowledge of her previous character. An irascible, excitable, or highly nervous woman will certainly make a bad nurse, and the most trivial causes might afterwards interfere with the quality of her milk. Particular attention should be paid to the nurse's own child, since its condition affords the best criterion of the quality of her milk[186]

Homeopathic and allopathic *daktar* Annadacharan Khastagir's (Assistant-Surgeon) similarly titled book *A Treatise on the Science and Practice of Midwifery* also mentioned similar medical criteria for what was considered good quality breast milk and selection of an appropriate wet nurse. In his book, he discussed nursing of infants and the gender of the child interchanged between *sishu* or infant and *cheley* or boy child.[187] He argued that the '*dhatri* or wet-nurse's milk becomes unsuitable for a child if she is infected with blood-related diseases like syphilis, scrofula, phthisis, etc.', the '*dhatri* needs to be around the same age as the parturient woman; if this is not possible she should not exceed 30/35 years or be under 16 years of age'. Aside from examination of breasts and nipples as well as the child of the wet nurse, even her breast milk was to be bluish white and if 'examined under a microscope it will be teeming with milk corpuscles or milk granules will be visible'. The quality of breast milk was also directly correlated with the temperament of the wet nurse who was not supposed to be 'violent, quick tempered, or uncontrollably frenzied'.[188]

Shri Hemantakumari Debi's elaborate essay titled '*Santan-Palan*' published in the Brahmo women's magazine *Bamabodhini Patrika* in 1916 elaborated on how mothers and wet nurses alike should not breastfeed if they are agitated, menstruating or pregnant, especially if the baby is within the first six months and solely reliant on breast milk.[189] Nripendranath Seth pointed out that if a mother is angry, her agitated mental state affects the quality of the breast milk and causes ailments in children. A disorderly, uncontrolled, wild mental state, in turn, also created *apakari* or 'harmful' breast milk. He added that the cheap and perverted literature which was usually read on a daily basis also corrupted her mental equilibrium. In a Rousseaunean logic, Seth argued, however, that mothers from lower classes were economically deprived but closer to nature, producing 'purer' breast milk and lesser numbers of 'diseased' children than the 'respectable'/*bhadra* classes and/or castes who adopted a '*babuyani*' or '*babu*-like', luxurious lifestyle.[190] Medical practitioners have been particularly attentive to the temperament of the mother and wet nurse alike in both European and Bengali medical manuals. Besides detailed medical criteria for hiring wet nurses, as also mentioned in the previous chapter, the 'economy of the borrowed breast'[191] often demanded the inhuman criteria of giving up nursing her own baby for the wet nurse – it is argued here that such observations were not merely based on *colonial difference*. As this was also a common assumption among Bengali *daktars* as late as the 1930s – gynaecologist and obstetrician to the Calcutta Medical Hospital, J. C. Chatterjee's medical criteria for the selection of a wet nurse are cited in detail as follows:

> Doctor's and nurse's duty is to use all their influence with patients to persuade them always to nurse their babies, unless strong reason exists for not doing so. There is no true substitute for breast milk. Some infants thrive on properly regulated artificial food but a large number perish annually or grow up into delicate children, for want of breast feeding. . . . In hospitals, infants may be fed for several weeks on milk drawn with a breast pump from another woman who have more milk than their babies' need. Sometimes the woman may nurse her own and also another baby.
>
> The selection of a wet nurse is a serious responsibility upon the medical man. The following are the essentials of a wet nurse.

> (1) She must be perfectly healthy and free from every disease which can be communicated to the infant.
> (2) Her age should be between twenty and thirty five years of age.
> (3) Her breasts must be firm with well-shaped nipples and contain abundance of milk.
> (4) Her . . . infant must be about the same age or slightly older than the infant she is going to nurse must be thriving well upon her milk and *she must be prepared to give up nursing it.*
> (5) Her character must be *good* for admitting in a patient's house.
> (6) She should have a good physique, with sound teeth, cleanly in habits. So the physician must make *a complete physical examination* of the mother and her child before selecting a wet nurse.
>
> It is difficult to secure the services of a *respectable* woman or a wet nurse. Be very careful against frauds such as substitution of another child for her own and so misleading the medical man. A syphilitic child should not be nursed by a wet nurse. A prospective wet-nurse whose antecedents are not thoroughly known to the doctor should be submitted to the Wasserman test in all cases, also her child.
>
> (emphasis added)[192]

Such recommendations for detailed bodily examinations seem to be quite puzzling considering, as Sujata Mukherjee argues, the '[o]ne prevalent practice in Hindu society which seemed to obstruct delivery of proper medical care' was 'avoidance of any contact between women patients and doctors'.[193] Assistant-Surgeon Koilash Chunder Bose highlighted that '[t]he custom for Hindu ladies is to instruct others [male members] about their ailments. The rule is to communicate through a maidservant, her mother, or guardian'.[194] With such a climate of opinion about 'modesty', it is particularly relevant to note that whereas the lactating *dai's* breasts were meant to be open to examination for hiring purposes, *daktar* and famous obstetrician,[195] Kedarnath Das confirmed that usually this was not the case when examining the breasts of 'Indian women':

> Examination of the Breasts. – This is undertaken only as a corroborative evidence when other signs are not absolutely definite. We generally spare this in our patients specially Indian women – as they have strong prejudice against exposing their breasts. It is better to examine the breasts covertly, while pretending to listen to the heart. In this way not only do we satisfy the modesty of our

patients but also avoid suspicions in unmarried women or Hindu widows.[196]

This chapter explored 'clean'/'dirty' midwifery together with previously underexplored detailed medical criteria for hiring a wet nurse in Bengali medical manuals. It examined how socio-religious and medical discourses naturalised, sacralised and purified the mother's breasts, breast milk and breastfeeding. Classical and contemporary medical discourses have been touched upon to reveal that there were similar medical ideas about breastfeeding across temporal and transnational boundaries. Commonsensical and naturalised connections about the mother and wet nurse's body, mother love and effective breastfeeding have also been questioned. It also aimed to offer an alternative argument, moving beyond the dominant historiographical worldview about *colonial difference* in European physicians' advice about the detailed bodily examination of the Indian wet nurse as also discussed in the previous chapter. This study delved into various aspects of why and how midwifery, motherhood and wet nursing were medically crafted by regimenting mothering of infants in everyday lives to eradicate disease, both physiological and cultural.

Notes

1 Meredith Borthwick, *The Changing Role of Women in Bengal, 1849–1905* (Princeton: Princeton University Press, 1984), p. 153
2 Ibid., p. 155.
3 For a detailed discussion see Introduction, p. 18n4.
4 For an elaborate discussion on 'clean midwifery', caste, childbirth and related issues, 'Chapter Eight Preventive Medicine Part I. The Problems of Childbirth' in Margaret Ida Balfour and Ruth Young, *The Work of Medical Women in India with a foreword by Dame Mary Scharlieb* (London: Humphrey Milford Oxford University Press, 1929), pp. 123–140. The phrase 'clean midwifery' has been cited from Balfour and Young, *The Work of Medical Women in India*, p. 140; also Lt.-Col. E.E. Waters, 'Chapter II. Opinions of Provinces. I. – Bengal Presidency', in *Improvements of the Conditions of Childbirth in India Including a Special Report on the Work of the Victoria Memorial Scholarships Fund During the Past Fifteen Years and Papers Written by Medical Women and Qualified Midwives* (Calcutta: Superintendent Government Printing, India, 1918), p. 10.
5 For instance, Dr. Y. Sen, F.R.F.P. & S. (Glasgow), Women's Medical Service, Raj Dufferin Hospital, Bettiah, in 'Chapter VI. Papers Continued: Drs. G.J. Campbell, Wallace, Sen, George', in *Improvements of the Conditions of Childbirth in India*, p. 129; also it is a phrase used in Mridula Ramanna, *Health Care in Bombay Presidency 1896–1930* (Delhi: Primus, 2012), p. 123. On *dais* and their assistants as 'cord-cutters', see Supriya Guha, 'A History of the Medicalisation of Childbirth in Bengal in the Late Nineteenth and Twentieth Centuries', Unpublished PhD Thesis, 1996, University of Calcutta, pp. 114–116.
6 On the sociological concept of 'medicalization', see Introduction, p. 17n1.

7 For a detailed discussion on 'clean' versus 'dirty' midwifery, see Chapter 5 of this book.

8 See for example, Ruth Perry, 'Colonizing the Breast: Sexuality and Maternity in Eighteenth-Century England', *Journal of the History of Sexuality*, Special Issue, Part 1: The State, Society, and the Regulation of Sexuality in Modern Europe, vol. 2, no. 2, 1991, pp 204–34.

9 This phrase has been quoted from Waters, 'Chapter II. Opinions of Provinces. I. – Bengal Presidency', p. 10.

10 Lt.-Colonel R. P. Wilson, I.M.S., Superintendent, Campbell Medical School Calcutta in *Improvements of the Conditions of Childbirth in India, p. 9.* Similar opinion expressed in Waters, 'Chapter II – Opinions of Provinces. I. – Bengal Presidency', in *Improvements of the Conditions of Childbirth in India*, p. 11. Cecelia Van Hollen points out that the general climate of opinion was that 'the best way to achieve desired changes is through education so that the public comes to desire change of its own will'. She argues, using a Foucauldian approach, that this marked 'a change from juridical power to discursive power that has been a hallmark of the discourse of civil society'. This was also a post-Mutiny change in colonial policy 'to rule effectively'. Cecelia Van Hollen, *Birth on the Threshold Childbirth and Modernity in South India* (Berkeley: University of California Press, 2003), p. 48. Here she is referring to Michel Foucault, *Discipline and Punish: The Birth of the Prison*. Translated from the French by Alan Sheridan (New York: Pantheon Books, 1978).

11 Geraldine Forbes, *Women in Colonial India. Essays in Politics, Medicine, and Historiography* (New Delhi: Chronicle Books, 2005), pp. 84–88, 91.

12 Sean Lang, 'Drop the Demon *Dai:* Maternal Mortality and the State in Colonial Madras, 1840–1875', *Social History of Medicine*, vol. 18, no. 3, 2005, p. 368.

13 Maneesha Lal, 'The Politics of Gender and Medicine in Colonial India: The Countess of Dufferin's Fund, 1885–1888', *Bulletin of the History of Medicine*, vol. 68, no. 1, 1994, p. 31.

14 For example, in 1888, at least 50 missionary physicians were working in India which comprised 'approximately two-thirds of India's total number of "lady doctors".' Countess of Dufferin's Fund, *Fourth Annual Report of The National Association for Supplying Female Medical Aid to the Women of India* (Calcutta: Superintendent of Government Printing, 1889), pp. 39–41 cited in Lal, 'The Politics of Gender and Medicine in Colonial India', p. 32.

15 Letter From the Inspector-General of Hospitals, Indian Medical Department, to The Secretary to the Government of Bengal, Judicial Department, Letter Number 266, 22 June 1871, General Department Proceedings, September 1871, West Bengal State Archives [hereafter WBSA]. Dr. Chevers is Dr. Norman Chevers, Principal of the Calcutta Medical College. Under 'Proceeding 8 Resolution by His Honor the Lieutenant – Governor of Bengal, – (dated Fort William, the September 12, 1871), it was stated that '[t]he Lieutenant – Governor is not very sanguine of success, which to be complete requires not only the training of a certain number of dhaies in practical midwifery, but also their general admission for ordinary confinements in private native houses'. Proceeding 8 Resolution by His Honour the Lieutenant – Governor of Bengal, – (dated Fort William, the 12th Sept 1871)', General Department Proceedings, September 1871, WBSA.

16 'Report of the Medical College Hospital for the Year 1870' in Letter From the Inspector-General of Hospitals, Indian Medical Department To The

Secretary to the Government of Bengal, Judicial Department, Letter Number 266, 22 June 1871, General Department Proceedings, September 1871, WBSA.

17 Ibid.

18 Ibid.

19 'Annual return of out and in-patients at the Medical College Hospital, Calcutta, for the year ending 31st December 1870' in Letter From the Inspector-General of Hospitals, Indian Medical Department To The Secretary to the Government of Bengal, Judicial Department, Letter Number 266, 22 June 1871, General Department Proceedings, September 1871, WBSA.

20 Paraphrased from 'Annual return showing the number of Midwifery Cases and Diseases of Women and Children treated in the Lying-in Wards of the Medical College Hospital, for the year ending 31st December 1870' in Letter no. 266, dated 22 June 1871, from the Inspector – General of Hospitals, Indian Medical Department, forwarding the report and returns of the Medical College for the year 1870, General Department Proceedings, September 1871, WBSA. Moreover, following the establishment of the Countess of Dufferin Fund in 1885, Dufferin hospitals usually got the credit for treating women, even though many women were treated by civil surgeons at the dispensaries and general wards as earlier, see Ambalika Guha, *Colonial Modernities Midwifery in Bengal, c. 1860–1947* (London: Routledge, 2018), p. 78.

21 'Proceeding 46 Dated Calcutta, the 24th Feb 1873 Resolution – By the Government of Bengal' cited from section on 'Proceedings 45&46 Resolution on the reports on the working of the scheme of training native women in practical midwifery during the past year', General Department Proceedings, February 1873, WBSA.

22 Sujata Mukherjee, *Gender, Medicine, and Society in Colonial India Women's Health Care in Nineteenth- and Early Twentieth-Century Bengal* (New Delhi: Oxford University Press, 2017), p. xxii.

23 Training Native Women in Midwifery File 63 Proceeding 7 Order Number 1031, dated Fort William, the 28th November 1873 From Campbell Brown, Surgeon-General, Indian Medical Department, To- The Secretary to the Government of Bengal Judicial Department, General Department Proceedings, December 1873, WBSA.

24 Ibid.

25 On the persistence of home births and mostly lower classes and castes and complicated cases having been sent to hospitals, see Meredith Borthwick, *The Changing Role of Women in Bengal, 1849–1905* (Princeton: Princeton University Press, 1984), p. 156. Also, similar argument in Mukherjee, *Gender, Medicine and Society in Colonial India*, p. 77. At the turn of the century women seeking hospitalised treatment had increased although the number of Hindu middle-class women, as compared to Muslim women, remained low – Chandrika Paul, 'The Uneasy Alliance, The work of British and Bengali women medical professionals in Bengal, 1870–1935' in Guha, *Colonial Modernities*, pp. 77, and p. 101n65. Increased hospitalised treatment of women was visible within a decade of the foundation of the Dufferin Fund, for example, in 1895, approximately 107,000 women were treated which is an increase over the previous year (1894) of approximately 27,000 – see The Bengal Branch of the Dufferin Fund', *The Indian Lancet*, vol. 7, March 1896, p. 255 cited in Guha, *Colonial Modernities*, p. 101n66.

26 Mukherjee, *Gender, Medicine, and Society in Colonial India*, p. 84.

27 On ritual pollution associated with childbirth, see Borthwick, *The Changing Role of Women in Bengal*, pp. 153–156; also on childbirth see Patricia Jeffery, Roger Jeffery, and Andrew Lyon, *Labour Pains and Labour Power. Women and Childbearing in India* (New Delhi: Manohar, 1989).

28 *Abridgement of the Report of the Committee Appointed by the Right Honorable the Governor of Bengal for the Establishment of a Fever Hospital and for Inquiring Into Local Management and Taxation in Calcutta* (Calcutta: 1840), p. 64 cited in Ishita Pande, *Medicine, Race and Liberalism in British Bengal. Symptoms of Empire* (New York: Routledge, 2010), p. 144.

29 Mukherjee, *Gender, Medicine, and Society in Colonial India*, p. xxiii.

30 For a detailed discussion, see Guha, *Colonial Modernities*, pp. 68–69. Guha bases her arguments on WBSA, *General Committee of the Fever Hospital and Municipal Improvements*, Miscellaneous Evidences and Papers, Appendix F, No. 27, 1839, pp. 87–88 cited in Guha *Colonial Modernities*, pp. 68–69. For details on Gupta, see Deepak Kumar, 'Medical Encounters in British India, 1820–1920', *Economic and Political Weekly*, vol. 32, no. 4, 1997, pp. 166–170 in Guha, *Colonial Modernities*, p. 98.

31 Guha, *Colonial Modernities*, pp. 70–71.

32 WBSA, General Department, Education Branch, Proceedings 8–11, 12–13, 18–22, February 1868 cited in Guha, *Colonial Modernities*, pp. 70–71.

33 Meer Ushruff Ally, *Handbook of Midwifery in Bengalee* (Calcutta: Das and Sons, 1869), pp. 186–189. His name has been spelt accordingly.

34 Meer Ushruff Ally, *Diseases of Children in Bengalee Balchikitsa* (Calcutta: Das and Sons, 1870), pp. 1–7.

35 Ally, *Diseases of Children in Bengalee*, p. 1 (of Preface, pp. 1–2).

36 Frederick Corbyn, *Management and Diseases of Infants Under the Influence of the Climate of India Being Instructions to Mothers and Parents in Situations Where Medical Aid Is Not to Be Obtained and a Guide to Medical Men, Inexperienced in the Nursery and the Treatment of Tropical Infantile Disease.* Illustrated By Coloured Plates. (Calcutta: Thacker and Co., 1828), p. 15 cited in Saha, 'Milk, 'Race' and Nation', p. 150.

37 Ibid.

38 Ally, *Handbook of Midwifery in Bengalee*, p. 2. For details see Annada Charan Khastagir, *A Treatise on the Science and Practice of Midwifery with Diseases of Children and Women Manab-Jatna Tattva, Dhatribidya, Nabaprasuto Sishu o Stri Jatir Byadhi-Sangraha* (Calcutta: Author, 1878 second ed., first ed. 1868).

39 Kshirodaprasad Chattopadhyay, L.M.S., *Dhatribidya Subikhyato Daktar W. S. Playfair Sahiber A Treatise on the Science and Practice of Midwifery.* Granther Anubad [*Midwifery Famous Doctor W. S. Playfair Sahib's A Treatise on the Science and Practice of Midwifery.* Book Translation (Two Volumes) authorised and selected by the Vernacular Textbook Committee (Bhowanipur, 1886). In his Preface to *Midwifery* Volume I, Chattopadhyay argued that he had translated the book following instructions by A. Croft, Director of Public Instruction and founder of the Vernacular Textbook Committee, to translate Playfair's *A Treatise on the Science and Practice of Midwifery* among others, according to the list cited in the Calcutta Gazette (1881). The dedication right at the start of Chattopadhyay's *Midwifery* Volume I clearly dedicates his book to the Countess of Dufferin 'For Her Zeal In the Spread of Medical Education Amongst The Native Ladies of India'.

40 William Smoult Playfair, *A Treatise on the Science and Practice of Midwifery* with Notes and Additions by Robert P. Harris, M.D. With Two Plates and

One Hundred and Eighty-Two Illustrations (Philadelphia: Henry C. Lea, Second American from the Second and Revised London Edition, 1878, first ed. 1876).

41 Supriya Guha, '"The Best Swadeshi": Reproductive Health in Bengal, 1840–1940', in Sarah Hodges (ed), *Reproductive Health in India. History, Politics, Controversies* (Hyderabad: Orient Longman, 2006), p. 153.

42 Borthwick, *The Changing Role of Women in Bengal*, p. 16.

43 Saratkumari Deb, *Āmār sangsār* (Calcutta, 1942), p. 2 cited in Borthwick, *The Changing Role of Women in Bengal*, p. 160.

44 Shib Chunder Deb, *The Infant Treatment* First Part *Sishu Palan* Pratham Bhag (Calcutta: reprint 1864; first edition 1857), Preface, p. 1.

45 Borthwick, *The Changing Role of Women in Colonial Bengal*, p. 161.

46 Guha, *Colonial Modernities*, p. 36.

47 Jodu Nath Mukerje, *Dhatri Sikkha A Guide to the Dhaees or Native Midwives And to the Mothers Written in the Form of a Dialogue in Two Parts* Part 1 (Chinsura: Printed by Greesh Chunder Bhuttacharje, Chitsaprokash Press; third ed. 1875, first ed. 1867), pp. 1–2.

48 Waters, 'Chapter II – Opinions of Provinces. I. – Bengal Presidency', p. 10.

49 Ibid.

50 Ibid.

51 Also, members of voluntary organisations like the Saroj Nalini Dutt Memorial Association (SNDMA), established in 1925, at the district and village levels also offered trained midwifery services. Mukherjee, *Gender, Medicine, and Society in Colonial India*, p. 86.

52 Mukherjee, *Gender, Medicine, and Society in Colonial India*, pp. 76–77.

53 *The Countess of Dufferin's Fund – the Sixth Annual Report of the National Association for Supplying Female Medical Aid to the Women of India, Burma Branch, for the Year 1892* (Calcutta: Office of the Superintendent of Government Printing, 1893), pp. 13–14 cited in Mukherjee, *Gender, Medicine, and Society in Colonial India*, p. 77, 92n44.

54 See Geraldine Forbes and Tapan Raychaudhuri (eds), *From Child Widow to Lady Doctor: The Memoirs of Dr. Haimabati Sen* Translated by Tapan Raychaudhuri. Introduced by Geraldine Forbes (New Delhi: Lotus Collection, Roli Books, 2000), p. 245n11. Haimabati Sen had eight pregnancies and five children. For details on Sen's life, see Mukherjee, *Gender, Medicine and Society*, pp. 58–59; Indrani Sen, 'Resisting Patriarchy: Complexities and Conflicts in the Memoir of Haimabati Sen', *Economic and Political Weekly*, vol. 47, no. 12, 2012, pp. 55–62. For a detailed discussion of Sundari Mohan Das' childcare advice, see Chapter 5 in this book.

55 Forbes and Raychaudhuri, *The Memoirs of Dr. Haimabati Sen*, pp. 245–248.

56 Kumari Jayawardena, *The White Woman's Other Burden Western Women and South Asia During British Rule* (New York, Routledge, 1995), p. 76.

57 Maneesha Lal, 'The Politics of Gender and Medicine in Colonial India: The Countess of Dufferin's Fund, 1885–1888, *Bulletin of the History of Medicine*, vol. 68, no. 1, 1994, pp. 31, p. 49.

58 Ibid.

59 Mary Scharlieb, *Reminiscences* (London: Williams-Norgate, 1924), p. 41 in Jayawardena, *The White Woman's Other Burden*, p. 75.

60 Van Hollen, *Birth on the Threshold*, p. 42. On organisational structure and main objectives of the Dufferin Fund – see Harriot Dufferin, 'The National Association for Supplying Female Medical Aid to the Women of India', *Asiatic Quarterly Review*, vol. 1, 1886, pp. 260–261 in Lal, 'The Politics of Gender and Medicine

in Colonial India', p. 35; also see The Countess of Dufferin's Fund, *Fifty Years' Retrospect India 1885–1935* (London: The Women's Printing Society Ltd., 1935), p. 5, File: Countess of Dufferin's Fund, PP/MIB//C/4, Wellcome Library.

61 Van Hollen, *Birth on the Threshold*, pp. 42–43.

62 Ibid., p. 43.

63 Samiksha Sehrawat, *Colonial Medical Care in North India Gender, State and Society c. 1840–1920* (New Delhi: Oxford University Press, 2013), p. 185; also on central government aid, Ibid., pp. 184–185. On state subsidy for the W.M.S. from 1913 onwards, see The Countess of Dufferin's Fund, *Fifty Years' Retrospect India*, pp. 11–13.

64 For a detailed discussion on this subject, see Ranjana Saha, 'Motherhood on display: The child welfare exhibition in colonial Calcutta', *The Indian Economic and Social History Review*, vol. 58, no. 2, 2021, pp. 249–277.

65 Van Hollen, *Birth on the Threshold*, p. 43.

66 Guha, 'A History of the Medicalisation of Childbirth', pp. 114–116; Supriya Guha, 'Midwifery in Colonial India The role of traditional birth attendants in colonial India', *Wellcome History*, Issue 28, Spring, 2–3, WellcomeTrust, pp. 2–3, (Accessed 5 October, 2014). www.wellcome.ac.uk/stellent/groups/corporatesite/@msh_publishing_group/documents/web_document/wtx024905.pdf.

67 Guha, 'Midwifery in Colonial India', p. 2.

68 Ibid, p. 2.

69 Ibid.

70 Dr. Y. Sen, F.R.F.P. & S. (Glasgow), Women's Medical Service, Raj Dufferin Hospital, Bettiah. in 'Chapter VI. Papers Continued: Drs. G.J. Campbell, Wallace, Sen, George', in *Improvements of the Conditions of Childbirth in India*, pp. 126–127.

71 Ibid., pp. 126, 134.

72 Ibid., p. 129.

73 Hasan Suhrawardy, M.D., F.R.C.S.I., L.M. (Rotunda), District Medical Officer Lillooah, E.I.R., 'The Care of the Expectant Mother and Newborn Infant', in *Health and Child Welfare Exhibition, Calcutta, 1920* (Calcutta: Bengal Secretariat Book Depot, 1921), p. lxiv.

74 Charu Gupta, *The Gender of Caste. Representing Dalits in Print* (Ranikhet, Permanent Black in association with Ashoka University, 2016), p. 47.

75 Ibid., p. 46.

76 Ibid., p. 45.

77 Sen, in 'Chapter VI. – Papers Continued', p. 127.

78 Gupta, *The Gender of Caste*, p. 46; Saha, 'Motherhood on display', p. 261.

79 Balfour and Young, *The Work of Medical Women in India*, p. 131.

80 Ibid.

81 Ibid., pp. 131–132.

82 'Appendix 1 Maternal Mortality in Childbirth in India' in Balfour and Young, *The Work of Medical Women in India*, p. 190.

83 Balfour and Young point out that the mortality figures are lower in Calcutta than in Bombay and Madras as the cases sent to hospitals in Calcutta were not included. For more details, see ibid., p. 190.

84 It had adopted the same definition for 'maternal death' as was initially used by the Department of Health for Scotland few years earlier to mean 'Maternal deaths which occurred during pregnancy or within four weeks after the termination of pregnancy, or later if illness originated during pregnancy, childbirth or the puerperium'. M. I. Neal Edwards, *Report of an Enquiry into the Causes of Maternal Mortality in Calcutta Field Investigators:*

I. M. Massick, M.R.C.P., W.M.S., S. Pandit, M.B., B.S., D.M.C.W., W.M.S., F.M. Shaw, M.B., B.S. and Two Statistical Notes by Satya Swaroop M.A. (Delhi, Manager of Publications, 1940), p. 1.

85 Ibid., p. 32.

86 M. I. Neal Edwards, *Report of an Enquiry into the Causes of Maternal Mortality in Calcutta* (Government of India, Manager of Publications, 1940), p. 34 cited in Guha, *Colonial Modernities*, p. 138.

87 Guha, *Colonial Modernities*, p. 126. Ambalika Guha mentions that in Calcutta as early as in 1908 maternal and child welfare services were begun by the Corporation and from 1915 trained 'corporation midwives' provided domiciliary midwifery services, Guha, *Colonial Modernities*, pp. 127–128.

88 Neal Edwards, *Report of an Enquiry into the Causes of Maternal Mortality in Calcutta*, p. 26. Regarding child marriage, Neal Edwards added that it often resulted in 'not immediately obvious' problems due to 'too early child-bearing', childcare and repeated pregnancies causing anaemia, haemorrhage, sepsis, tuberculosis, among others. Besides deaths associated with childbearing, Neal Edwards also pointed out that, a large number of Muslims died from tuberculosis while Hindus from eclampsia and albuminuria. See mainly Ibid., p. 20.

89 Maneesha Lal, 'Purdah as Pathology: Gender and the Circulation of Medical Knowledge in Late Colonial India', in Sarah Hodges (ed), *Reproductive Health in India History, Politics, Controversies* (Hyderabad: Orient Longman, 2006), pp. 85–114.

90 Supriya Guha, 'The Nature of Woman. Medical Ideas in Colonial Bengal', *Indian Journal of Gender Studies*, vol. 3, no. 1, p. 30.

91 Sehrawat, *Colonial Medical Care in North India*, pp. xxix, 103–108, 146. Also, see Lal, 'The Politics of Gender and Medicine in Colonial India', mainly pp. 38–48.

92 Guha, 'The Best Swadeshi', p. 163.

93 Neal Edwards, *Report of an Enquiry into the Causes of Maternal Mortality in Calcutta*, p. 92.

94 See p. 63n113 in Chapter 1 of this book.

95 M. I. Balfour Pronito (composed), *Bharater desi daider jonno dhatrisikkha* (Calcutta, Printed at the Baptist Mission Press, 1922), pp. 26–33, 37–38, Title Translation: Midwifery for the Indian indigenous midwives; also see Ranjana Saha, 'Milk, mothering & meanings: Infant feeding in colonial Bengal', *Women's Studies International Forum* 2017, 60, p. 99. Translation mine.

96 Ruth Young, M.B.E., B.Sc., CH.B, W.M.S., *Antenatal Work in India A Handbook for Nurses, Midwives, and Health Visitors*, Indian Red Cross Society Maternity and Child Welfare Bureau (Incorporating the Lady Chelmsford All-India League for Maternity and Child Welfare, and the Victoria Memorial Scholarships Fund), 1930, p. iii.

97 For details see Ibid., p. 9.

98 Ibid., p. 10.

99 Ibid.

100 Ibid., pp. 12, 17.

101 The phrase 'history of confinement' was in capital letters on the card. On the cards, the patient would have to provide details of her husband's name and his occupation, her age and age when she married, caste, preparations for and history of confinement, attendants engaged, and sex of the baby, for details see Ibid., pp. 105–6.

102 Ibid., p. 15; also see Saha, Motherhood on display, pp. 257–258.

103 Atsuko Naono, 'Educating Lady Doctors in Colonial Burma Missionaries, the Lady Dufferin Hospital, and the Local Government in the Making of Burmese

Medical Women', in Poonam Bala (ed), *Contesting Colonial Authority Medicine and Indigenous Responses in Nineteenth- and Twentieth Century India* (New York: Lexington Books, 2012), pp. 98, 103. The Burma Nurses and Midwives Act was passed in 1922 but it remained inactive for at least another decade whereby the influence of the *wan zwe*, mainly in rural areas, prevailed – Ibid., p. 110. By the mid-1930s, most provincial governments had passed legislation requiring registration of nurses and midwives with regulatory councils to keep a watchful eye, Forbes, *Women in Colonial India*, p. 95. In Burma, even though female seclusion and caste restrictions were absent and the numbers of male students in midwifery and obstetrics were on the rise, childbirth and midwifery remained an almost exclusively female realm of expertise due to the predominance of missionary female medical practitioners and the Dufferin Fund. Naono, 'Educating Lady Doctors in Colonial Burma, p. 108.

104 Ibid., p. 102.

105 Van Hollen, *Birthing on the Threshold*, p. 50.

106 Ashis Nandy, *The Intimate Enemy: Loss and Recovery of Self under Colonialism* (Delhi: Oxford University Press, 1983) in Van Hollen, *Birth on the Threshold*, p. 50; also see Nandy, *The Intimate Enemy*, pp. 11–15 cited in Lal, 'The Politics of Gender and Medicine in Colonial India', p. 46.

107 Mary Hancock, 'Home Science and the Nationalization of Domesticity in Colonial India', *Modern Asian Studies*, vol. 35, no. 4, 2001, p. 874.

108 Lang, 'Drop the Demon *Dai*', p. 368.

109 J. C. Chatterjee, *An Introduction to the Study of Midwifery* (Calcutta, 1930), p. 537.

110 Marilyn Yalom, *A History of the Breast* (London: Pandora An Imprint of Rivers Oram Press, 1998), p. 48. Unlike the full nourishing breasts of the *bhadramahila*/Indian mother/Mother India, Yalom points out that there was a plump Jesus at the Virgin Mary's small breasts which seemed 'unrealistically attached to the Virgin's body, almost like a small piece of fruit – a lemon, apple, or pomegranate – that had accidentally dropped onto the canvas'. This was supposedly meant to underscore her divinity by highlighting that she was unlike any other woman or it was supposed to comfort people amidst crop failures, malnutrition and the plague in fourteenth century Italy. Yalom, *A History of the Breast*, p. 40.

111 Yalom, *A History of the Breast*, p. 45. This led Protestant reformer John Calvin to comment cynically – 'Had the breasts of the most Holy Virgin yielded a more copious supply than is given by a cow, or had she continued to nurse during her whole lifetime, she scarcely could have furnished the quantity which is exhibited'. John Calvin, *Tracts and Treatises on the Reformation of the Church* Edited by Henry Beveridge. Volume I, (Grand Rapids, Mich.: WM. B. Eerdmans, 1958), p. 317 in Yalom, *A History of the Breast*, p. 45.

112 Yalom, *A History of the Breast*, p. 147.

113 Ibid., p. 120.

114 Ibid.

115 Ibid., p. 122.

116 Ibid., p. 126.

117 Ibid., p. 106

118 Ibid., p. 108.

119 Ibid.

120 Ibid., p. 109.

121 Ibid. Yalom argues that the historian of science, Londa Schiebinger has questioned Linnaeus' choice of the term 'mammals' as the characteristic milk-producing trait is but one trait and to be found only among one half the human beings. Londa Schiebinger, *Nature's Body Gender in the Making of Modern Science* (Boston: Beacon Press, 1993), pp. 40–41 cited in Yalom, *A History of the Breast*, pp. 108–109.
122 Valerie A. Fildes, *Wet Nursing A History from Antiquity to the Present* (Oxford, Basil Blackwell, 1988)., p. 111.
123 Ibid., p. 119.
124 Ibid.
125 Ibid.
126 Ibid., p. 113.
127 Ibid.
128 William Cadogan, *An Essay Upon the Nursing and the Management of Children, from their Birth to Three Years of Age* (London: 1748), pp. 24–25 in Fildes, *Wet Nursing*, p. 114. Unlike Anna Davin, both Valerie A. Fildes, and Anja Müller highlight how high infant mortality rates triggered an interest in medicalisation of motherhood and infant feeding especially from mid-eighteenth century onwards. See Anna Davin, 'Imperialism and Motherhood', *History Workshop*, vol. 5, no. 1, 1978, pp. 9–65; and Anja Müller ed., *Fashioning Childhood in the Eighteenth Century Age and Identity* (Aldershot: Ashgate Publishing, 2006).
129 Cadogan, *An Essay Upon the Nursing and Management of Children* in Fildes, *Wet Nursing*, p. 114.
130 Ibid., p. 116.
131 Ibid.
132 Ibid.
133 Yalom, *A History of the Breast*, p. 111.
134 Jean Jacques Rousseau, *Emile* Translated by Barbara Foxley and Introduction by André Boutet de Monvel (London: J. M. Dent & Sons Ltd., 1911), p. 5n1.
135 Ibid.
136 Ibid., p. 13.
137 Mary Seidman Trouille, *Sexual Politics in the Enlightenment Women Writers Read Rousseau* (Albany: State University of New York Press, 1997), p. 27.
138 This 'is particularly well illustrated by a passage on pp. 700–1, in which male readers are referred to as "we" or "us" [*on* or *nous*], while women readers are referred to as "you" [*vous*] or "they" [*elles*]'. Ibid., p. 323n31.
139 Yalom, *A History of the Breast*, p. 111.
140 Ibid., p. 109.
141 Perry, 'Colonizing the Breast', pp. 214–215.
142 Ibid., p. 214.
143 Ibid.
144 Ibid., p. 213.
145 Ibid., p. 209.
146 Ibid., p. 209; also see p. 218.
147 Ibid.
148 Nripendra Kumar Bose and Aradhana Debi, *NarNarir Jounobodh Jouno Khudha o Jounojiban* (Calcutta: Katyani Book Stall, 1934), pp. 241–242, Title Translation: Sexual Awareness, Sexual Appetite and Sexual Life of Men and Women; translation mine; also see Saha, 'Milk, mothering & meanings', p. 107. Translation mine.
149 Tanika Sarkar, 'Nationalist Iconography: Image of Women in 19th Century Bengali Literature', *Economic & Political Weekly*, vol. 22, no. 47, 1987,

pp. 2011–2012, also see Sarkar, 'Nationalist Iconography', pp. 2011–2012 cited in Saha, 'Milk, mothering & meanings', p. 104.

150 Sarkar, 'Nationalist Iconography, p. 2011.

151 Rahul Peter Das, *The Origin of the Life of a Human Being Conception and the Female According to Ancient Medical and Sexological Literature* (Delhi: Motilal Banarsidass Publishers Private Limited, 2003), p. 310, including p. 310n1077.

152 Ibid., p. 310.

153 Das discusses several editions of *Caraka Samhita* and *Susruta Samhita* as well as other texts in relation to breast milk in Ibid., pp. 310–311, also useful information on pp. 478–479.

154 Ibid., p. 310.

155 Kaviraj Kunja Lal Bhishagratna, M.R.A.S., *An English Translation of The Susruta Samhita* With a Full and Comprehensive Introduction, Additional Texts, Different Readings, Notes, Comparative Views, Index, Glossary and Plates in Three Volumes Vol. II. *Nidána-Sthána, S'árira-Sthána, Chikitsita-Sthána and Kalapa-Sthána* (Calcutta: Published by the Author, No. 10, Kashi Ghose's Lane, 1911), p. 71.

156 Ibid.

157 Ibid., p. 225.

158 Ibid., p. 226.

159 Ibid.

160 Ibid.

161 Ibid., pp. 70–72, 225–228.

162 Pratik Chakrabarti, *Western Science in Modern India Metropolitan Methods, Colonial Practices* (Delhi: Permanent Black, 2004), p. 188.

163 Kabiraj Sri Harimohan Dasgupta, *Ayurvediyo Dhatribidya Sangraha. Pratham Khando A Compilation of Ayurvedic Midwifery* Part 1 (Berhampur: Kabiraj Srinikhilranjan Sengupta Kabibhushan Berhampur Dhanantari Pharmacy, Bengali Year 1324, c.1917), n.p., first three pages, pp. 69–78, translation mine. Also, see Dasgupta, *A Compilation of Ayurvedic Midwifery* cited in Saha, 'Milk, mothering & meanings', p. 99; and Saha, 'Milk, "Race" and Nation', p. 158n3. Malavika Kapur argues that similarity of the 'psychic constitution' of wet nurse and child has been mainly stressed by *Kashyapa Samhita*. Malavika Kapur, *Psychological Perspectives on Childcare in Indian Indigenous Health Systems* With a foreword by B. V. Subbarayappa (New Delhi: Springer, 2016), p. 86.

164 Sukumari Bhattacharji, "Motherhood in Ancient India," *Economic and Political Weekly*, vol. 25, no. 42/43, 1990, p. WS50. Malavika Kapur points out the salience of the *Kashyapa Samihita* focused on paediatrics. She also discusses various *samskaras* like praying for birth of sons (*pumsavana*) and initiation of infant feeding with honey, ghee or clarified butter, and gold by the father of the child before putting the child to the mother's breast (*jatakarma*). Kapur, *Psychological Perspectives on Childcare in Indian Indigenous Health Systems*, pp. 199–200.

165 Valerie Fildes, *Breasts, Bottles and Babies A History of Infant Feeding* (Edinburgh: Edinburgh University Press, 1986), pp. 13–16. There were also many Islamic incantations to cure indigestion, excessive lactation, '*dudh tola*' or bringing up of milk by infants, and other problems of daily life like increasing milk supply of cows which were included in various books like Munshi Waazuddin Muhammad, *Islamiya Mantra* Volumes I and II (Calcutta: Muhammad Soleman and Brothers, 1910), pp. 28–29, 52. Rafiuddin Ahmed argues that Muslims often borrowed Hindu charms and rituals as remedies for ailments and warding off evil spirits. Regarding *Islamiya Mantra* specifically, he pointed out that it was an example of 'badly Islamized' Hindu incantations or *mantras* with 'Urduized Bengali replacing the Sanskritic style' and phrases

like 'Allahu', 'pir', 'Nabi' and so on were inserted in place of Hindu names. See Rafiuddin Ahmed, *The Bengal Muslims, 1871–1906: a quest for identity* (Delhi: Oxford University Press, 1981), p. 67.

166 Fildes, *Breasts, Bottles and Babies*, p. 13–15, 26–27, 85–91, 115–122; also see Fildes, *Breasts, Bottles and Babies* cited in Saha, Milk, mothering & meanings, p. 99. For advice on maternal breastfeeding and wet nursing (including duration of breastfeeding for an average of two years, and ideas about breast milk in connection with pregnancy) by Aristotle (384–322BC), Talmud (200–500AD), Soranus (98–117AD), Galen (130–200AD), and the *Koran* (sixth-seventh century AD), see Fildes, *Wet Nursing*, pp. 1–31. Fildes argues that most of these ideas remained unchanged until the nineteenth century, see Fildes, *Wet Nursing*, p. 25. Under the laws of Islam, milk relatives (determined by breastfeeding) and blood relatives were forbidden to marry – see S. Altorki, 'Milk-kinship in Arab society: an unexplored problem in the ethnography of marriage', *Ethnology*, vol. 19, 1980, pp. 233–44 cited in Fildes, *Wet Nursing*, pp. 28–29.

167 Mukhopadhyay, *Matrisiksha*, pp. 54–55 cited in Guha, ' "The Best Swadeshi', p. 143. He also outlined behavioural and dietary requirements for effective lactation, while also recommending boiled *Bharanda* (also known as Bagh Bharanda, Latin. Jatropha) leaves and branches as a galactagogue. Gangaprasad Mukhopadhyay, *Matrisiksha Arthat Garbhabasthay o Sutikagrihey Matar ebong Ballabastha Porjonto Santaner Sasthyarakkha Bishayak Upodesh* (Calcutta: United Press, second ed. 1902), pp. 77–78. Title Translation: Educating the Mother Meaning Healthcare Advice During Pregnancy and in the Lying-Room for the Mother and the Child Till Childhood. Translation mine.

168 See Sundari Mohan Das, *Sishu Mangal Pratham Sikkha* (Calcutta: Shri Premananda Das and Shri Jogananda Das, 1927), p. 48, Title Translation: Child Welfare First Education; and Sundari Mohan Das, *Saral Dhatri-Shikkha o Kumar-Tantra* (Calcutta: Oriental Enterprises Syndicate., third ed. 1922), p. 129; among many others. Translation mine.

169 Mukhopadhyay, *Matrishikkha*, pp. 54–56; also Mukhopadhyay, *Matrishikkha*, pp. 54–56 cited in Saha, 'Milk, mothering & meanings', p. 103.

170 Bharati Ray, 'Introduction' in Sukhendu Ray, Bharati Ray and Malavika Karlekar (eds), *The Many Worlds of Sarala Devi & The Tagores and Sartorial Styles* (New York: Routledge, 2017), p. 12.

171 Borthwick, *The Changing Role of Women in Bengal*, pp. 171–172.

172 Swapna M. Banerjee, 'Blurring Boundaries, distant companions: non-kin female caregivers for children in colonial India (nineteenth and twentieth centuries)', *Paedagogica Historica*, vol. 46, no. 6, 2010, p. 784.

173 Ibid., p. 778. In Bengal, with three types of households namely: 'the households of the European/British officials working in India, the wealthy households of the early aristocrats (*abhijat bhadralok*), and the households of the ordinary Bengali middle class (*madhyabitto grihastha*)' belonging to different backgrounds with variegated racial, economic, and socio-religious allegiances that determined the recruitment and work patterns of the domestic workers. Domestic service was not really 'a woman's job in colonial Bengal. Until 1930 domestic service was predominantly a male occupation in Bengal, and Calcutta had the highest percentage of domestic workers compared with other Indian cities'. Ibid.

174 Ibid. p. 788.

175 Ibid., p. 782. For a discussion on wet nurses' salaries, see Ibid., pp. 780, 783–784.

176 Ray, Ray and Karlekar, *The Many Worlds of Sarala Devi*, pp. 32, 35.

177 Haimabati Sen's notebook originally in Bengali, was finally translated and published only during grandchildren's time, about 80 years after her death. Sen discusses her Vernacular Licentiate in Medicine and Surgery (VLMS) degree from

Campbell Medical School together with both her professional and personal lives, see Sen, 'Resisting Patriarchy'.

178 Forbes and Raychaudhuri, *The Memoirs of Dr. Haimabati Sen*, pp. 57–58.

179 Rachana Chakrabarty argues that in Bengal, the chief women's organisation that fought for women's enfranchisement was the *Bangiya Nari Samaj* guided by 'Kumudini Bose, Kamini Roy, Mrinalini Sen and Jyotirmoyee Ganguly. Even though the initial resolution was defeated in the Bengal Legislative Council in 1921, it was passed in 1925 and women voted in 1926. See Rachana Chakrabarty, 'Women's Education and Empowerment in Colonial Bengal', in Hans Hägerdal (ed), *Responding to the West Essays on Colonial Domination and Asian Agency* (Amsterdam, Amsterdam University Press, 2009), p. 99. Kumudini Bose was a graduate of the Calcutta University and a member of the Bharat Stree Mandal, see Geraldine Forbes, *Women in Colonial India*, p. 70. Also, Kumudini Bose on women's place in the home and suffrage required for better functioning of the home, see Anupama Roy, *Gendered Citizenship Historical and Conceptual Explorations* (Hyderabad: Orient Longman Private Limited, 2005), pp. 164–165.

180 On breastfeeding by mother and wet nurse and detailed milk charts comparing nutritive values of mother's milk with different kinds of animal milk, see Kumudini Bose, 'Sishu Palan', *Ayurved*, vol. 4, no. 2, Bengali Year 1326 (1919), pp. 66–72. Translation mine.

181 Bose, 'Sishu Palan', p. 69.

182 On statistics of infant mortality, see Kumudini Bose, 'Sishu Palan', *Ayurved*, vol. 4, no. 1, Bengali Year 1326 (1919), pp. 18–23. *Sishu Palan* translates as 'Childrearing'. Translation mine.

183 The wet nurse was variously referred to as *dhatri* (midwife)/*dugdhabati dhatri* (wet nurse)/*stanadayini* (breast-giver)/*Upamata* (foster mother or wet nurse) in the Bengali medical and popular writings on infant feeding in colonial Bengal.

184 The midwife and wet nurse sometimes may have been one and the same person.

185 He was an extremely renowned obstetrician who was briefly Professor of Surgery at the Calcutta Medical College before returning to London.

186 W. S. Playfair, *A Treatise on the Science and Practice of Midwifery* with Notes and Additions by Robert P. Harris, M.D. (Philadelphia, Henry C. Lea, Second American edition, 1878, first ed. 1876), p. 538.

187 Khastagir, *A Treatise on the Science and Practice of Midwifery with Diseases of Children and Women*, pp. 197–199. Translation mine.

188 Ibid., p. 186. It is relevant to note that medical practitioner Basantakumar Choudhuri, about his experience as a physician about twenty years prior to when he was writing in 1925, stated that in a *koibarto* family in a remote rural area of Bengal, the baby had been left crying in a soiled, tattered sheet in a room for two days, and ritual pollution prevented anyone from wet-nursing the baby. The doctor took it upon himself to feed the baby animal milk and 'Horlicks-milk-food' but failed to save the baby. He also cited other medical cases related to infant feeding from his experience as a physician, alongside detailed analyses of the components of breast milk under a microscope, how breast milk changes over time in order to keep up with the nutritional needs of the infant, how to discern 'good' quality breast milk, and finally, 'rasayonik pariksha' or 'chemical examination' of the wet nurse's milk is necessary if someone is inexperienced in hiring a wet nurse. see Shri Basantakumar Choudhuri, 'Sishu Khaddya', *Swasthya Samachar*, vol. 14, no. 1, Bengali Year 1332, c.e. 1925, pp. 8–21. Sishu Khaddya translates as Infant Food. Translation mine.

189 Paraphrased from Shri Hemantakumari Debi, 'Santan-Palan', *Bamabodhini Patrika*, (Sraban-Kartik, 1323 Bengali year, 1916; cited in Basu, *Samayiki*, pp. 780–784. Translation mine.

190 Nripendranath Seth, L.M.S., 'Amader Sishu' or 'Our Children', *Sakhi*, Chaitra, Bengali Year 1307, c.e. 1900, in Basu, *Samayiki*, p. 686. Translation mine. Dalit women's capacity for hard labour, painless childbirth and effective breast-feeding was also a romanticised ideal, misused by subjecting her to an even heavier workload, see Gupta, *The Gender of Caste*, pp. 39–40.

191 Sara Suleri, *The Rhetoric of English India* (Chicago: University of Chicago Press, 1992)., p. 81.

192 J. C. Chatterjee, *An Introduction to the Study of Midwifery* (Calcutta, 1930), pp. 522–23, 537–538.

193 Mukherjee, *Gender, Medicine and Society in Colonial India*, p. 44.

194 Evidence of Koilash Chunder Bose, Indian Mirror, 13 August 1878 cited in Bothwick, *The Changing Role of Women in Bengal*, pp. 321–2 cited in *Mukherjee, Gender, Medicine and Society in colonial India*, p. 44.

195 Kedarnath Das is famous for his 'Bengal forceps' designed for the smaller pelvis of Bengali women. For details, see Guha, *Colonial Modernities*, pp. 89–90.

196 Kedarnath Das, *A Text-book of Midwifery for the Medical Schools and Colleges in India* (Calcutta: Thacker Spink & Co., 1921), p. 82.

3

'INDIAN MOTHERS' AND MODERN CHILDCARE

'Indian mothers'[1] and their tendency of nursing whenever the child cried were recurrent and malleable stereotypes, both championed and pathologised, in colonial and indigenous medical literature on childcare in colonial India. Asian and Pacific motherhood in colonial settings were often criticised for their ways of dealing with childbirth, cutting the cord, withholding of colostrum, feeding premasticated food and prolonged suckling of infants, among others.[2] Thus, 'modernizing maternity' involved not only the 'medicalization of pregnancy, birth and the postpartum period but also the discipline of mother love itself'. It aimed to ' "clean up" and rationalize birth' and bring the mother and child under medical surveillance of 'others' often separated by 'race' and 'class'.[3] Indian mothers were frequently represented as the 'Other' being 'rescued' by the benevolent Raj and European women as the 'maternal imperialists'.[4] On the other hand, it is pertinent to note that the colonised elite, usually the upper and middle class and/or caste mainly male and gradually female populations, 'attempts to write itself into history'[5] by discoursing on tradition, modernity and hygiene.

Childbirth, a dangerous experience with high risks of maternal and infant deaths, was further complicated by different customary beliefs and practices. According to Santi Rozario, ritual pollution, confinement and dietary restrictions were a part of the childbirth experience.[6] Women have been considered more susceptible to the attack of evil spirits than men mainly 'unmarried women, new brides, pregnant and postnatal women' whereby they are supposed to 'avoid the *nazar* (i.e. evil or greedy eye) of the *bhut*'.[7] The phrase 'bad air' also implies evil spirits (*bhut-pret* or *jin*) primarily blamed for causing different illnesses in the mother and infant.[8] In the context of colonial India, Geraldine Forbes highlights that birthing was considered to be 'ritually impure' making both the mother and the newborn child 'highly susceptible to both diseases and evil spirits'.[9] This chapter begins by going back in time to nineteenth-century Bengal and bringing back into focus the horrifying custom of the 'exposure of infants' associated with refusal of the breast by an infant due to supposed possession by evil spirits. Thereafter,

 DOI: 10.4324/9781003327837-4

it discusses the more everyday problems of 'prolonged lactation'[10] and 'over-nursing'[11] or 'constantly breastfeeding'[12] which became catchphrases for 'bad' mothering particularly in colonial Calcutta. Medical practitioners often blamed customary breastfeeding practices alongside the so-called ignorance of 'Indian mothers', older women of the household,[13] and *dais*[14] for the contemporary high infant and maternal mortality rates. Mothering had to be learned as not just anyone could be a 'good' mother. From the mid-nineteenth century onwards, particularly in Calcutta, childcare advice insisted that breastfeeding had to be a disciplined and regulated activity by the clock. The second section, therefore, explores the materialities of 'scientific' motherhood in colonial Calcutta – from mechanical clocks to select problematic aspects of maternal dress and diet together with imported baby foods, adulterated milk and milk-borne diseases amidst soaring infant mortality figures.

Customs, Prejudices and Breastfeeding

> This inhuman custom prevails principally in the northern districts of Bengal. If an infant refuse its mother's breast, and appear to decline in health, it is said to be under the influence of some malignant spirit. Such a child is sometimes put into a basket and hung up on a tree, where this evil spirit is supposed to reside; it is generally destroyed by ants or birds of prey, but sometimes perishes by neglect. If it should not be dead at the expiration of three days, the mother receives it home again, and nurses it, but this seldom happens.
>
> (see Figure 3.1)[15]

Company artist Mrs. Sophie Charlotte Belnos provided this horrifying illustration and description of the exposure of infants in her *Twenty Four Plates Illustrative of Hindoo and European Manners in Bengal* (1832). She began by prefacing:

> It is highly gratifying to me to be able to adduce in favour of its fidelity such testimonies as those contained in the Letters subjoined in the Preface, from the HONORARY SECRETARY to the ROYAL ASIATIC SOCIETY, and the RAJA RAMMOHUN ROY, whose opinions of the Work must carry great weight, when the undeniable capacity of both these gentlemen to form an accurate judgement on its merits, from their personal acquaintance with the inhabitants of India is considered.[16]

She added credibility to her lithographic drawings as 'true representations of nature' and 'real scenes alluded to of that unhappy country' as described

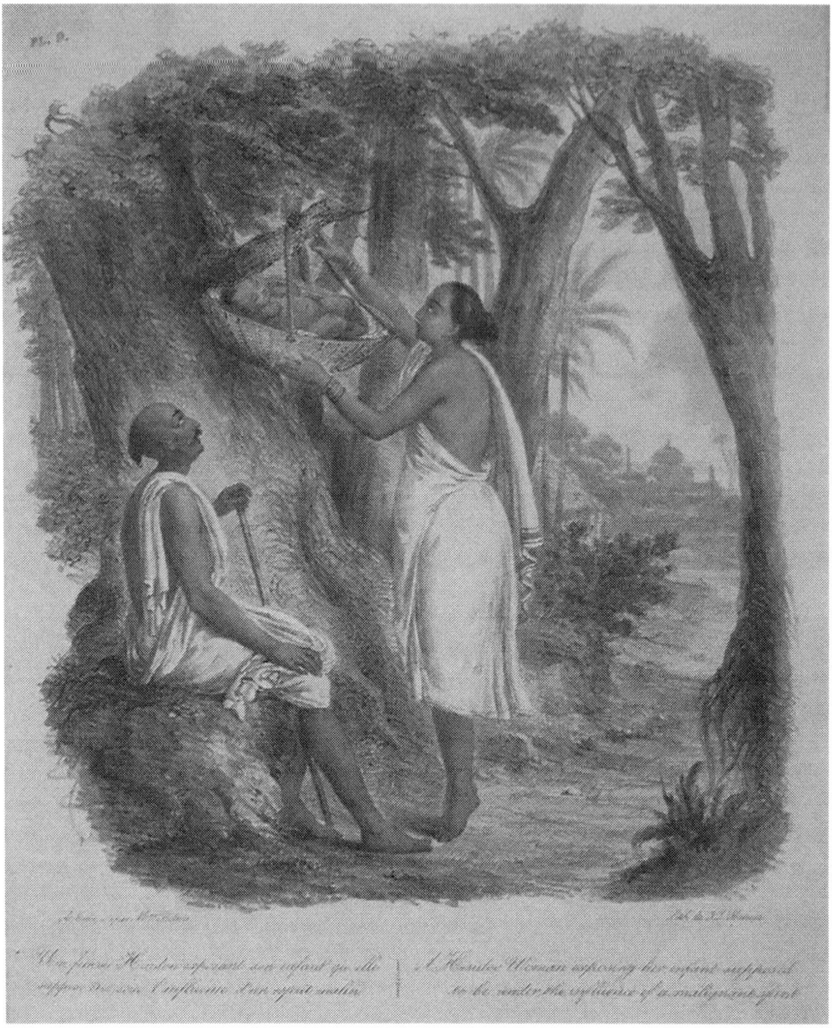

Figure 3.1 'A Hindoo Woman Exposing Her Infant Supposed to be Under the Influence of a Malignant Spirit'.

Source: Mrs. S. C. Belnos and A. Colin, *Twenty Four Plates Illustrative of Hindoo and European Manners in Bengal*, plate 9; and Saha, 'Milk, Mothering & meanings' [with permission from the British Library (London), and the *Women's Studies International Forum* Journal].

by famous Brahmo reformer Raja Rammohun Roy.[17] Moreover, Honorary Secretary of the Royal Asiatic Society Graves C. Haughton believed that 'they portray the every day scenes of life' and 'afford the person who has never visited the East, a faithful picture of the prominent characteristics of the Hindu and European population of India'.[18] William Joseph Wilkins in his *Modern Hinduism* (1887) also corroborated the validity of such a custom as follows:

> If the room sacred to Sasthi, in which the young mother is placed, is bare and uncomfortable, the means of restoration of her devotees are most painful too. A drink called jhāl (hot) is made of pepper, chillies, &c., and given her to drink; and even in the hottest months of the year a fire is lighted, near which she is made to lie; and until the fifth day after the birth of the child no attempt is made to clean this place. . . . If a child refused the breast, it was supposed to be possessed by a devil, and exposed in a basket tied to the branches of a tree for three days. At the expiration of this time it was taken down; if it survived the test, which was a most rare occurrence, it was taken back to its mother; but generally it was dead, and this was taken as a confirmation of the suspicion about its possession. It is said that the great Hindu reformer Chaitanya was thus exposed, and would most probably have shared the fate which others have suffered had not a Brāhman happened to pass at the time, who asserted that the infant was an incarnation of Vishnu, and for this reason he was restored to his home.[19]

The Vedic *Jatakarman* ceremony to keep evil spirits away was performed prior to putting the child to the breast, and also according to later Puranas and Dharmasastras, *Sasthi* puja performed on the sixth day after childbirth in the lying-in room to ward off evil spirits that harm small children.[20]

In 1869, an eye-witness account of the exposure of an infant following the ritualised practice of exorcism with charms and spells in the *Hindu Hitoishinee* blamed indigenous mothers for their belief in witchcraft and the consequent exposure of infants:

> The *Hindoo Hitoishinee* of the 17th July hopes Government will prohibit the Rojas (exorcists) from following the profession in the Mofussil. These men pretend to be possessed of charms and incantations by which they are able to expel evil spirits from children. *Their power, and the evil done by them, are greatly enhanced by the belief of native mothers, that the maladies to which infants are subject are the result of witchcraft. . . . We were once eye-witnesses of an instance in which an infant only five days old refused nourishment, which was followed by a swelling of the stomach.* In accordance with the current belief the advice of Doctors was refused and a Roja was summoned. On his appearance the child was placed in the lap of its mother who was made to sit on the floor with hair dishevelled. The Roja proceeded to make several evolutions round the patient with tufts of flaming straw. Burnt mustard seed was

> then sprinkled on the body of the child, and the hot seeds falling on its body made it shriek with agony; this was interpreted as a favorable sign. . . . *The patient is left carelessly on the ground in some clear spot for some time; after which, if life still remain, it is placed in a basket and hung on a tree sometimes for two or three days together in the sun and rain.* Here death relieves the exorcist of further trouble. Under these circumstances it cannot be denied that this foul practice be prohibited; and as Hindoo Society will not take measures against it, the Government should.[21]
>
> (emphasis added)

Surgeon-Major Norman Chevers, Principal of the Calcutta Medical College and the author of significant handbooks on medical jurisprudence in India, elaborated about the 'barbarity' of the customary practice of exposure of infants who refused the breast.[22] He corroborated his argument by citing a trial at Backergunge, in 1855, involving 'a babe of a few days old . . . in a basket, suspended from a tree. The prisoners (Hindus) were the parents'.[23] The Sessions Judge remarked that the exposure of infants who become 'afflicted with peculiar fits' was 'a very common custom in parts of this district. . . . I should think that the child is, on such occasions, utterly abandoned by its parents; but . . . the parents affirm that they fed the child'.[24] The Judges of the Nizamut Adawlut emphasised that the seriousness of the charge – that the prisoners had exposed their infant on a branch of a tree and had abandoned it there to die – was not proven. On the contrary, the parents declared that they were following their regional customary practices and thereby 'they had so placed the child in the hope of preserving its life'.[25] It is pertinent to note that police reports in early nineteenth-century Bengal categorised 'exposure of infants' under Class I 'Offences against the person'. Under sections 317 and 318 of the Indian Penal Code of 1860, however, 'exposure of infants or concealment of birth' began to appear as a joint category under Class II. 'Serious offences against the Person', whereas Class I came to include 'Offences against the State, Public tranquility, Safety and Justice' – as visible in late nineteenth- and early twentieth-century police reports for the Bengal Presidency.[26] Chevers further elaborated on this custom by citing from various kinds of sources like French traveller and merchant Jean Baptiste Tavernier's (1605–1689) *Travels in India* Volume II pointed out that:

> Tavernier says:- "When a woman is brought to bed, and the child will not take the teat, they carry it out of the village, and putting it in a linen cloth, which they fasten by the four corners to the boughs of a tree, they there leave it, from morning till evening. By this means, the poor infant is exposed to be tormented by the crows, insomuch that there are some who have their eyes picked out of their heads;

> which is the reason that, in Bengalla, you shall see so many of these idolaters that have but one eye, and some that have lost both." [!] "In the evening, they fetch the child away, to try whether he will suck the next night; and, if he still refuse the teat, they carry him to the same place next morning, which they do for three days together; after which, if the infant after that refuses to suck, they believe him to be a devil, and throw him into the Ganges. Sometimes some charitable people among the English, Hollanders, and Portugals, compassionating the misfortune of those children, will take them away from the tree, and give them good education."[27]

Chevers clarified, however, that this practice should not 'be mistaken for Infanticide' in many cases, as it 'appears to be a practice of very ancient standing' and often the goal was, as mentioned earlier, 'preserving' an infant's life.[28] He also acknowledged that an entire gamut of practices was also related directly to infanticide due to the exposure of infants to unsuitable environments like the well, jungle, sand, and river due to a variety of reasons like non-preference for the female child, poverty, and illegitimate offspring in various parts of India.[29] The female infant was often drowned in a vessel containing milk as Cooverjee Rustomjee Mody argued in the piece he wrote in response to the '"Advertisement that appeared in the Government Gazette of 8th March, 1848" inviting Essays against the practice of Female Infanticide'. He pointed out that milk, 'the food of the new-born babe', was often used to drown female infants, alongside other means, for instance, opium was also rubbed on the nipples before breastfeeding mainly among Rajpoots with the intention to kill the female child.[30]

Satadru Sen counters Partha Chatterjee's argument about Indian patriarchy having zealously shielded the inner spiritual domain of the home and the zenana from the colonial state.[31] Instead, Sen argues that they opened their doors to colonial intervention in order to perpetuate patriarchal control, sometimes 'after pruning its excesses', and also to prove that their own homes were 'beyond reproach'.[32] Sen highlights that female infanticide was treated as an 'epidemic' by colonial administrators whereby doctors gained an entry into and a say in 'the home and the natal chamber'.[33] He cites Lalita Panigrahi's argument that Mughal law distinguished between infanticide and murder.[34] However, by 1795, 'colonial law (Regulation XXI of the Bengal Code) had recognized the phenomenon; this law, however, required that infanticide be punished as murder'.[35] The colonial state, with the help of census recordings of male and female births and deaths categorised by region and community alongside surveillance through European officials sometimes right down to the traditional *dais* hired to ideally keep a watchful eye in the zenana, targeted entire communities as 'infanticidal communities'[36] under the terms of the Act for the Prevention of Female Infanticide (1870).[37] It is of particular interest to note as Sen points out that *dais* were also instructed to report whether the girl child had been breastfed or not for 'the assumption that a baby that had been breastfed would not be killed'.[38]

Chevers also cited a heart-wrenching case of death by drowning of a boy child in a well by his indigent mother who had no breast milk as follows:

> In June 1853, a Hindu woman was tried at Bhaugulpore, for the murder of her male child, five or six months old. . . . The woman pleaded guilty, and stated that, not having milk for her infant, she threw it into the well. She was proved to be in very indigent circumstances, and not to have had milk for her infant. One of the eye witnesses to this effect had been the temporary wet-nurse to the deceased, and had given it milk late in the evening of the day of its death. . . . This ignorant, simple woman's evident poverty, and want of sustenance for her child, were humanely taken as extenuating circumstances, and she was sentenced to imprisonment for life.[39]

It is relevant to note that 'Want of breast milk' as a cause of death regularly appeared in the administration reports of late nineteenth-century Calcutta. The causes of deaths for different communities were classified into five classes, namely: (I) Zymotic Diseases, (II) Constitutional Diseases, (III) Local Diseases, (IV) Developmental diseases and (V) Violent deaths. These classes were further categorised into different orders, for instance, zymotic diseases were divided into four orders namely: (1) Miasmatic Diseases, (2) Constitutional Diseases, (3) Dietic Diseases and (4) Parasitic Diseases. 'Want of Breast Milk' was constructed as a medicalised and pathologised enumerative category for colonial administrative purposes listed under Class (I) Zymotic Diseases Order (3) Dietic Diseases. This was outlined clearly, together with other causes of death, in several tables for different communities listed specifically as Non-Asiatics, Mixed Race, Hindoos, Mahomedans, and Other Class, and finally a cumulative table of 'All Nations' in cases of both urban and suburban Calcutta in, for instance, the *Administration Report of the Commissioners of Calcutta for 1893–94* Part II (Table 3.1).[40]

Another problem – connected with breastfeeding in colonial India – was that of prolonged lactation.[41] Both indigenous and European medical practitioners usually cautioned about the problem of prolonged lactation beyond the weaning period as harmful for both mother and child. Dr. Y. Sen, F.R.F.P. & S. (Glasgow), of the Women's Medical Service, Raj Dufferin Hospital, Bettiah, noted that infant mortality in Calcutta due to abdominal ailments is very low as very few babies were artificially fed.[42] However, she used the 'Report on the Municipal Administration of Calcutta for the year 1916–17' to emphasise that the problem of prolonged lactation coupled with socio-economic factors like poverty, insanitary surroundings, and the strain of premature and frequent pregnancies tended to 'weaken and

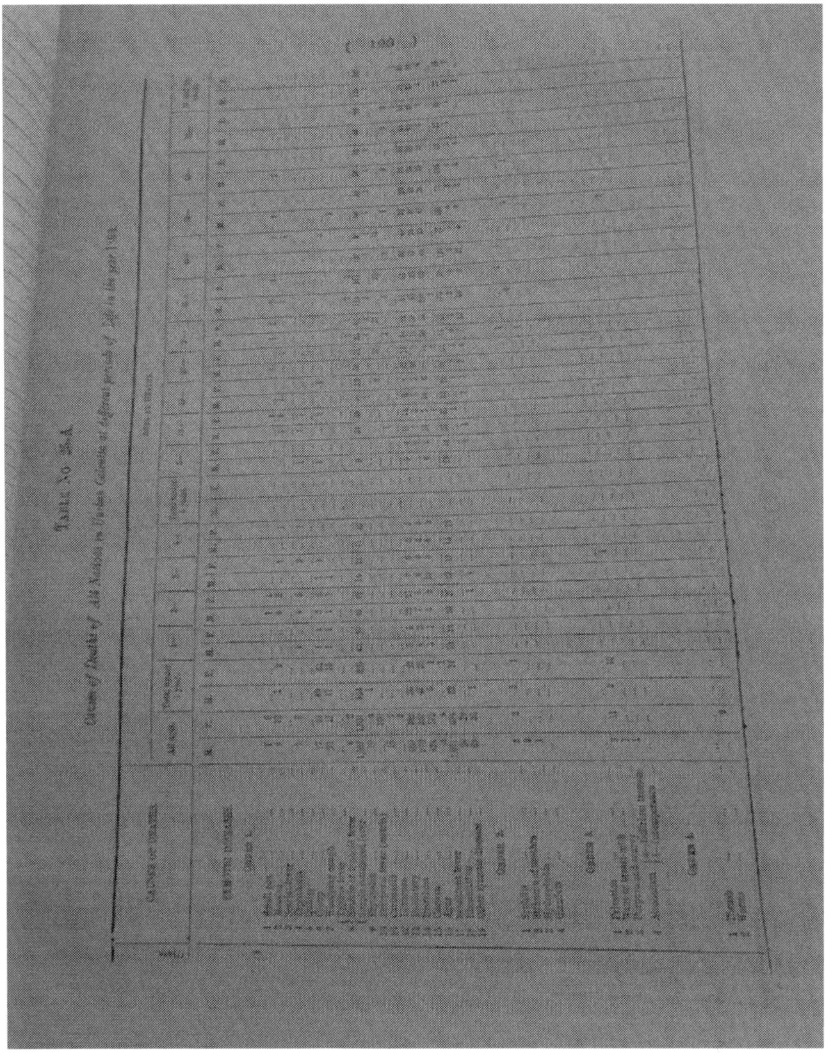

Table 3.1 'Causes of Deaths of All Nations in Urban Calcutta at Different Periods of Life in the Year 1893'.

Source: Administration Report of the Commissioners of Calcutta for 1893–94 Part II, Table 25-A, p. 193 [with permission from the British Library].

debilitate the mother, and puny sickly babies are the result'.[43] For Chevers, however, prolonged lactation beyond the weaning period was only detrimental for the health of the mother alone. He also highlighted that lactation was a key factor in determining delivery and abortion cases. He acknowledged that '[p]regnancy frequently occurs during lactation among women of all races and classes in India'.[44] In a detailed footnote in his book, he discussed prolonged lactation in Bengal, Bombay and Burma beginning with a description by Reverend William Ward of Serampore:

> Ward says that a Hindu woman suckles her child, if she have only one, till it is five or six years old; and that it is not uncommon to see such children standing and drawing the mother's breast. Dr. De Crespigny mentions that, at Butnagherry (Bombay Presidency), children are kept at the breast, often until they are three and four years of age, with a view to prevent pregnancy. Some years ago, a woman, born and brought up in India, but apparently of pure European blood, was admitted to my ward suffering from unmistakable evidences of starvation. This was due to her obstinate pertinacity in suckling a strong active girl of five. She ultimately sunk. Dr. Waring mentions that nothing is more calculated to excite surprise in the mind of a medical man, newly arrived in Burmah, than to witness the lengthened period to which lactation is carried, with apparent impunity, at least as far as the infant is concerned. No certain period is fixed, the general rule being to suckle one child, until the mother is several months advanced in pregnancy with her next; but even this rule is not strictly adhered to. He has, in more than one instance, seen two children – one a sturdy young urchin of five or six years old, and the other an infant of as many months – engaged in drawing sustenance from the mother at the same time. Three years is by no means an uncommon time at which to wean a child, but instances have come under, his notice, of which notes were made at the time, in which lactation was prolonged to four years and six months, to five years, and to six years respectively; the last-mentioned varied the amusement of sucking by an occasional whiff of a cigar! This prolonged lactation does not appear to affect the child in any way – a finer set of children cannot be seen; but it tells wonderfully upon the constitution and outward appearance of the mother.[45]

Prolonged lactation was not just an instance of so-called Indian pathology, however. Valerie F. Fildes argues that it was not such an alien concept in Europe either because:

> The age recommended by physicians and surgeons . . . was frequently based upon the recommendations of ancient authorities. . . . As late as the 1740s, medical authorities were still basing their advice on the length of suckling advised by authorities such as . . . Galen. . . . The median ranged from 24 to 21 months in the 16th and 17th centuries, to 10 months in the 18th century . . . from the

> late 17th century prolonged suckling attracted disapproval of medical writers. Early weaning was not mentioned in the 16th century but by the 18th century this had become a more viable proposition due to the availability and acceptability of artificial feeding. Factors to be considered when weaning a child early included the health of the nurse or mother, the state of her milk and the health of the infant.[46]

It is relevant to note, going back to 1830s Britain, that British physician Edward Morton's book *Remarks on the Subject of Lactation* (1831) went to the extreme of directly correlating 'idiocy' together with hydrocephalus and other diseases to 'protracted lactation'. He also located the problem of 'protracted lactation' within the realm of 'prejudice' and old wives tales:

> The belief so generally prevailing, that the longer a child is suckled the stronger it will become, is a prejudice, like many others concerning women and children, which has been handed down from mother to daughter for ages, and has thereby become so universally entertained and so deeply rooted in the minds of females, that even medical men scarcely venture to question its propriety. My own experience, however, compels me to declare, that there is not a more erroneous or mischievous doctrine . . .. As a general rule, at nine months after birth the child ought to be entirely weaned. . . . In two cases where suckling was protracted to three years, the subjects of this baneful practice did not equal in size an ordinary child of half their age. One of them became idiotic, and afterwards died of Hydrencephalus, under my care; the other was affected with Tabes Mesenterica, – the result I did not witness – but believe the disease terminated fatally.[47]

Finally, in colonial India, the tendency to 'constantly breastfeed' among Indian, including Bengali mothers, was often naturalised and glorified in colonial and nationalist medical literature.[48] However, this same custom of breastfeeding 'all the time' by responding to the child's cries was also pathologised as faulty breastfeeding which justified medicalising and disciplining breastfeeding by the clock. In colonial Bengal, meticulous medical advice to the *bhadramahila* mother on infant feeding as a disciplined and regulated activity by the clock, 'numeralization'[49] of the infant diet including charts on how much mother's milk a newborn should consume,[50] and 'humanisation' of animal milk (often by adding sugar, water, etc.) is visible in Bengali medical advice on childcare.[51] It is pertinent to note that medical treatises often addressed the management of the health of a boy child, a *cheley*, the *only* future citizens of the nation.[52] As briefly discussed in the previous chapter, Meredith Borthwick argues that Shib Chunder Deb, an administrator and 'not a doctor', published his childcare manual titled *The Infant Treatment* First Part in 1857, which is one of the oldest Bengali childcare manuals created generally on 'English prototypes'.[53] To elaborate here, he recommended clocked infant feeding and he also ensured that his son was fed 'by the clock'.[54] Deb advised that the infant must be put to the mother's breast within eight to ten hours of birth to cleanse the bowels. He advised against '*sarbada*' or constant breastfeeding in order to produce 'good' breast milk and, in turn, a healthy child. He also sometimes allowed mothers the choice to decide whether or not the baby needed a feed. Successful breastfeeding was supposed to depend on the digestive system of the child as well as the lactating woman's bodily strength and the nutritional levels of her breast milk which varied from one woman to another. Furthermore, he pointed out that if the mother was unable to breastfeed, a doctor was the only person capable of evaluating and hiring a suitable *dai*. As the wet nurse's physical appearance did not always prove to be a good yardstick to gauge her diseases or the 'goodness' of her milk, he recommended that examination of her breast milk and her child was necessary. He also warned that in case the *dai* does not produce enough milk, then her tendency would be to breastfeed her own child properly first. In this regard, he recommended strict surveillance on the wet nurse by the mother and the need to replace her immediately if such a situation arose. Deb used both the words '*balak*' (boy child) and '*sishu*' (child) interchangeably in his book.[55]

The gender of the child addressed in Bengali medical treatises is, therefore, also problematic. Scientific and medical guidance for maternal and child welfare were often presented as matter of fact, objective suggestions. The underlying logic was that because it is based on science, it is automatically already justified, unquestionable and commonsensical. Not to follow such advice would be counterintuitive, foolish and detrimental for the health of the family, community and the nation. This apparent objectivity also seems to have extended to the gender of the child.

Materialities of Modern Motherhood? Clocks, Corsets and '*Cheleder Khabar*'

> Amongst Indian mothers the tendency of over-nursing the baby is very great. The baby is always at the breast, and is put to it whenever it makes the least noise.[56]
>
> Discipline does not mean harshness as so many Indian mothers are apt to think. . . . In all houses where it can be afforded and understood, a clock should be regarded as an indispensable piece of the furniture.[57]

This section neatly dovetails Bruno Latour's argument that a 'whole supplementary work' of 'sorting out, cleaning up and dividing up' was necessary for 'a modernization that goes in step with time'.[58] This section explores previously unexplored sources that puts a spotlight on the material culture of 'scientific' motherhood advice from the role of modern clocks, which is, thereafter connected to a discussion about dress and diet, particularly imported baby foods (many referred to baby foods as '*cheleder khabar*' or food for boys in Bengali) and the problem of adulterated foodstuffs which together reveals the intersections between medicine, modernity, motherhood, colonialism and anti-colonial nation-building. Here I am primarily interested in Bengali *daktars* who insisted on reducing infant mortality through regular breastfeeding as a disciplined and regulated activity by the clock.[59] As also mentioned in the Introduction, my main argument is that breastfeeding advice offered an opportunity for Bengali *daktars* to introduce clock time into the home as well as anti-colonial nation-building through subject formation of the Bengali middle class by discoursing about the modern and medicalised self-disciplining regimen. By mainly using gender as an anchor, it also sheds light on the different meanings attached with the birth of girl and boy children along with the matter-of-factness associated with the visibility of the male child in most childcare manuals and baby food advertisements.

In famous Bengali *daktar* Hasan Suhrawardy's (MD, F.R.C.S.I) description, the parturient *bhadramahila* was usually 'incarcerated' in the lying-in room and 'given hot fomentations on her body' and 'made to drink decoctions of various "heating" vegetables and dried fruits from three weeks to forty days'.[60] During the confinement period, the baby was 'never brought out of the *souri* or *atoor*, as this room of horrors is called, for fear of the evil eye, the *dain* or village witch and the evil spirits'.[61] He asked 'how under such conditions mothers have ever escaped cent. per cent. mortality and why our very manhood has not been exterminated or dwarfed to the lowest possible ebb by the blight of these harrowing surroundings'.[62] He stated, therefore, that 'Preventive Medicine, the Science of Eugenics and Child – welfare' as 'propaganda for the protection of our children and regeneration of our country' is 'a sacred duty for every thoughtful Indian . . . the best Swadeshi and Nationalist movement'.[63]

Suhrawardy explained the merits of putting the child to the mother's breast right after birth and clocked breastfeeding together with, as you might recall from the brief excerpt at the start of this section, the problem of 'over-nursing':

> The child should be put to the breast not later than 8 to 12 hours after its birth, but if the child is wakeful it might be put to the breast at once although there is no nourishment in it. It is good for both the mother and the child, the stimulus of sucking reflexly contributes to the contraction of the womb, and by helping involution stops any tendency to bleeding. It is good for the infant as it gives it warmth, and the thick milk called colostrum acts as a gentle

> purgative and helps expulsion of the black contents of the bowels known as 'meconium' without interfering with the absorption of the useful material. It also acts beneficially as a 'secretogen' that is to say, it stimulates into activity the glands of the infant's digestive system and prepares them to digest and assimilate its milk food. It is therefore apparent how useful it is to put the infant to the mother's breast soon after its birth. . . . The feeding of the infant is important. It should be put to the breast about three times in the first 24 hours and after that every three hours – say at 6 A.M., 9 A.M., 12 Noon, 3 P.M., 6 P.M., 10 P.M. If a regular routine about feeding is kept up, proper sleep and sufficient nourishment is ensured for the child and a restful night for the mother, which is very essential for her health, and for the well-being of the infant she is nursing. It is a great mistake to feed an infant each time it cries. . . . *Amongst Indian mothers the tendency of over-nursing the baby is very great.* (emphasis added)[64]

Mechanical clocks signifying precision and discipline became pivotal to the very making of the modern materialities of Indian motherhood in colonial Calcutta. Both British and Bengali doctors advised against feeding every time the child cried. Around this time, in her manual, *Maternity and Infant Welfare* (1922), renowned medical practitioner, Ruth Young (M.B.E., B.Sc., CH.B., W.M.S.), pointed out that she was influenced by the very popular Dr. Truby King's *The Expectant Mother* and *Feeding and Care of Baby*.[65] Young advised, as also mentioned in the brief excerpt at the start of this section, that '[d]iscipline does not mean harshness as so many Indian mothers are apt to think'. She emphasised that clocks and routine were central to the medical instruction and disciplining of 'Indian mothers' and her (male) child.[66] Undercurrents of 'Darwinist notions of the struggle for existence as an essential part of the survival of the race'[67] are also visible when Young discussed that, in India, most infants were born 'feeble and die after a few weeks or months of life', while those who survived 'remain weak, constantly ill, and pass from childhood spent in struggles against disease, to adolescence and *manhood* where they are *unfit to face the struggle for existence*' (emphasis added).[68] She believed that '[b]abies who are taken up or fed whenever they cry', or those who are not properly 'trained' in 'self-control' from birth, develop various 'irregular habits'.[69] However, such advice on disciplining was not just for Indian mothers alone – renowned medical practitioner of Delhi and Lahore, Mildred Staley (M.B., L.M.), pointed out in case of the European mother (and her male child) – 'A well trained infant will not give so much trouble as one who is accustomed to be rocked off to sleep, picked up when *he* cries, and generally encouraged in the *fussy egoism* so natural to young children' (emphasis added).[70] Young also elaborated, in case of 'Indian mothers', that '[r]egularity in times of feeding, etc., cannot be expected if mothers have no idea of the passage of time; it cannot be done by guess-work'. She emphasised that '[f]athers and husbands should be enlightened as to the necessity of clocks and encouraged to buy them for their wives'.[71]

Bengali advice on conjugality and motherhood, including regular breast-feeding, intersected with 'global bourgeois notions of respectability, domesticity, and order' which were 'incorporated to routinise copulation, reproduction and childcare with the help of clock time'.[72] These also provided, as Mary Hancock argues, discursive 'elite nationalist maps for female agency in the fields of citizenship, motherhood, rationalized home management'.[73] Clocks became a 'status symbol' and 'people increasingly timed activities they would never have thought of timing'.[74] Meredith Borthwick informs us that, in case of Bengal, particularly progressive Brahmo Bengali *bhadralok* lifestyle was expensive and '[t]heir expectations and aspirations were always higher than their means'[75] – for instance, in the *Indian Mirror* advertisements from the 1870s, '[c]locks ranged from 40 to 100 rupees, and watches varied from 35 for a "railway guard" keyless watch to 200 for one in a gold case'.[76] As mentioned earlier, the 'whole supplementary work' of 'cleaning up and dividing up' was necessary for keeping modernisation 'in step with time'.[77] Socio-cultural, moral, material and *natural* entities were systematically ordered as belonging to the same time to construct 'modern temporality' as an 'irreversible arrow' of 'progress' or 'decadence'.[78] The paraphernalia of modernity therefore extended to, for instance, the 'reformed dress' of the 'new woman'[79] – including chemise, jacket, *cādar* (a shawl-like wrap), petticoats and shoes – which were sometimes more expensive than 'a simple sari'.[80] She was also advised in domestic manuals to learn skills of how to 'keep accounts' and it was 'a quality sought after in the new housewife'.[81]

Dipesh Chakrabarty alerts us that 'memsahib-like behaviour' was, however, central to Bengali men and women's anxieties, often voiced in their literary and medical writings at the time as they constructed the 'new woman'. As Kundamala Devi's article from Brahmo women's magazine *Bamabodhini Patrika* cautioned as early as in 1870: 'Oh dear ones! If you have acquired real knowledge, then give no place in your heart to memsahib-like behaviour. This is not becoming in a Bengali housewife'.[82] Chakrabarty's arguments about the Bengali 'modernity of tradition' highlights that Alakshmi (anti-Lakshmi) together with '[s]everal negative terms' like '*bibi* (the feminine form for babu, a dandy), *memsahib* (European women), *boubabu* (a housewife who behaves like a babu), *beshya* (slut) etc.' implied 'assertiveness on the part of women and its undesirability'.[83] These 'figures of imagination' were used to 'demonise the "free" and "private" (female) individual whom the European writers on conjugality idealised'.[84] Projit Bihari Mukharji emphasises that *daktars* also strove for the creation of ideal 'national constitutions' and sometimes explicitly pointed out '*Bangali Shaheb nohey*' which literally translates as the Bengali is not like a *sahib*.[85] This discussion neatly dovetails Suhrawardy's anxieties about Indian women's 'partiality' towards the 'useless fashion' of the West from wearing corsets to high-heeled and pointed shoes as follows:

> In the matter of *clothing*, the Indian women score over their Western sisters, whose figure is distorted and breathing hampered by whalebones and tight-laced dress. The costume of Indian women are generally loose and quite suitable, as it allows space for the growth of the child and give freedom to the mother's breathing mechanism sufficient to compensate for the increased upward pressure of the womb on her chest. In some provinces in India, the women are in the habit of tying their saris below the navel and are therefore likely to get a pendulous belly should be given support by means of a fold of *chaddar* or special elastic abdominal bandages may be used. This condition is uncomfortable at all times, and by helping displacement of the growing wombs gives rise to difficulty in labour, hence it should not be allowed to persist. In some cases a maternity corset may be useful, but an Indian woman had better be left uninitiated to the use of corsets and also high heeled and pointed shoes for which, I am afraid, some of them are showing a partiality. The former interferes with the freedom of breathing and the latter has a tendency of throwing back the spine in order to establish equilibrium. As the spine of the pregnant woman is already curved forward it should not be burdened with further stress from useless fashion. . . . During pregnancy, the breasts of a woman grow in size and weight and require attention. As a result, there is generally a dragging pain, it should be supported by means of a broad bandage or piece of cloth. The use of the Oriental bodices, known as *shalooka, angia* and *mahram kurti* are useful as a means of providing support.[86]

Suhrawardy's particular reference to the 'maternity corset' maybe further clarified by referring to Rebecca Gibson's delineation of the corset in a different context as 'a simple way to stiffen and shape the front of the garment with a busk – a long, straight, stiff length of material' – which 'went through many changes in form such as the additions of sets of stays (side stiffeners, often called bones, that radiate from the busk around the sides of the body)' to '*specialty corsets such as ones designed to accommodate pregnancy and nursing*' (emphasis added). Gibson goes back in time to the early nineteenth century to highlight that an 'Europeanized' individual across social hierarchies might have 'worn a corset when living' as evident from the skeleton of an 'Indian from Bombay [Mumbai], a domestic servant who died under home care at the l'hospice Beaujon, in Paris, in 1839' – 'MNHN-HA-784, from India. Coronal dimension: 19.5. Sagittal dimension: 17. Ratio of coronal to sagittal dimensions: 1:.87. Age at death, 36–45'. She argues that it exhibits 'deformation from corseting'. She points out that she had 'a cylindrical rib cage' and her bottom ribs had been rounded inward towards the centre line together with 'small-angled spinous processes' – thereby revealing that she had been part and parcel of the traffic in ideas and people across the '"civilized" world' and that women 'who came under that métier had the proper shape'.[87]

Locating the negative bodily effects of corsets specifically on European women and girls in 'tropical' India, Staley in her *Handbook for Wives and Mothers in India* (1908) provided the following detailed instructions:

> [T]he corset, as usually worn in the heat of India, is a most pernicious article of dress. It overheats the region it covers, prevents evaporation from the damp garments beneath, and renders the internal organs therefore liable to chills. It also impedes the circulation and lungs, preventing waste materials from being thrown off properly, and so assists in the production of the dyspepsia, anaemia, and nervous disorders so common in the country. In addition, corsets, if worn tight, tend to displace internal organs. When worn in hot weather, they should be of some porous material and without steel supports . . . the mother has to 'breathe for two,' and clothing should be at least three inches larger than the waist to ensure that there is no pressure anywhere. Corsets should be discarded now, and it is best to give up all attempts at possessing a 'waist' from the beginning of pregnancy. Stays . . . may press on the breasts, injure their glandular structure, and compress the nipples flat with the surface. In place of corsets there is an excellent invention called the 'Emancipation' bodice, which can be obtained from the large English outfitters. . . . For girls, thick stiff 'stay-bodices' into which the lower garments are buttoned are most unsuitable. . . . A well-fitting flannel bodice acts far better, and can be worn till the girl leaves school. Or one of the close fitting 'emancipator' bodices, or other soft substitute for stays, can be worn. The 'backache' from which so many women suffer may be often directly traced to its right cause by finding that the muscles of the back are feeble and wasted, having been prevented from developing through years of girlhood by the use of stays. . . . Other evil results of stays for growing girls are spinal curvature, from weakness of the back muscles, and anaemia or poverty of blood from the lungs being compressed.[88]

Mary Morris argues that the very term 'stays' meaning 'bindings in women's corsets' is particularly revealing in terms of how women's dress and physical mobility were intimately linked – 'Someone who wore stays wouldn't be going very far'.[89] American consul at Bombay, Henry D. Baker, presented a counterintuitive argument that European women in India were also known for their 'fondness of outdoor sports, especially horseback riding and lawn tennis'.[90] Moreover, in his description, a large number of them belonged to 'military social circles in which open-air amusements constitute a leading feature' – there was

> an especial demand for corsets suitable for riding and other athletic exercises. These, however, are changed for more elaborate corsets for social functions in the afternoon and for the evenings, when social custom in India prescribes full dress'.[91]

Baker also confirmed Suhrawardy's fears about some Indian women's 'partiality' towards corsets by pointing to a most recent interesting development in 'the corset trade of India' – 'in which the United States has the most important share' – that

> native women of high caste – known as purdah women, because they keep their faces covered with purdahs, or thick veils, and live a life of seclusion from the male sex – are beginning to wear corsets, the same as their European sisters.[92]

Most Indian women, except the already mentioned 'high-caste purdah women', however, 'do not wear corsets and probably never will' considering them 'a most extravagant and uncomfortable luxury'.[93]

Writing around the same time, travel writer Mrs Elizabeth Cooper although alluding to the popularity of being 'more English in manner than are the English' among the Indian elite noted instead that the 'French corset' and 'French slippers' were in vogue during her visit to early twentieth-century Calcutta:

> In the cities the rich families are sending their daughters to private schools, and the Oriental home is the happy hunting ground for the English governess . . . as it seems to be the main object in life of the educated Indian, both man and woman, to be *more English in manner than are the English themselves*. . . . In Calcutta I went to a reception given by a great Indian lady. With the exception of the costumes worn by the pretty dark-eyed Bengalis, and the absence of men, I would have thought I was in an English house. . . . *Most of the ladies wore high-heeled French slippers, and many of them had their beautifully draped saris twined around bodies held in place by the French corset, which must have been most uncomfortable for these people, used to untrammelled freedom in regard to their dress.*
>
> (emphasis added)[94]

Reversing the colonial gaze, Krishnabhabini Das' travelogue *Iṃlaṇḍe baṅgamahilā* (Bengali Woman in England), published in 1885 and based on her eight years' experience of living in England, offered a critique of the highly gendered notion of beauty in the metropolis:

> [I]t is astonishing how many artificial things English women use to enhance their beauty. By wearing things like corset and crinoline, the posture and the gait can be altered so much that it is impossible to determine who is really beautiful and who is just a camouflaged beauty.[95]

Moreover, English women 'even tolerate pain that distorts their natural physique. I have heard that at one point, to display narrow waistlines, they would tie it so tightly that while walking down the road, they would even faint'.[96] Commenting on her own attire as she sailed for England, Das exclaimed 'where is my veil today? . . . even my acquaintances will not be able to recognize me and might even bow to me or be afraid of me and keep a distance thinking me as a memsahib'.[97]

Indian attitudes to European clothes were, however, varied and, in areas with a strong British presence like Calcutta, western clothes were likely to be more readily available and adopted.[98] Particularly for men, British clothing also represented 'all the values which the British boasted: superiority, progress, decency, refinement, masculinity'.[99] Thus, if Indians wanted to participate in western civilisation, then 'wearing the correct clothes was surely one means of doing so'.[100] The clothing dilemmas of the Indian elite were also tied to their clamour for *swadeshi* and self-identity as expressions of their increasing uneasiness with colonialism.[101] Indira Chowdhury argues that growing nationalist demands also included negotiations with colonial stereotypes which resulted in the 'process of resignification' in the form of an 'Indian' modernity which homogenised what was 'Indian' while it glossed over underlying tensions particularly of gender, class, caste, and community.[102] Himani Bannerji specifically points out that, from the 1860s onwards, together with the gradual growth in cultural nationalism, a small section among the elite dressed in gowns and experimented with saris.[103] She explains that 'saris won the day', however, due to the 'elision between feminine shame/modesty and *deshiata*, or "nationalist" cultural authenticity, which includes a restrained female sexuality' and a 'moral-sartorial' project with an 'insignia of virtue and vice'.[104] As Brahmo educationist Jyotirmoyee Gangopadhyay's (M.A.) article 'Sari or Gown' in the popular Bengali women's magazine *Bharati* highlighted that although

> [t]here was a time when the new promoters of women's emancipation, both male and female, adorned themselves in western clothes. . . . [W]e have many proofs of the fact that educated men

and women did not wish to wear western clothes, since they conveyed an anti-nationalist mentality.[105]

On the other hand, it is pertinent to note that across racial and class hierarchies, there also exists a fluidity of embodied historical contexts and cultural geographies of the 'lived garment'[106] like the gown or the sari particularly in the case of Vicereine of India, Lady Mary Curzon (1898–1905). She had her maternity dress designed with 'sari material' which although unusual perhaps, also reflects, as Nupur Chaudhuri argues, that British women variously embodied wider processes of transculturation and hybridity, rather than racial exclusiveness, in colonial India.[107] Lady Curzon specifically acknowledged, as Nicola J. Thomas points out, that her bodily changes due to pregnancy required hiding inside maternity dresses designed for a display of 'propriety' in performance of imperial 'public duty'.[108]

An Indian mother in a sari and holding a baby, as Srirupa Prasad emphasises – the 'Indian cultural repertoire'[109] – was a dominant presence in many drug and baby food advertisements including tonics for curing women's ailments across colonial India. It is pertinent to note that in advertisements that promised to make 'women fertile and bless them with children', there was definitely an 'affective strategy – the deployment of mother – child bonding to invoke a special connection with the consumer product'.[110] The tonic Rad-Jo, supposed to 'minimise pains of pregnancy' and promote 'easy birth' and lactation, was advertised, for instance, in the *Directory of the City Health & Baby Week 1931*, Madras, with a picture of an Indian mother in a sari and holding a baby (Figure 3.2).[111] Prasad deploys Jackson Lears' trope of 'imperial primitivism'[112] as particularly applicable in the 'household targeted advertisements'.[113] In this regard, it is pertinent to note that Patricia R. Stokes, arguing in the context of twentieth-century Germany, points out that Rad-Jo, manufactured and marketed by Vollrath Wasmuth, had as its primary ingredient supposedly used by 'native' African women during deliveries, a plant extract 'Jogonie, for what it was named' which meant a return to Nature and 'exoticism'.[114] The 'Indian cultural repertoire' was also present in the advertisement for the tonic Lodhra in the same *Directory* (Figure 3.3). Sarah Hodges argues that Kesari's Lodhra was one of 'the most high-profile, widespread and long-running campaigns in the Tamil and English-language press' to various means of public transport like Madras tramcars.[115] It had doctors' recommendations with personal anecdotes: for example, Dr. Mrs. Anna Thomas, Superintendent Health and Infant Welfare, Bangalore Cantt., claimed that it had been 'beneficial' for her 'weak' and 'emaciated' sister while it was also strategically marketed as a challenge to the 'so-called foreign patent medicines' which have 'failed in many of my patients' (Figure 3.3).[116] Besides this particular advertisement 'Lodhra for Ladies' Health', there was another advertisement 'Lodhra for Ladies' Troubles & Disorders' on the previous page of the *Directory*.

It was, however, deliberately dissociated from the 'Indian cultural repertoire'. Instead, it had a picture of the upper body of a European lady wrapped in possibly an exotic palm leaf hinting at problems relating to female sexuality and gynaecology in 'tropical' India with the header: 'Queen of Tonics' (Figure 3.4). This coincides with Hodges' argument that these 'tonics for complaints peculiar to ladies' present a large gray area of 'possible subterfuge in meanings'.[117] Douglas E. Haynes emphasises that besides the fact that these seemed to be 'modern' and 'scientific', the significance of such advertisements, particularly those encased in 'vernacular capitalism', was 'self-medication'. Using these tonics claiming to cure women's diseases often had the advantage of being not just affordable but, more importantly, 'discrete'. Such advertising permitted 'a certain anonymity on the part of the middle-class consumer that was missing when he or she relied on the medical specialist, whether "biomedical" or "indigenous".'[118]

Both 'race' and gender were central to baby food advertisements in colonial India. Usually a 'white' child was often portrayed as Indian, possibly to signify a universal Caucasian yet culturally neutral baby in a 'nuclear, modern family as an ideal'.[119] 'A smiling blonde baby boy sitting on a scale was featured atop this advertisement for vita-milk, an enriched milk substance imported to the subcontinent'. It further stated that '"In the ancient times and throughout the land of India, parents used to have to consult a vaid if their children were not growing". In modern India, they just had to feed the child vita-milk'. Rachel Berger highlights that both Ayurveda and biomedicine were sometimes deployed making evident the tension between the two traditions. This also coincides with Prasad's argument that the medically plural nature of drug and food markets based on tropes used for market control like Indian/foreign, modern/traditional and civilised/uncivilised alongside the medical systems of Allopathy, Homeopathy, Ayurveda, and Unani competed with each other.[120] Vita-Milk (Figure 3.5) was advertised at the start of Director of Dairy Research, Government of India, W. L. Davies' *Indian Indigenous Milk Products* as: An Important Factor! Vita-Milk is the *only* food which plays an important part in baby's diet . . . to build strong bones, sturdy limbs and sound teeth and is easily digestible. *Ask your doctor or nurse about Vita-Milk. They will surely tell you that it is the milk for your baby.* It is known for: Freshness, Mixed Carbohydrates and Inert Gas Packing (emphasis added).[121]

As also mentioned in Chapter 1 of this book, it is pertinent to note that the discourses on artificial milk, medicine and modernity also incorporated a 'discourse on "vitalism"' – the way in which imported baby food advertisements combined the 'ideal' of 'purity' of one place to the lack thereof in the 'hot climate of India'.[122] As also in the case of baby-food advertisements like Mellin's Food and Nestle Milo Food in Chapter 1 of this book, 'mechanization' was a 'guarantee' of the 'superiority' and 'purity' of baby food products.[123] In Chapter 1, I had also discussed the Mellin's 1922 calendar captioned in

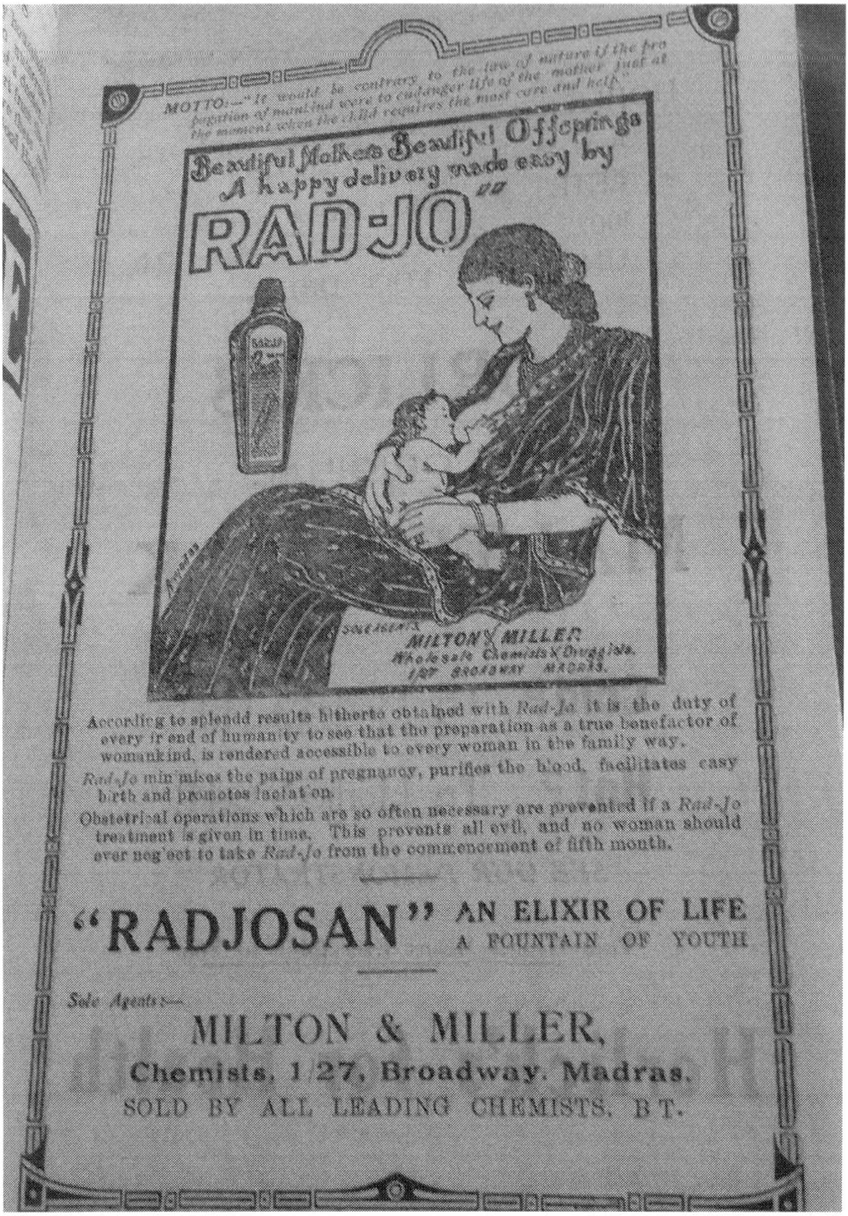

Figure 3.2 Advertisement of Rad-jo.

Source: Directory of the City Health and Baby Week 1931, n.p. [with permission from the British Library].

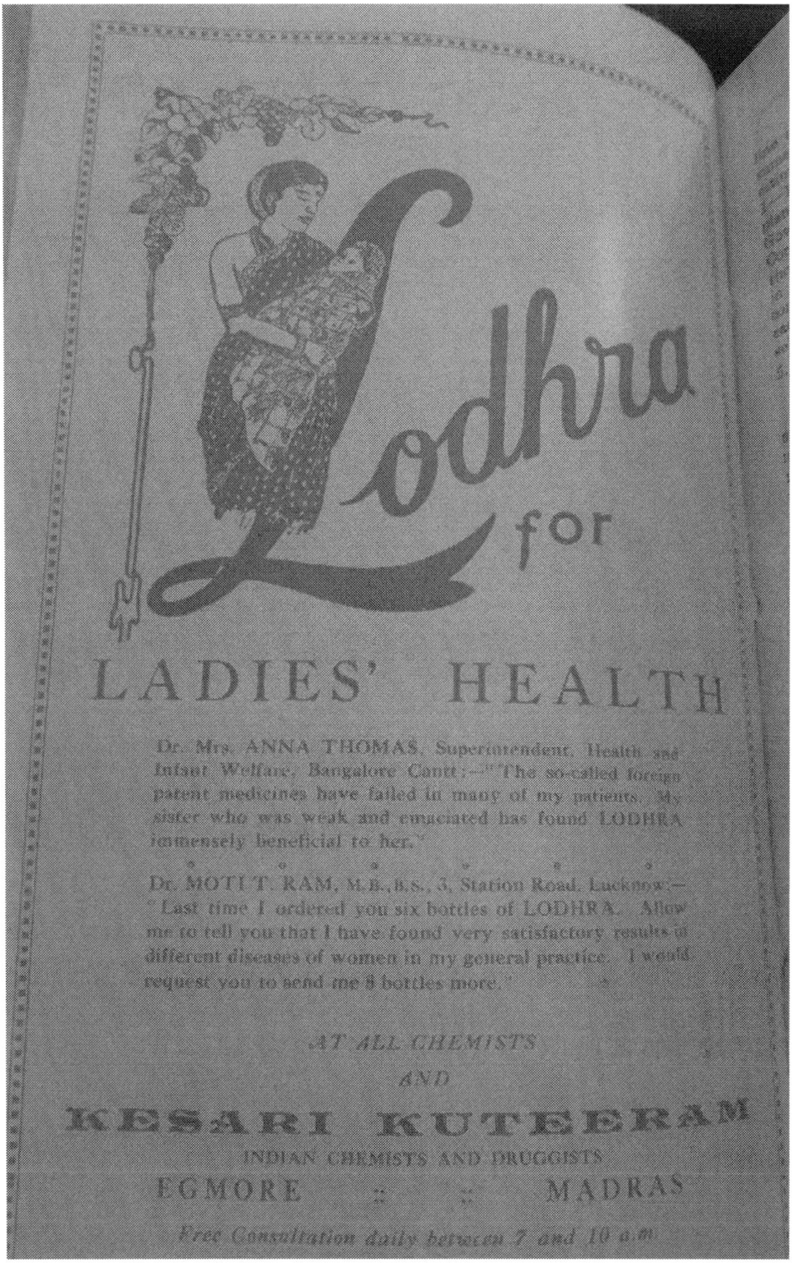

Figure 3.3 'Lodhra for Ladies' Health Source'.

Source: Directory of the City Health and Baby Week 1931, n.p. [with permission from the British Library].

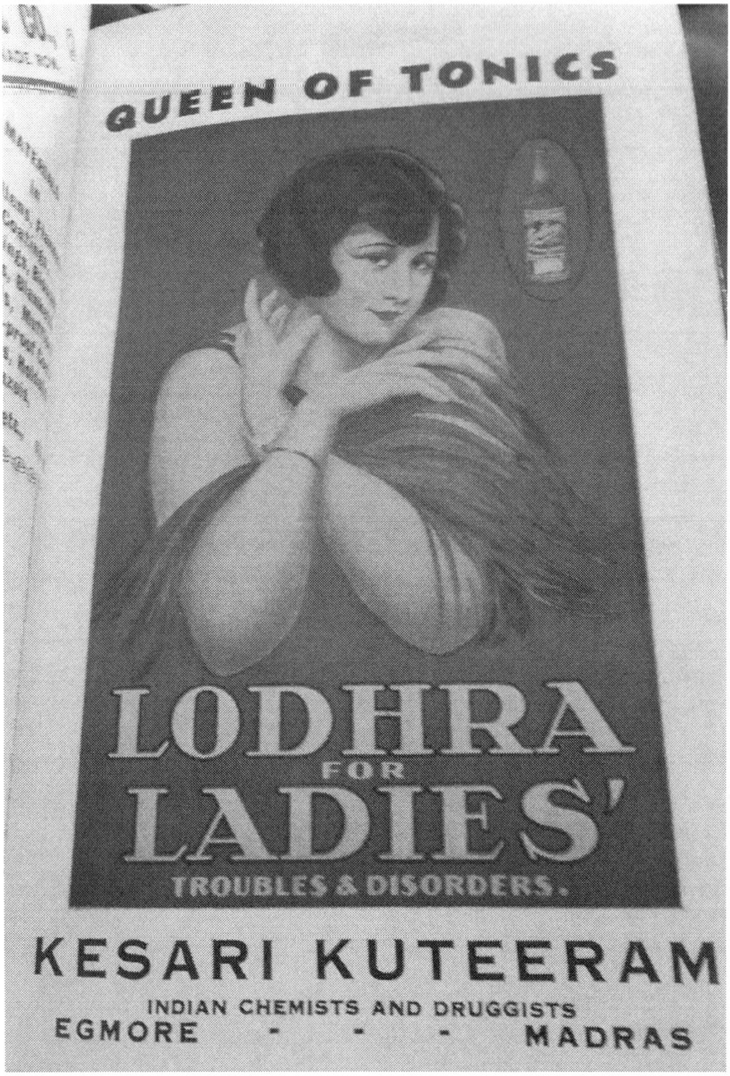

Figure 3.4 'Lodhra for Ladies' Troubles & Disorders'.

Source: Directory of the City Health and Baby Week 1931, n.p. [with permission from the British Library].

both English and Bengali and illustrated with a young Lord Krishna playing the flute thereby highlighting how imported baby food advertisements were often Hinduised, and thereby located amidst 'codes of local culture',[124] in colonial Calcutta (Figure 1.1). Madhuri Sharma points out that a baby boy who looks like a 'white' (British) child was central to the advertisement of

Glaxo baby food in *Abhyudaya*, September 14, 1929.[125] She explains that European firms often ensured that 'codes of local culture', like using Sanskrit phrases in advertisements, 'assimilated them to their own symbols so as to draw on features with a universal appeal'.[126] She emphasises that European products also dominated English newspapers and periodicals.[127] They also had the financial resources to flood vernacular newspapers with both visual and print advertisements.[128] Besides the enormous significance of the 'codes of local culture' in baby food advertisements of the 1920s, I argue here that, particularly, during the First World War, 'the most profitable overseas Glaxo business'[129] had also both strategically universalised and marketed the war-effort with a promise to make 'mothers of the empire'[130] and 'vigorous future citizens'[131] in a colonial setting like Calcutta. 'The Future of the Empire lies in the arms of every Nursing Mother' – the caption headed a huge advertisement of Glaxo, advertised as both a baby food and a galactagogue (substance promoting lactation), with a pretty (possibly 'white') baby girl that played in one corner while, in the other, a (possibly 'white') boy-child held up the Scout's salute and a British flag.[132] This particular Glaxo advertisement also referred to British medical and municipal authorities' testimonies to forcefully authenticate Glaxo baby food. There was also an underlying objectivity and matter-of-factness associated with the purposeful visibility of the male child in relation to nation-and-empire-building which often ran across many contemporary advertisements of baby foods and galactagogues (materials promoting lactation) in colonial India.

The making of the 'Fat baby of advertisement' – and their concomitant problem of rickets from patent foods – was expressed emphatically by Bengali *daktar* Srijukta J. N. Ray (M.B.) in his article 'Saishabiyo Khaddya O Pattha Prodan' published in the Bengali year 1324 (1917) in the popular medical periodical *Chikitsa-Prokash*.[133] During and after the First World War, infant mortality as a public health problem became a central motif across Bengali periodicals and newspapers.[134] At the time, there were excessive infant deaths in colonial Calcutta.[135] Another Bengali periodical dedicated to raising health awareness, *Swasthya Samachar*, began one of its issues in the sixth month (Ashwin) of the Bengali year 1326 (1919), with a full-page illustration titled 'Bharatey Proti Minutey Charti Kariya Sishu Morey' which translates as 'In India four babies die every minute'. I argue that this illustration is particularly unnerving as it is forthright and accusatory giving a speaking voice of demands to infants themselves to right their wrongful infant deaths. It needs to be located amidst the post-War global context of the 'save the babies' movement, particularly in the shadows of wartime loss of life and the influenza pandemic, coupled with growing Indian nationalist enthusiasm for self-government in 1919. Following are my translations of the Bengali captions from this particular image – above the image on top read: 'In Calcutta 5107 Babies Died last year' (in 1918) while below it boldly stated 'Mourning Black-flag-bearing Babies' Campaign'. Each black

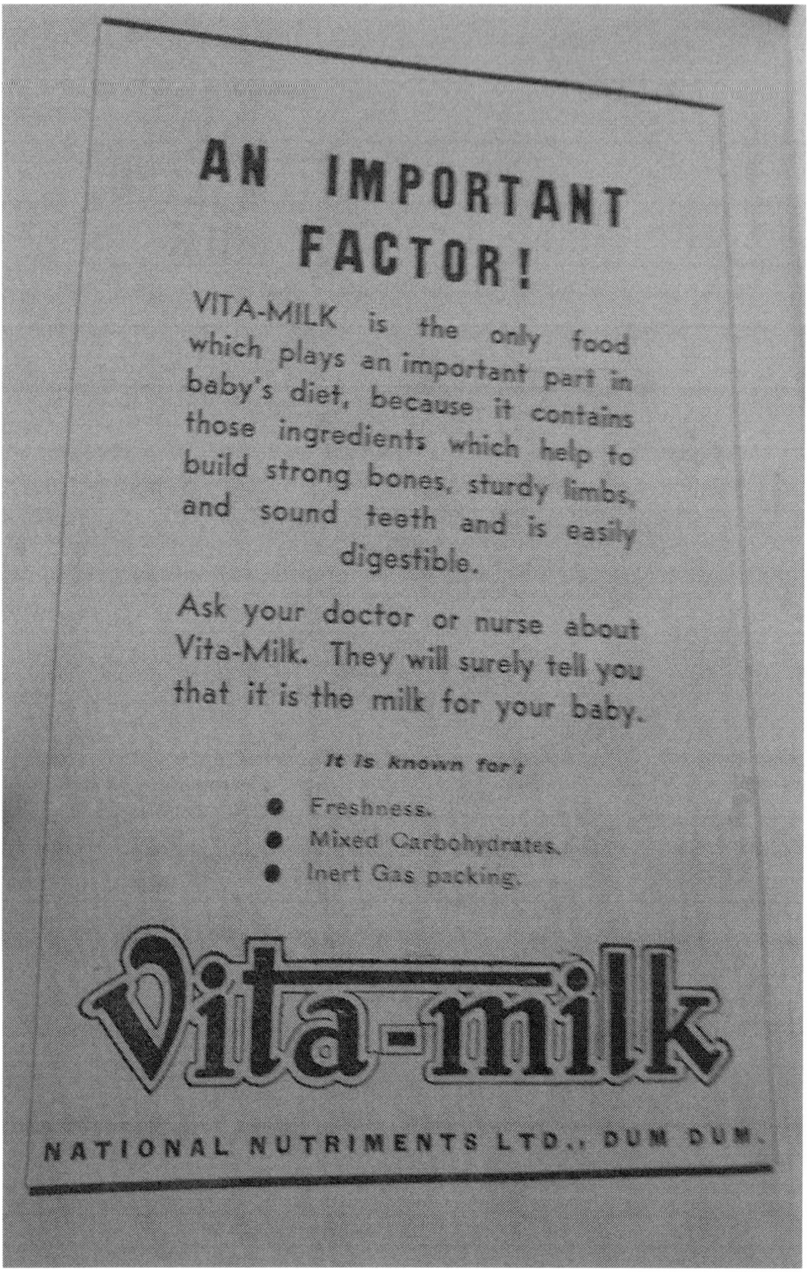

Figure 3.5 Advertisement of Vita-Milk.

Source: W. L. Davies' *Indian Indigenous Milk Products* [with permission from the British Library].

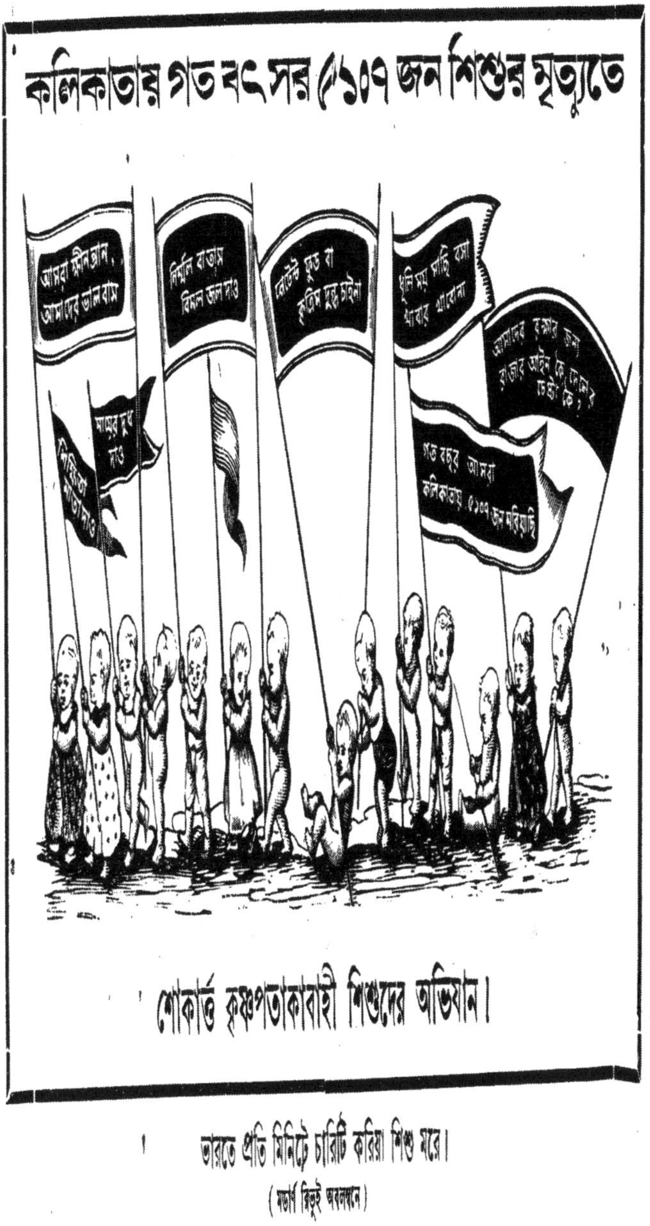

Figure 3.6 'Bharatey Proti Minutey Charti Kariya Sishu Morey'.

Source: Swasthya Samachar, vol. 8, no. 6, 1919, n.p. Illustration Title Translation: 'In India four babies die every minute'. This was published in the sixth month of Ashwin in the Bengali year 1326 (1919) [with permission from the CSSSC Hiteshranjan Sanyal Archives, Kolkata].

flag carried a specific demand (from left to right): 'We Are Frail, Love Us'; 'Give Educated Mothers', 'Give Mother's Milk', 'Give Clean Air and Pure Water', 'Do Not Want Patent Food or Artificial Milk', 'Will not Eat Dirty Food Which Had Flies Sitting on It', 'Last Year 5107 of Us Died in Calcutta', and finally, 'To save us where is the Raja's code of laws, where is the Nation's effort' (Figure 3.14).[136]

The same issue of *Swasthya Samachar* carried an article titled 'Bongey Sishu Mrittyur Karon' which translates as 'Causes of Infant Mortality in Bengal' by Calcutta litterateur Sri Manindralal Basu. In the section 'Matar Dugdhoi Sishur Sarbosreshto Ahaar' (Mother's Milk is Baby's Best Food), with before and after illustrations, he clearly marked out the transition of a particular baby boy from artificial milk (*kritrim dugdha*) to breastfeeding. The painful sight of a baby wasting away in Figure 3.7 'Dated 13 Sraban Age 4 Months Weight 2 Ser'[137] is captioned in Bengali captions translated as follows: (on top): 'A mother was unable to breastfeed as she became very ill following childbirth; after having artificial milk the baby gradually became diminished and weak with low vitality'.[138] Below read: 'The doctor advised that artificial milk has to be stopped. At last a *dhatri* (wet nurse) breastfed and saved the life of the boy-child'.[139] On the following page, we are welcomed by a well-poised, strong, alert and plump baby looking directly at the reader in Figure 3.8 'That Boy Dated 20 *Poush* Weight 7 Ser' which is captioned below as 'Drinking mother's milk ensures digestion occurs easily; it is germ-free; no stomach ailments; and aids bone and flesh formation'.[140]

The very notion of childhood which translates as *chelebela* (boyhood) in Bengali coincides with Sibaji Bandyopadhyay's significant argument on the invisibility of the girl child and her lack of girlhood together with the 'good'/'bad' (male) child explored through an investigation of Bengali children's literature.[141] At the time, many also referred to baby foods as '*cheleder khabar*' (food for boys) in Bengali – like *daktar* Rames Chandra Ray (Licentiate in Medicine and Surgery, L.M.S.) in his article 'Kochi Cheleder Khabar' (which translates literally as 'Food for Very Young Boys'). Ray blamed scanty lactation on lack of fresh air and city lifestyle which necessitated daily use of imported baby foods.[142] Similarly, Assistant Surgeon and Teacher of Medical Jurisprudence and Hygiene at Campbell Medical School, Calcutta, Devendranath Roy (L.M.S.), in local parlance, also referred to artificial foods in a very matter of fact manner as '*cheleder khabar*' or 'food for boys'.[143] He also stressed on medical consultation before feeding infants any artificial foods available in the market.[144] He also provided a detailed yet concise chart on 'humanisation' of milk and specific timings for artificial feeding by the clock.[145] Like most of Bengali childcare advice, often gender-neutral terms like *sishu* or 'baby' were used interchangeably with *cheley* or boy child which was usually tied up with the centrality of patriotic sons in anti-colonial nation-building. For instance, Roy provided the following breastfeeding advice for mothers:

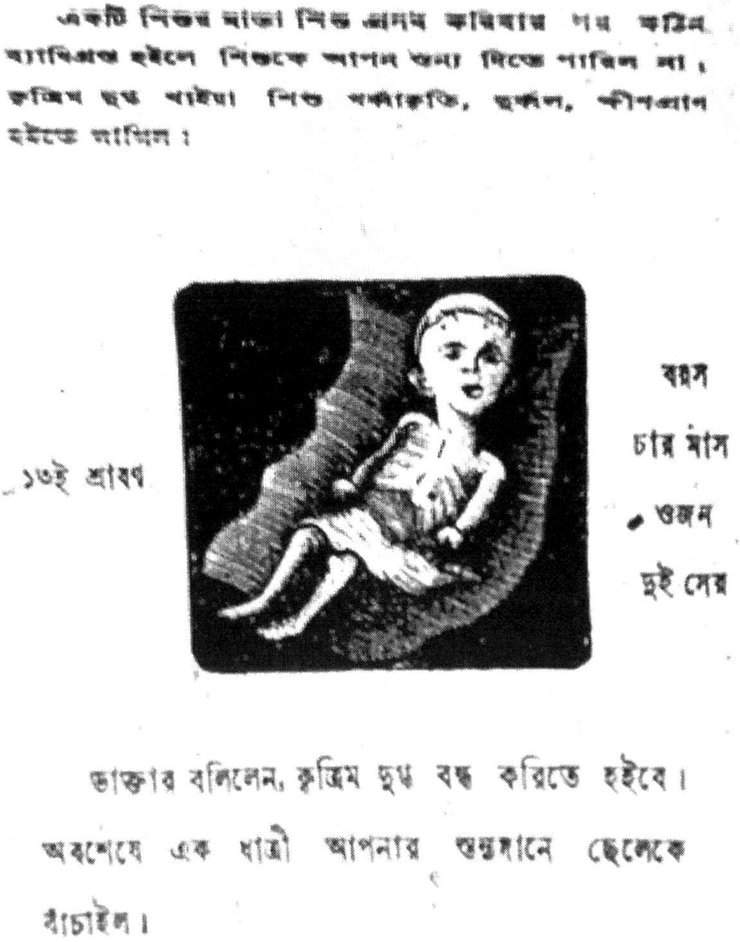

Figure 3.7 Dated 13 Sraban Age 4 Months Weight 2 Ser.

Source: Sr Manindralal Basu, 'Bongey Sishu Mrittyur Karon', *Swasthya Samachar*, vol. 8, no. 6, Ashwin Bengali Year 1326, 1919, p. 139, enlarged image [with permission from the CSSSC Hiteshranjan Sanyal Archives, Kolkata].

> If . . . difficult illness, and her body is weak, then she should not suckle the *boy child*. If the parturient woman is healthy, she must breastfeed her *son*. Before breasts bear milk, the *boy child* should be put to the breast. In that case whatever stool is there in his stomach gets purged. Then when milk has arrived, then he

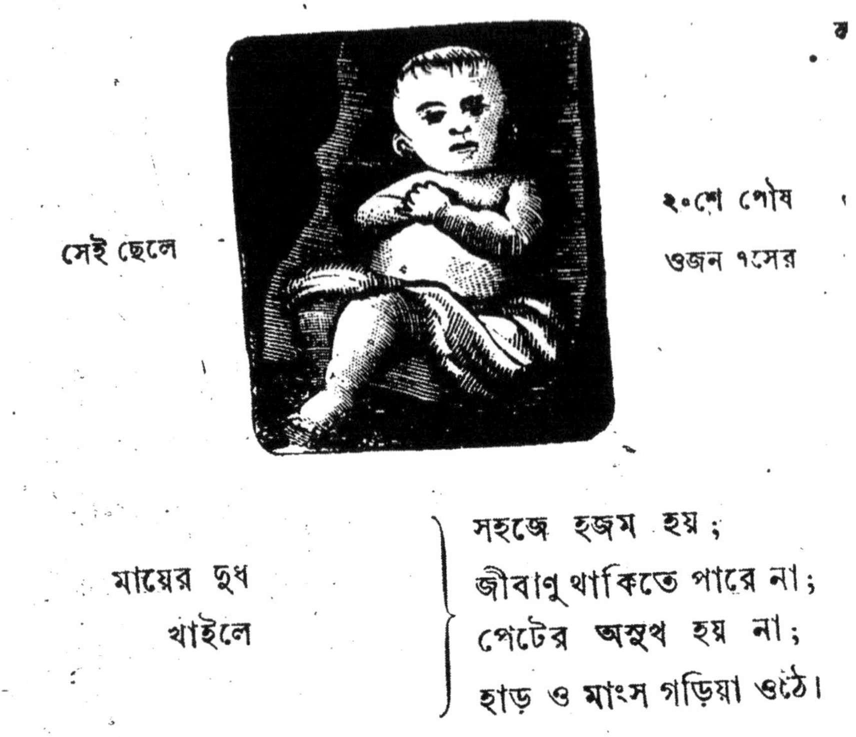

Figure 3.8 'That Boy Dated 20 *Poush* Weight 7 Ser'.

Source: Sri Manindralal Basu, 'Bongey Sishu Mrittyur Karon', *Svasthya Samachar*, vol. 8, no. 6, Ashwin Bengali Year 1326, 1919, p. 140, enlarged image [with permission from the CSSSC Hiteshranjan Sanyal Archives, Kolkata].

> must be fed every two hours, it is not good to feed before this interval. In this manner, she must feed every three hours after one week. After 10 at night, there should be no breastfeeding for six hours. Then parturient woman can sleep a little bit, and the *boy child* also sleeps then. Do not use only one breast, need to interchange.
>
> (emphasis added)[146]

Besides the purposeful visibility of the male child in relation to nation-and-empire-building across English and Bengali newspapers, periodicals and/or handbooks discussed so far, it is also relevant to acknowledge that in India, often due to different meanings attached with the birth of girl and boy children, the birth of a girl child was not always welcome. Thus, boys and girls are often related with different ritual celebrations and childrearing practices. Writing in the late nineteenth-century Calcutta, Shib Chunder Bose had similarly pointed out that the birth of a girl child was often followed by sorrow and silence rather than the noise of the conch and celebrations. However, he attempted to console his readers by arguing that the mother despite a slight delay, did begin to love and care for her girl child, 'as if it were a boy'.[147]

The female child faced 'various forms of alimentary subordination' – 'as infants they are breast-fed for a shorter duration than are boys', 'their *annaprashan* ceremonies (a ceremony in which the infant is first fed rice)' are less extravagant than their brothers, and 'they are routinely fed less well than male children'.[148] Parama Roy builds on the argument put forward by Amartya Sen and Sunil Sengupta that poverty or external constraints are not the only culprits and an increase in income needed to be accompanied by 'nutritional intervention through supplementary feeding' required in order to alleviate dietary biases within the household in favour of the male child in rural Bengal.[149] Roy emphasises that '[l]ittle heed is taken moreover of lactating mothers' increased dietary needs, breast-feeding being thought of as "natural" and "costless"; when malnourished women breast-feed their infants, it is therefore at the expense of their own health, time, and energy'.[150] Thus, Indian mothers might have breastfed infants however, as Rai Kailash Chandra Bahadur's lecture on 'Infantile Mortality: Its Causes and Its Prevention' in the *Proceedings of the Second All India Sanitary Conference* held in Madras in 1912 pointed out, there was also the often neglected problem of the 'insufficiency of the Bengali diet which became fatal for both the pregnant and lactating women'.[151]

'Gastropolitics' in diet was central to the everyday existence of women, especially in a middle-class Bengali household.[152] Roy highlights that 'caste Hindu women's function as symbolic and literal providers (*Annapurna*, *Lakshmi*) rather than consumers of food' is problematic as it was primarily associated with cooking and serving rather than with eating as well as in the very structure of meals as men and children are served first with the best servings.[153] There are also hierarchies among women in this 'gastropolitical order'.[154] It is ' secondariness at mealtimes' and 'a diet of less desirable and leftover foods' along with fasts and other forms of 'alimentary asceticism', especially the dietary restrictions of Hindu widows, which has given hunger a decisive role in their everyday lives.[155] Female foeticide and infanticide might account for the disparate sex ratios of females to males in India; however, these forms of 'nutritional (and medical) denial' also contribute markedly to high rates of female mortality.[156] Roy also cites Tanika Sarkar's insightful argument about how such prescriptions and proscriptions on diet often became internalised by women even when 'no one was present to watch her'.[157]

Judith Richell argues that, in the case of colonial Burma, a part of British India till 1937 and thereafter a separate British protectorate until independence in 1948, the diet of the lactating women was most often 'restricted by cultural beliefs'.[158] Here it was believed, however, that vegetables, fruits and proteins like eggs and meat might harm the baby.[159] The desire to have smaller babies was another factor responsible for maternal malnutrition in Burma.[160] As 'birth weight probably also helps determine the quantity of the mother's breast milk; the production of a larger, stronger baby results in a larger lactation capacity'.[161] The popularity of the salt fish and rice diet among Burmese mothers, therefore, resulted in poor lactation and malnutrition of the infants. This, coupled with the habit of feeding infants chewed rice, a superstitious practice as rice was believed to have mystical properties,[162] affected the fate of the baby from '*in utero* stage up to its first birthday'.[163] Infant mortality rate (IMR) 'is a measure of the health and prosperity of a community'[164] – however, as Richell highlights, in Burma, infant mortality was not recorded according to age up to 1920 while a third of the deaths escaped registration.[165] Richell provides the average official IMR in Burma for 1931 to 1939 which 'is almost identical with the rate for 1901 to 1910 as both are almost 200 per 1000'.[166] She also highlights, that in India,

> the probability of dying in the first year of life declined after 1920 from the highest values of 301 per 1,000 live births (1911–20) for males and 284 for females (1901–11), to 190 and 175, respectively, in 1941–50.[167]

Bombay Municipal Analyst, Lemuel Lucas Joshi's (BSc, M.D.) 'Table 1 Statement showing the rate of infant mortality per 1000 births in some of the Principal Indian Cities' between 1904 and 1913 provided estimates on the high infant deaths in the major cities in early twentieth-century colonial India.[168] The influence of 'germ theory'[169] is palpable in Joshi's argument as he argued that 'pathogenic microbes' in 'impure water' used to adulterate milk has been proved to be the cause of cholera in Calcutta.[170] He emphasised that the 'physical and chemical properties' and 'nutritional value' of adulterated milk were compromised which made it 'physiologically unsuitable' for infants leading to 'debility' as a common symptom which included malnutrition, feebleness, rickets, among others.[171] Joshi also pointed out that for milk-borne diseases like typhoid and small outbreaks of enteric fever in Bombay and Calcutta – tracing the links between cases of the disease and milk supply sources were often quite difficult.[172] However, this was no deterrent to outlining the main milk-borne diseases, especially as they related to the city's milk supply, infant feeding and infant mortality figures. Diseases resulting from 'bad milk' were diphtheria, rickets, Malta fever (through goats' milk), typhoid fever, as well as gastro-intestinal disorders including ordinary diarrhoea and dysentery, cholera, tuberculosis, and so on.[173] He attributed the 'slaughter of the innocents'[174] in India to a number of complex factors mainly 'bad milk' adulterated by 'filthy water', 'dirt', and 'disease'[175]; poverty, negligence, 'ignorance' of mothers, insufficient food for nursing mothers and consequently poor milk for their babies,[176] the 'illiterate' and 'meddlesome' midwife, and so on.[177] He believed that meddlesome midwives coupled with poverty and maternal ignorance were usually responsible for infant mortality in colonial India as there was 'a large proportion of infants in India who are breast-fed'[178] and 'neglect of children' by Indian mothers was 'seldom wilful'.[179]

Surgeon-General Charles Pardey Lukis, Director General of the Indian Medical Service (I.M.S) was one of the three representatives of the Government of India at the first English-speaking Conference on Infant Mortality in 1913 held at Caxton Hall, Westminster in London, U.K.[180] His notion of the knowledge/power dynamics between the metropolis/colony is somewhat visible in his greetings at the Conference as he acknowledged that:

> You will see that the Government of India has taken a great interest in this movement, and if we do not take any large part in your discussions I hope you will realize that this is not from want of interest, it is merely from the fact that we come here to obtain information rather than to impart it.[181]

Lukis pointed out that '[t]he Indian woman was a model wife and mother, and if she erred in the management of feeding of her child, it was merely through ignorance, and not from want of maternal affection'.[182] Cecelia Van Hollen argues that the idealisation of the 'Indian woman' as 'moral' was based on 'colonial and nationalist perceptions of upper-class, upper-caste propriety' which significantly differed from constructions of Indian womanhood in other colonial contexts where the 'Indian woman' was, for instance, an indentured labourer treated with considerable disdain as in Fiji and Malaya.[183] Lukis also added that maternal ignorance 'with regard to the feeding and care of the infant' often resulting from child marriage, premature motherhood and 'primitive methods of midwifery' alongside 'severe physical labour which Indian women of the poorer classes' performed were responsible for the 'excessive infantile mortality in India', 'under 1 year of age'.[184] He emphasised that 'primitive' midwifery caused tetanus in infants and maternal deaths which 'indirectly increased the infant mortality by depriving the children of their natural nourishment'. He argued that '[i]t must be remembered that owing to the unsatisfactory nature of the diet substituted for their mother's milk, the death of the mother or the drying up of her milk practically sealed the fate of the child'.[185]

Furthermore, Lukis blamed human agency as the main problem sanitary reformers faced in India:

> the illiteracy of the majority of the population – 90 per cent. of whom live a life of fatalism – their innate dislike to any innovation, their ignorance and their disregard of even the most elementary rules

> of domestic hygiene, all combine to build up an almost insurmountable barrier in the path of rapid progress in sanitary reform.[186]

He added that, fortunately, Indians boiled their milk and Indian cattle did not suffer from tuberculosis and in rare cases if the source of contamination was traced back to the milk, it was because the 'tubercle bacilli of human origin' had been passed on as a 'result of the carelessness of native milkmen'.[187] He argued that, in India, efforts to provide 'efficient control of the milk supply, or to render polluted milk innocuous by pasteurization, or to substitute dried milk in lieu of a doubtful supply of the fresh article' were hampered – first, because 'the cow is looked upon as a sacred animal, and second that caste prejudices prevented the taking of food prepared by outside agencies, or which had been touched by persons of another caste'.[188]

In his book, *The Milk Supply of Calcutta*, Rai Bahadur Chunilal Bose (MB), Chemical Examiner, Calcutta, also pointed out that even the problem of the adulteration of milk was closely associated with the Hindus who considered the cow and its products, including cow dung as a 'purifying substance' instead of a contaminant.[189] Charu Gupta argues that the cow was sacralised through a Hinduised understanding of 'cow as mother' (Gau-Mata) which together with the nationalist iconography of *Bharatmata/Mother India* called for the devotion of strong and healthy patriotic Hindu sons to the motherland and the 'Aryan race'.[190] Bengali middle-class ideas about what was 'pure'/'unadulterated'/'untouched' actually had several layers of meaning.[191] Prominent figures, like the famous nationalist and Brahmo, Calcutta *daktar* Sundari Mohan Das, who also gave an elaborate lecture 'Ravages of Putana' at the Health and Child Welfare Exhibition in Calcutta in 1920 discussed later in Chapter 5 of this book, were involved in the battle against adulterated food which was most often embodied by the 'effeminate', 'emaciated' and 'dyspeptic Bengali babu'.[192] Responding to the problem of food adulteration in detail, for instance, S. B. Ghose (M.B.), Chemical Analyst with the Municipal Corporation of Calcutta, in an article 'Food Adulteration in Calcutta' in the *Calcutta Medical Journal* in 1907, complained about the fact that what was sold as barley was 'a mixed starch composed of cassava and sago meal'. It 'is universally sold either as pure barley powder or arrowroot at the fancy of the seller. . . . These mixed starches are also sold in tins as foods for infants and invalids at 2 to 3 annas a pound'. About '[t]he milk which is obtained in Calcutta as cow's milk', he highlighted that it 'is a mixed fluid, not only of different breeds of animal, but is largely intermixed with buffalo milk. The adulterant which is being chiefly used is water' which is 'positively polluted'. He blamed the insufficient legal provisions that failed to control food adulteration which led to the high mortality rates in Calcutta.[193]

Saurabh Mishra points out that a series of anti-adulteration bills were passed regionally in the late nineteenth century starting with a bill for the municipalities in Calcutta in 1866 and thereafter 'the first substantial law against adulteration that was passed in Bengal in 1886' were all a result of middle-class agitation.[194] From a 'thin trickle' to a 'virtual deluge' of legislation against adulteration was visible in early twentieth century with almost every province passing its own bills beginning with the

> United Provinces Prevention of Adulteration Act in 1912 (subsequently amended in 1916 and 1930), followed by similar bills in Madras (1918 and 1928), Central Provinces (1919 and 1928), Bengal (1919 and 1925), Bombay (1925 and 1935), and Punjab (1919 and 1929).[195]

Mishra highlights the centrality of milk in 'middle-class anxieties' about 'food purity' mainly related to the upper caste Hindu vegetarian diet alongside the idealisation of earlier 'Aryan' practices and the contributions of Ayurveda in 'modern' research on nutrition.[196] Mishra also cites Sudeshna Banerjee's argument that, at the time, the Bengali middle-class concern about nutrition was also visible in its letters and essays in periodicals about the low nutritive value and negative consequences of adulterated milk and milk products due to a 'high strung sensitivity' to the rising child mortality rates.[197] Extending Banerjee and Mishra's arguments here, it is argued that the adulteration of milk and various foods affected both infant and maternal well-being as simple digestible foodstuffs like milk, barley, and other similar foods also constituted the lactating mother's daily diet following childbirth.[198]

In conclusion, this chapter brought back the focus on customs and prejudices related to breastfeeding practices which came to be labelled as 'bad' mothering. It discussed how a 'whole supplementary work' of 'sorting out' and 'cleaning up' was necessary in order to create moral/cultural/material entities as a part of the systematicity of modern motherhood. This was used to tackle the lack of discipline of Indian mothers in childcare to the anxiety-ridden politics of the mother's dress and diet. It argued that 'ideal' mothering of infants as clocked childcare, a learned duty to community-nation-and empire-building gradually became integral to the making and makeup of the systematised paraphernalia of modern motherhood in colonial Calcutta. In particular, it brought back the focus on modern clocks central to Bengali and English advice manuals and periodical essays instructing Indian mothers about clocked breastfeeding of their infants. Coinciding with the global mothercraft movement, the emphasis was on 'regularity' in childcare and it was considered indispensable to the rejuvenation of 'racial' and national health and vigour. Using gender as an anchor, this chapter also questioned the purposeful visibility of the male child, particularly in childcare advice, and addressed the problem of adulteration of milk and other foods central to maternal and infant diet.

Notes

1 'Indian mothers' along with the child's cries, clocks and routine were regular themes in European and indigenous advice literature on infant feeding in colonial India. On a discussion about the goddess-like *bhadramahila* and clocked breastfeeding of infants, see Ranjana Saha, 'Milk, "Race" and Nation: Medical Advice on Breastfeeding in Colonial Bengal', *South Asia Research*, vol. 37, no. 2, 2017, pp. 147–165, especially pp. 154–157; see also Meredith Borthwick, *The Changing Role of Women in Bengal, 1849–1905* (Princeton, NJ: Princeton University Press, 1984), pp. 172–175.
2 Margaret Jolly, 'Introduction Colonial and postcolonial plots in histories of maternities and modernities', in Kalpana Ram and Margaret Jolly (eds), *Maternities and modernities Colonial and postcolonial experiences in Asia and the Pacific* (Cambridge: Cambridge University Press, 1998), pp. 1–4.
3 Jolly, 'Introduction', p. 4.
4 Barbara N. Ramusack, 'Cultural missionaries, maternal imperialists, feminist allies British women activists in India, 1865–1945', in Nupur Chaudhuri and Margaret Strobel (eds), *Western women and imperialism complicity and resistance* (Bloomington and Indianapolis: Indiana University Press, 1992), pp. 119–136.
5 Srirupa Prasad, *Cultural Politics of Hygiene in India 1890–1940 Contagions of Feeling* (New York: Palgrave Macmillan, 2015), p. 17.
6 Santi Rozario, 'The dai and the doctor: discourses on women's reproductive health in rural Bangladesh', in Kalpana Ram and Margaret Jolly (eds), *Maternities and modernities Colonial and postcolonial experiences in Asia and the Pacific* (Cambridge: Cambridge University Press, 1998), p. 148.
7 Rozario, 'The dai and the doctor'.
8 Rozario, 'The dai and the doctor', pp. 150–151.
9 Geraldine Forbes, *Women in Colonial India. Essays in Politics, Medicine, and Historiography* (New Delhi: Chronicle Books, 2005), p. 84.
10 Norman Chevers, *A Manual of Medical Jurisprudence for India Including the History of Crime Against the Person in India* (Calcutta: Thacker, Spink & Co., 1870), p. 747.
11 Hasan Suhrawardy, M.D., F.R.C.S.I., L.M. (Rotunda), District Medical Officer Lillooah, E.I.R., 'The Care of the Expectant Mother and Newborn Infant', in *Health and Child Welfare Exhibition, Calcutta, 1920* (Calcutta: Bengal Secretariat Book Depot, 1921), p. lxiii.
12 Constant or always breastfeeding whenever the child cried was pathologised in order to be medically disciplined by clocks in contemporary European and indigenous medical literature on childcare – see mainly Frederic Truby King, *Feeding and Care of Baby* (London and Calcutta: Macmillan and Co., 1913), Young, *Maternity and Infant Welfare A Handbook for Health Visitors, Parents, and Others in India* (Calcutta: The Lady Chelmsford All-India League for Maternity and Child Welfare, second ed. 1922), pp. 96–97, and on clocked feeding of infants and dos and don'ts of hiring a *dai* or wet nurse, Shib Chunder Deb, *The Infant Treatment* First Part *Sishu Palan* Pratham Bhag (Calcutta: reprint 1864; first edition 1857), pp. 40–58, among others.
13 In colonial Bengal, family usually denoted joint family based on idea of '*ekannavarti* (sharing the same kitchen)' – see Bharati Ray, 'Introduction', in Sukhendu Ray, Bharati Ray and Malavika Karlekar (eds), *The Many Worlds of Sarala Devi A Diary & The Tagores and Sartorial Style A Photo Essay* (London: Routledge, 2017), p. 4n9.

14 In colonial Bengal, *dai* refers to both the traditional midwife and wet nurse as discussed in the previous chapter. They were often lower class and/or caste Hindus and Muslim women, among others – for instance, they were often hired from the 'Dome and the Bagthee caste' – Sujata Mukherjee, 'Medical Education and Emergence of Women Medics in Colonial Bengal', Occasional Paper 37, Institute of Development Studies, Kolkata, August 2012, pp. 17, 27.

15 Mrs. S. C. Belnos, 'Preface' in Mrs. S. C. Belnos and A. Colin (eds), *Twenty Four Plates Illustrative of Hindoo and European Manners in Bengal Drawn on the Stone by A. Colin From Sketches by Mrs. Belnos* (London: Smith and Elder Cornhill, 1832), plate 9, n.p.; also see Ranjana Saha, 'Milk, mothering & meanings: Infant feeding in colonial Bengal', *Women's Studies International Forum*, vol. 60, 2017, pp. 97–110, here p. 102.

16 Belnos, 'Preface' in Belnos, and Colin, *Twenty Four Plates Illustrative of Hindoo and European Manners in Bengal*, n.p.

17 Letter dated 5 March 1832, Place: 48, Bedford Square, From Rammohun Roy to Mrs. Belnos cited in Belnos and Colin, *Twenty Four Plates Illustrative of Hindoo and European Manners in Bengal*, n.p. Also see Belnos and Colin, *Twenty Four Plates Illustrative of Hindoo and European Manners in Bengal*, n.p. cited in Bikas Karmakar and Ila Gupta, 'Unraveling the Social Position of Women in Late-Medieval Bengal: A Critical Analysis of Narrative Art on Baranagar Temple Facades', Rupkatha *Journal on Interdisciplinary Studies in Humanities,* Special Conference Issue, vol. 12, no. 5, 2020, p. 8.

18 Ibid.

19 William Joseph Wilkins, *Modern Hinduism Being An Account of the Religion and Life of the Hindus in Northern India* (London: T. Fisher Unwin, 1887), pp. 8, 434. Also, William Ward, mentions how in the fifteenth century Chaitanya was once hung in a tree as a baby when he refused his mother's breast. Ward also believed that 'Voiragees and other mendicants, who make a merit of possessing no worldly attachments, sometimes hang up a child in a pot in a tree, or, putting it in a pot, let it float down the river. Persons of other casts may do it, but these the most frequently'. For details see William Ward, *A View of the History, Literature, and Religion, of the Hindoos: Including a Minute Description of their Manners and Customs and Translations from their Principal Works* In Two Volumes Volume II The Second Edition: Carefully Abridged and Greatly Improved (Serampore: Mission Press, 1815), p. 173. Also, see Ward, Volume II, Third Edition, p. 123 (no further details given) cited in Chevers, *A Manual of Medical Jurisprudence for India*, pp. 760–761. However, here Chevers seems to have also cited Mrs. S. C. Belnos' description of this custom without referring to her specifically.

20 See Sukumari Bhattacharji, 'Motherhood in Ancient India', *Economic and Political Weekly*, vol. 25, no. 42/43, 1990, pp. WS50–WS51. On the use of mustard seeds in the *Jatakarman* ceremony, see Ibid., p. WS50.

21 Report on Native Papers for the Week ending the 24th July 1869 in *Supplementary Volume of Report on Native Papers, Bengal, 1869–1895* (Imperial Record Department, 1914), NAI. On exorcism and the evil eye, William Crooke, *An Introduction to the Popular Religion and Folklore of Northern India* (Allahabad: Printed at the Government Press, North-Western Provinces and Oudh, 1894); Sudhir Kakar, *Shamans, Mystics and Doctors A Psychological Inquiry Into India and Its Healing Traditions* (New York: Alfred A. Knopf, 1982); among others.

22 Chevers, *A Manual of Medical Jurisprudence for India*, pp. 760–763.

23 Nizamut Adawlut Reports, May 4, 1855, p. 498 cited in Chevers *A Manual of Medical Jurisprudence for India*, p. 761.

24 Ibid.

25 Ibid.
26 For instance, *Report on the Police of the Lower Provinces of the Bengal Presidency for the Year 1873* By Colonel J. R. Pughe (Calcutta: Bengal Secratariat Press, 1874), *Annual Report on the Police Administration of the Town of Calcutta and Its Suburbs for the Year 1912* By Sir Frederick Halliday (Calcutta: The Bengal Secretariat Book Depot, 1913), among others.
27 Chevers, *A Manual of Medical Jurisprudence for India*, p. 760. For details also see Jean Baptiste Tavernier, *Travels in India* In Two Volumes Volume II. Translated from the original French edition of 1676 with a biographical sketch of the Author, Notes, Appendices, Etc. by V. Ball. (London: Macmillan and Co, 1889), pp. 214–215.
28 Chevers, *A Manual of Medical Jurisprudence for India*, pp. 760–761.
29 Ibid., pp. 750–763.
30 Cooverjee Rustomjee Mody, *An essay on female infanticide: to which the prize offered by the Bombay Government, for the second best essay against female infanticide among the Jadajas and other Rajpoot tribes of Guzerat, was awarded* (Bombay: Printed by order of Government, at the Bombay Education Society's Press, 1849), pp. 1, 2, 7. Also, see Mody, *An essay on female infanticide*, p. 11 in Chevers, *A Manual of Medical Jurisprudence for India*, p. 229.
31 On Partha Chatterjee's argument about home, family and colonialism, Partha Chatterjee, 'The Nationalist Resolution of the Women's Question', in Kumkum Sangari and Sudesh Vaid (eds), *Recasting Women. Essays in Colonial History* (New Delhi: Kali for Women, 1989), pp. 233–253.
32 Satadru Sen, 'The Savage Family: Colonialism and Female Infanticide in Nineteenth-Century India', *Journal of Women's History*, vol. 14, no. 3, 2002, p. 54.
33 Ibid., p. 70.
34 Lalita Panigrahi, *British Social Policy and Female Infanticide in India* (Delhi: Manoharlal, 1972), p. 5 in Sen, 'The Savage Family', p. 55.
35 Panigrahi, *British Social Policy*, p. 18 in Sen, 'The Savage Family', p. 55.
36 Sen, 'The Savage Family', p. 60.
37 On *dais* as state agents, see Ibid., p. 66–69.
38 Sen, 'The Savage Family, p. 68. Sen also points out that there were exceptional levels of leniency expressed by the colonial state towards women who committed female infanticides (these infants were given birth by married women or widows). See Sen, 'The Savage Family', p. 61.
39 Nizamut Adawlut Reports, Volume III, Part 1 of 1853, p. 807 (no further details given) cited in Chevers, *A Manual of Medical Jurisprudence for India*, p. 626; also see Government and Bhyro Ghose versus Musst. Tilkee and Fakeer, Chowkeedar in *Report of Cases Determined in the Court of Nizamut Adawlut, From July to December 1853*. With an Index. Volume III, Part I (Calcutta: Thacker, Spink & Co., 1855), pp. 807–809.
40 '*Causes of Deaths of All Nations in Urban Calcutta at different periods of Life in the year 1893*', in *Administration Report of the Commissioners of Calcutta for 1893–94* Part II, Appendices. Table 25-A (Calcutta: Printed at the Municipal Press, 1894), p. 193
41 See also Sanjam Ahluwalia, *Reproductive Restraints Birth Control in India 1877–1947* (Ranikhet: Permanent Black. 2008), pp. 151–152; and for instance, in the context of the Belgian Congo, see Nancy Rose Hunt, '"Le bébé en brousse": European Women, African Birth Spacing, and Colonial Intervention in Breast Feeding in the Belgian Congo', in Frederick Cooper and Ann Laura Stoler (eds), *Tensions of Empire Colonial Cultures in a Bourgeois World* (Berkeley: University of California Press, 1997), pp. 287–321.

42 Dr. Y. Sen cited in 'Chapter VI. – Papers Continued: Drs. G. J. Campbell, Wallace. Sen, George', *in Improvements of the Conditions of Childbirth in India Including a Special Report on the Work of the Victoria Memorial Scholarships Fund during the past Fifteen Years and Papers Written by Medical Women and qualified Midwives* (Calcutta: Superintendent Government Printing, India, 1918), p. 129.
43 Sen in 'Chapter VI', pp. 128–129.
44 Chevers, *A Manual of Medical Jurisprudence for India*, p. 747.
45 'Medical Notes on the Burmese', *Indian Annals of Medical Science*, No. 1, October 1853, p. 97 cited in Chevers, *A Manual of Medical Jurisprudence for India*, p. 747n*.
46 Valerie A. Fildes, *Breasts, Bottles and Babies A History of Infant Feeding* (Edinburgh: Edinburgh University Press, 1986), pp. 352, 370.
47 Edward Morton, *Remarks on the subject of lactation: containing observations on the healthy and diseased conditions of the breast-milk, the disorders frequently produced in mothers by suckling: and numerous illustrative cases, proving that, when protracted, it is a common cause, in children, of hydrencephalus, or water in the brain and other serious complications* (London: Longman, Rees, Orme, Brown, and Green, 1831), pp. 10, 61.
48 Borthwick highlights that wet-nursing was also a prevalent practice among wealthy Bengalis. Borthwick, *The Changing Role of Women in Bengal*, p. 172.
49 See Projit Bhihari Mukharji, *Nationalizing the Body. The Medical Market, Print and Daktari Medicine* (Delhi: Anthem Press, 2012), p. 125.
50 Durga Das Gupta, 'Sishuder Khadyer Pariman', *Swasthya*, vol 2, no. 7, pp. 153–55 cited in Ibid., p. 125–6.
51 For details, see second section of this chapter together with Chapter 5.
52 This excerpt has been cited from Jodu Nath Mukerje, *Dhatri Sikkha A Guide to the Dhaees or Native Midwives And to the Mothers Written in the Form of a Dialogue in Two Parts Part 1* (Chinsura: Printed by Greesh Chunder Bhuttacharje, Chitsaprokash Press; third ed. 1875, first ed. 1867), pp. 1–2. His name is spelt here as in the third edition of his book, *Dhatri Sikkha*.
53 Borthwick, *The Changing Role of Women in Bengal*, p. 161.
54 Saratkumari Deb, *Āmār sangsār* (Calcutta: 1942), p. 2 cited in Ibid., p. 175.
55 For details on breastfeeding and selection of a *dai*, see Deb, *The Infant Treatment*, pp. 40–58, see especially pp. 54–56; also Deb, *The Infant Treatment*, 40–58 cited in Saha, 'Milk, mothering & meanings', p. 103.
56 In this section Materialities of Modern Motherhood? Clocks, Corsets and '*Cheleder Khabar*', I would like to express my deepest gratitude to Dr. Kaveri Qureshi for her invaluable guidance and insightful comments. Hasan Suhrawardy, 'The Care of the Expectant Mother and Newborn Infant', in *Health and Child Welfare Exhibition, Calcutta, 1920* (Calcutta: Bengal Secretariat Book Depot, 1921), p. lxiii.
57 Ruth Young, *Maternity and Infant Welfare A Handbook for Health Visitors, Parents, and Others in India*, (Calcutta: The Lady Chelmsford All-India League for Maternity and Child Welfare, second ed. 1922), p. 96–97.
58 Bruno Latour, *We Have Never Been Modern* Translated by Catherine Porter (Cambridge: Harvard University Press, 1993), p. 72.
59 For a detailed discussion on regular breastfeeding, patent foods and child's cries, see for example, Dr. Srijukta J. N. Ray (M.B.), 'Saishabiyo Khaddya O Pattha Prodan', *Chikitsa Prokash*, vol 10, no. 9, Bengali Year 1324, pp. 358–372. The title translates as food for infants and giving a wholesome diet. Translation mine.
60 Suhrawardy, 'The Care of the Expectant Mother and Newborn Infant', p. lxiv
61 Ibid.
62 Ibid., p. lxv.
63 Ibid., pp. lx–lxi; on merits of regular breastfeeding, Ibid., p. lxxvi; also see Ibid., pp. xii–xiii cited in Supriya Guha, '"The Best Swadeshi": Reproductive Health

in Bengal, 1840–1940', in Sarah Hodges ed., *Reproductive Health in India. History, Politics, Controversies* (Hyderabad: Orient Longman, 2006), p. 139.

64 Suhrawardy, 'The Care of the Expectant Mother and Newborn Infant', p. lxxvi.

65 Young, 'Preface to the First Edition', *Maternity and Infant Welfare*, p. iii.

66 Also, see detailed discussion on the subject in chapter 5 of this book.

67 Anna Davin, 'Imperialism and Motherhood', *History Workshop*, vol. 5, no. 1, 1978, p. 10. Davin points out that, in Britain, eugenists drew both on ideas of 'the survival of the fittest' put forward by Francis Galton and Karl Pearson, and Mendelian theories of heredity by the end of the nineteenth and beginning of the twentieth century – see Ibid., p. 57n2.

68 Ruth Young, *Antenatal Work in India A Handbook for Nurses, Midwives, and Health Visitors* [Indian Red Cross Society Maternity and Child Welfare Bureau (Incorporating the Lady Chelmsford All-India League for Maternity and Child Welfare, and the Victoria Memorial Scholarships Fund), 1930], p. 6. Also, on antenatal work, see for example, Dr. A., Headwards, 'Ante-Natal Work', in *Report of Maternity and Child Welfare Conference Held at Delhi. February 4th–8th 1927* (Delhi: The Lady Chelmsford All-India League for Maternity and Child Welfare, 1927), pp. 101–103.

69 Young, *Maternity and Infant Welfare*, p. 96.

70 Mildred Staley, *Handbook for Wives and Mothers in India* (Calcutta, Thacker, Spink & Co., 1908), p. 226.

71 Young, *Maternity and Infant Welfare*, p. 97. Reference to the male child was also common in Bengali women's magazines like the *Bamabodhini Patrika*, for example, ShriHemantakumari Debi, 'Santan-Palan', *Bamabodhini Patrika*, Sraban-Kartik 1323 Bengali year, 1916 in Pradip Basu (ed), *Samayiki Purano Samayik Patrer Prabondho Sankalan Ditiyo Khanda: Griha o Paribar* (Kolkata, Ananda Publishers Private Limited, 2009), pp. 779–793. Title Translation: Journal on Current Topics Collection of Old Essays from Periodicals Second Volume: Home and Family.

72 Ranjana Saha, 'Motherhood on display: The child welfare exhibition in colonial Calcutta', *The Indian Economic and Social History Review*, vol. 58, no. 2, 2021, pp. 253–254.

73 Mary Hancock, 'Home Science and the Nationalization of Domesticity in Colonial India', *Modern Asian Studies*, vol. 35, no. 4, 2001, p. 874 cited in Saha, 'Motherhood on display', p. 254.

74 Fiona Dykes, *Breastfeeding in hospital mothers, midwives and the production line* (New York: Routledge, 2006), p. 12.

75 Borthwick, *The Changing Role of Women in Bengal*, p. 188.

76 Ibid., p. 189 (no further details given).

77 Bruno Latour, *We Have Never Been Modern* Translated by Catherine Porter (Cambridge: Harvard University Press, 1993), p. 72.

78 Ibid., p. 73.

79 As Partha Chatterjee points out, the 'new woman' was supposed to have been literate and 'modern' but only to a limited extent in order to be a 'good' wife and mother/sugrihini, the guardian of 'tradition', with godly, 'feminine (spiritual) virtues'. For a detailed discussion, see Chatterjee, 'The Nationalist Resolution of the Women's Question', p. 246.

80 Borthwick, *The Changing Role of Women in Bengal*, pp. 188–189. On trousers and saris worn by Parsi women, 'Patra', *Bamabodhini Patrika*, vol. 8, no. 1, 1904, n.p. in Borthwick, *The Changing Role of Women in Bengal*, pp. 249–250. Also, on Keshub Chunder Sen's suggestions of Brahmo reform in dress at the Bharat Ashram – see Ibid., p. 251, and on women's objections to such new

types of expenses on clothing, Harasundari Datta, *Swargiya Srinath Datter*, pp. 158–160 (no further details given) cited in Ibid., p. 251.

81 Borthwick, *The Changing Role of Women in Bengal*, p. 190.

82 Kundamala Debi, "Bidya sikhile ki grihakarmma karite nai?" *Bamaganer racana*, BP, 6, 86 (October 1870), n.p. in Borthwick, *The Changing Role of Women in Bengal*, p. 105 cited in Dipesh Chakrabarty, 'The Difference: Deferral of (A) Colonial Modernity: Public Debates on Domesticity in British Bengal', *History Workshop*, No. 36, Colonial and Post-Colonial History (Autumn, 1993), p. 9. The title translates as 'If you are Educated Then Are You Not Supposed to do Housework?'. Translation mine.

83 Chakrabarty, The Difference', pp. 9, 11.

84 Ibid., p. 11.

85 Durga Das Gupta, "Bangali Saheb Nahe", *Swasthya*, vol. 5, no. 2, 1901, 36–37 cited in Projit Bihari Mukharji, *Nationalizing the Body The Medical Market, Print and Daktari Medicine* (Delhi: Anthem Press, 2012), p. 114.

86 Suhrawardy, 'The Care of the Expectant Mother and Newborn Infant', p. lxviii. Suhrawardy also voiced concerns about the use of 'comforters' – '[a] nother great abuse is the use of chusni or dummy teats or "baby comforters" for keeping a crying infant quiet. It is extremely harmful . . . and . . . *spoils the looks of the child. In a female child it is a serious matter in Indian society*' (emphasis added). Moreover, he added – 'the infant's life may be cut short by the introduction of microbes, as often the "dummy teat" or "comforter" which has fallen off the infant's mouth is put back by the ayah after wiping and drying it with her dirty fingers and dirtier clothes' Ibid., p. lxxvi-lxxvii.

87 Rebecca Gibson, *The Corseted Skeleton A Bioarchaeology of Binding* (Cham, Switzerland: Palgrave Macmillan imprint published by Springer Nature Switzerland AG, 2020), pp. 94–96.

88 Staley, *Handbook for Wives and Mothers in India*, pp. 17, 18, 121, 294–5.

89 Mary Morris, 'Women and Journeys. Inner and Outer', in M. Kowalewski (ed), *Temperamental Journeys. Essays on the Modern Literature of Travel* (Athens: University of Georgia Press, 1992), p. 25 cited in Sukla Chatterjee, *Women and Literary Narratives in Colonial India Her Myriad Gaze on the 'Other'* (New York: Routledge, 2019), p. 30.

90 United States Bureau of Foreign and Domestic Commerce, Henry D. Baker, American Consul at Bombay and Other Consular Officers, *British India with notes on Ceylon, Afghanistan, and Tibet* (Washington: Government Printing Office, 1915), p. 262.

91 Ibid.

92 Ibid., p. 261.

93 Ibid., p. 263.

94 Elizabeth Cooper, *The Harim and the Purdah Studies of Oriental Women* (New York: The Century Company, 1915), pp. 138–139; see also Elizabeth Cooper, *The Harim and the Purdah Studies of Oriental Women* (London: T. Fisher Unwin Ltd., 1915), pp. 138–139 cited in Indrani Sen, *Memsahibs' Writings Colonial Narratives on Indian Women* (Hyderabad: Orient BlackSwan Private Ltd., 2012, Orient Longman 2008), pp. 275–276.

95 Krishnabhabini Das, *Kṛṣṇabhābinī Dāser Iṃlaṇḍe baṅgamahilā*. Sampādanā o bhūmikā Sīmantī Sen; Mukhabandha Pārtha caṭṭopādhyāẏ. [Krisnabhabini Das' *A Bengali Woman in England*.] Editor and Introduction Simanti Sen; Preface Partha Chatterjee (Calcutta: Stri, 1885, 1996, first ed.). p. 77, cited in Chatterjee, *Women and Literary Narratives in Colonial India*, p. 42n43.

96 Krishnabhabini Das, *Englande Bangamahila* (Kolkata: Satyaprasad Sarbadhikari from J.N. Banerjee & Son, Banerjee Press, 1885), n.p., translated by and in Jayati Gupta, *Travel Culture, Travel Writing and Bengali Women, 1870–1940* (London: Routledge, 2021), p. 64.

97 Das, *Kṛṣṇabhābinī Dāser Iṃlaṇḍe baṅgamahilā*, p. 7 cited in Chatterjee, *Women and Literary Narratives in Colonial India*, p. 29. Chatterjee alerts us that Das might have donned gowns in England but when she 'returned from England after eight years with very little of the impact of English life and living left in her' and following her husband's death, she followed strict codes of widowhood back in India. Ibid., p. 37.

98 Emma Tarlo, *Clothing Matters Dress and Identity in India* (London: Hurst & Company, 1996), p. 44

99 Ibid., p. 45.

100 Ibid.

101 Ibid., p. 61.

102 Indira Chowdhury, *The Frail Hero and Virile History Gender and the Politics of Culture in Colonial Bengal* (Delhi: Oxford University Press, 1998), p. 3. On 'limited or controlled emancipation' of women or *stri swadhinata*, Sumit Sarkar, 'The Women's Question in Nineteenth Century Bengal', in Kumkum Sangari and Sudesh Vaid (eds), *Women and Culture* (Bombay: Research Centre for Women's Studies, 1994), p. 106; see also Ibid., p. 82.

103 Himani Banerji, *Inventing Subjects Studies in Hegemony, Patriarchy and Colonialism* (New Delhi, Tulika, 2001), pp. 119.

104 Ibid., pp. 103–4, 119.

105 Jyotirmayee Gangopadhyay, 'Gown o Sari' [Gown or Sari) in *Bharati,* Aswin Bengali Year 1330 (1924), pp. 1055–1056 cited in Ibid., p. 120. For a detailed discussion on Jyotirmoyee Gangopadhyay, also referred to as Jyotirmoyee Ganguli, see her discussion on child marriage in Chapter 4 of this book.

106 Nicola J. Thomas, 'Embodying imperial spectacle: dressing Lady Curzon, Vicereine of India 1899–1905', *Cultural Geographies*, vol. 14, no. 3, 2007, p. 395.

107 Nupur Chaudhuri, 'Shawls, Jewelry, Curry and Rice in Victorian Britain' in Thomas, 'Embodying imperial spectacle', pp. 387–388; also see Nupur Chaudhuri, 'Shawls, Jewelry, Curry and Rice in Victorian Britain', in Nupur Chaudhuri and Margaret Strobel (eds), *Western Women and Imperialism Complicity and Resistance* (Bloomington and Indianapolis: Indiana University Press, 1992), p. 235.

108 Thomas, 'Embodying imperial spectacle', p. 377. On her use of 'altered sari' fabric together with notions of 'colonial order' and her sense of an 'imperial dress code', see discussion in Ibid., pp. 378–379.

109 Prasad, *Cultural Politics of Hygiene in India*, p. 109.

110 Ibid.

111 Ibid. In fact, a combination of advertisements for imported baby foods like Cow & Gate, Mellin's Food, and Lactogen were all present in the *Directory of the City Health and Baby Week 1931* (Madras: The City Health and Baby Week Committee, 1931), n.p.

112 Jackson Lears, *Fables of Abundance A Cultural History of Advertising in America* (New York: Basic Books, 1994), p. 146. Also see Prasad, *Cultural Politics of Hygiene in India*, p. 108, and p. 129n46.

113 Prasad, *Cultural Politics of Hygiene in India*, p. 10. Moreover, Anne McClintock argues that until 1964, 'the verb to domesticate also carried as one of its meanings the action "to civilize".' Karen Hansen, ed., *African Encounters With Domesticity* (New Brunswick: Rutgers University Press, 1992), p. 23 in A. McClintock, *Imperial Leather Race, Gender and Sexuality in the Colonial Contest* (New York: Routledge, 1995), p. 35. Also, see 'Commodity racism' and 'commodity spectacle' took place through advertising of various products

including baby foods, which functioned as an embodiment of the convergence of Victorian middle-class ideals of domesticity and imperialism. McClintock, *Imperial Leather*, pp. 31–36, 207–231. Also see McClintock, *Imperial Leather* in Prasad, *Cultural Politics of Hygiene*, p. 129n46.

114 See Patricia R. Stokes, 'Purchasing comfort, patent remedies and the alleviation of labour Pain in Germany between 1914 and 1933', in P. Betts and G. Eghigianed (eds), *Pain and prosperity reconsidering twentieth-century German history* (Stanford: California: Stanford University Press, 2003), pp. 78–86.

115 Sarah Hodges, *Contraception, Colonialism and Commerce Birth Control in South India, 1920–1940* (New York: Routledge, 2016, 2008 Ashgate ed.), p. 133.

116 *Directory of the City Health and Baby Week 1931*, n.p.

117 Hodges, *Contraception, Colonialism and Commerce*, p. 133.

118 Douglas E. Haynes, 'Vernacular Capitalism, Advertising, and the Bazaar in Early Twentieth-Century Western India', in Ajay Gandhi, Barbara Harris-Whites, Douglas E. Haynes and Sebastian Schwecke (eds), *Rethinking Markets in Modern India Embedded Exchange and Contested Jurisdiction* (Cambridge: Cambridge University Press, 2020), p. 124.

119 Rachel Berger, *Ayurveda Made Modern Political Histories of Indigenous Medicine in North India 1900–1955* (New York: Palgrave MacMillan, 2013), pp. 103–104.

120 Prasad, *Cultural Politics of Hygiene*, pp. 13, 110.

121 W. L. Davies, *Indian Indigenous Milk Products* (Calcutta: Thacker, Spink & Co., 1940), n.p.; also Davies, *Indian Indigenous Milk Products*, n.p. cited in Saha, 'Milk, mothering & Nation', p. 105

122 Prasad, *Cultural Politics of Hygiene in India*, p. 108.

123 Ibid.

124 Madhuri Sharma, 'Creating a consumer Exploring medical advertisements in colonial India', in Biswamoy Pati and Mark Harrison (eds), *The Social History of Health and Medicine in Colonial India* (London: Routledge, 2009), pp. 215.

125 Ibid., pp. 215–216.

126 Ibid. p. 215.

127 Ibid., p. 214.

128 Ibid.

129 Alec Nathan, February 1930 D 1/5 cited in R. P. T. Davenport-Hines and Judy Slinn, *Glaxo A History to 1962* (Cambridge: Cambridge University Press, 1992), p. 117. During the First World War, Glaxo was marketed to India from New Zealand, for details see Davenport-Hines and Slinn, *Glaxo*, pp. 117.

130 Ibid.

131 Ibid.

132 *The Statesman and Friend of India*, Calcutta, 17 March, 1918, p. 20. While this advert features a boy scout's salute, on girl guides in India see Kristine Alexander, *Guiding Modern Girls Girlhood, Empire and Internationalism in the 1920s and 1930s* (Vancouver: UBC Press, 2017).

133 Dr. Srijukta J. N. Ray (M.B.), 'Saishabiyo Khaddya O Pattha Prodan', *Chikitsa-Prokash*, vol. 10, no. 9, 1324, p. 369. In the original text, advertisement was spelt as 'odvertisement'.

134 On infantile diseases like diarrhoea, Dr. SriNarendranath Das (L.M.S.), 'Saishabiyo Atisar – Infantile Diarrhea' *Chikitsa-Prokash*, vol 10, no. 11, 1324, pp. 413–19. On childrearing, particularly infant mortality figures in major Indian cities and infant feeding by the 1920s, see discussion in Dr. SriNarendrakumar Das (M.B., M.C.P.S.), 'Sishu Mangal O Sishu Chikitsa' Part 1, *Chikitsa-Prokash*, vol. 19, nos. 6, 7, Bengali year 1333, pp. 224–227; and Dr. SriNarendrakumar Das (M.B., M.C.P.S.), 'Sishu-Mangal O Sishu-Chikitsa' Parts 1 & 2, *Chikitsa-Prokash*, Bengali Year 1333, vol. 19, nos. 9, pp. 355–356.

On infant malnutrition see Captain H. Chatterjee (L.R.C.P.S, Edin), 'Saishobiyo Aparipushtota', *Chikitsa-Prokash*, vol 17, no. 10, 1331, pp. 396–399.

135 For vital statistics of birth and death registration and diseases in Bengal prior to the 1920s, see for instance, Lieutenant-Colonel F. C. Clarkson, *Forty-First Annual Report of the Sanitary Commissioner for Bengal Year 1908* (Calcutta: The Bengal Secretariat Book Depot, 1909). On infant mortality, see L.S.S. O'Malley, *Census of India, 1911. Volume VI City of Calcutta. Part I: Report* (Calcutta: Bengal Secretariat Book Depot, 1913); on influenza in 1918, W.H. Thompson, *Census of India, 1921. Volume VI City of Calcutta Part I. Report* (Calcutta: Bengal Secretariat Book Depot, 1923), pp. 55–56; on public health figures, including birth rates and vaccination statistics in Bengal, see for example, C.A. Bentley, *Bengal Public Health Report Reports of the Bengal Sanitary Board and the Chief Engineer Public Health Department for the Year 1929* (Calcutta: Bengal Secretariat Book Depot, 1930).

136 'Bharatey Proti Minutey Charti Kariya Sishu Morey', Source: Swasthya Samachar, vol. 8, no. 6, 1919, n.p. Illustration Title Translation: 'In India four babies die every minute'. This was published in the sixth month Ashwin in the Bengali year 1326 (1919) – (Online source, accessed date: 25.11.2022) https://digi.ub.uni-heidelberg.de/csss/Svasthya_Sama char/Svasthya_Samachar_Vol_008.pdf. In Bengali, translations are mine. A detailed article with infant mortality statistics across India was also published in this issue. Urgent appeals on behalf of children were also voiced at the time, for example, right at the start of the official report of the Health and Child Welfare Exhibition 1920. See 'An Appeal on Behalf of the Children of Bengal' cited in *Health and Child Welfare Exhibition*, np. It was priced at 'Price Re.1–4'. This has been cited in Chapter 5 in this book.

137 Bengali caption translation: 'Dated 13 Sraban Age 4 months weight 2 Ser' in Sri Manindralal Basu, 'Bongey Sishu Mrittyur Karon', *Swasthya Samachar*, vol. 8, no. 6, 1919, p. 139. Title Translation: 'Causes of Infant Mortality in Bengal'. Online source: Accessed Date: 25.11.2022. https://digi.ub.uni-heidelberg.de/csss/Svasthya_Samachar/Svasthya_Samachar_Vol_008.pdf. This was published in the sixth month Ashwin of the Bengali calendar in the Bengali year 1326. (1919). Sraban is the fourth month in the Bengali calendar. Ser is basically one seer which was slightly under one kilogram. Translations mine.

138 Ibid.

139 Ibid.

140 Bengali caption translation: 'That boy Dated 20 Poush Weight 7 Ser' Source: Basu, 'Bongey Sishu Mrittyur Karon', p. 140. Online Source Accessed Date: 25.11.2022. https://digi.ub.uni-heidelberg.de/csss/Svasthya_Samachar/Svasthya_Samachar_Vol_008.pdf. Poush is the ninth month in the Bengali calendar. This implies that the incident might have taken place in the previous year. Translations mine.

141 See Sibaji Bandyopadhyay, *Gopal-Rakhal Dwandasamas, Upanibeshbad o Bangla Sishusahitya* (Calcutta: Papyrus, 1999); *Aabar Shishushikha* (Kolkata: Anustup, 2005); and Sibaji Bandyopadhyay, *Bangla Shishusahityer Chhoto Meyera by Sibaji Bandyopadhyay* (Kokata: Ganghil, 2007). On child marriage as a stark exemplification of the absence of girlhood, see discussion in the following chapter.

142 Rames Chandra Ray (L.M.S.), 'Kochi Cheleder Khabar', *Svasthya Samachar*, vol. 8, 1919, pp. 204–206; also see Ray, 'Kochi Cheleder Khabar', *Svasthya Samachar*, vol. 8, 1919, pp. 204–205; and Ray, "Cheleder Khabar", *Mashik Basumati*, 1928, n.p. cited in Ishani Choudhury, 'In Search of Proper Diet For Kids: Concerns Regarding Children's Food As Reflected In Bengali Periodicals of The Early Twentieth Century'; *The International Journal of Social Sciences and Humanities Invention*, vol. 3, no. 1, 2016, p. 1794.

143 Devendranath Roy, (L.M.S.), *Garhastha Sastharakkha ebong sachitro Dhatrisikkha Domestic Hygiene and Guide to Bengali Midwives (with illustrations)*, (Calcutta, S. K. Lahiri & Co, 1904), p. 226.
144 Roy, *Garhastha Sastharakkha*, p. 226. p. 226.
145 Homeopathic and allopathic practitioner Khastagir's *A Treatise on the Science and Practice of Midwifery* also discussed nursing of infants and the gender of the child interchanged between *sishu* or infant and *cheley* or boy child. Annadacharan Khastagir, *A Treatise on the Science and Practice of Midwifery with Diseases of Children and Women Manab-Jatna Tattva, Dhatribidya, Nabaprasuto Sishu o Stri Jatir Byadhi-Sangraha* (Calcutta: Author, 1878 second ed., first ed. 1868), pp. 197–199.
146 Ibid., p. 165. Translation mine.
147 Shib Chunder Bose, *The Hindoos as they were A description of the Manners, Customs and Inner Life of Hindoo Society in Bengal* With a prefatory note by the Rev. W. Hastie, B.D., Principal of the General Assembly's Institution, Calcutta (Calcutta, w. Newman and Co., 1881), p. 24.
148 Parama Roy, 'Women, Hunger and Famine: Bengal, 1350/1943', in Bharati Ray (ed), *Women of India: Colonial and Post-Colonial Periods* (New Delhi: Published by Professor Bhuvan Chandel, 2005), p. 393. It is a part of Series on History of Science, Philosophy and Culture in Indian Civilization Volume IX, Part 3, General Editor D.P. Chattopadhyaya.
149 Amartya Sen and Sunil Sengupta, 'Malnutrition of Rural Children and the Sex Bias', in Devaki Jain and Nirmala Banerjee (eds), *Tyranny of the Household: Investigative Essays on Women's Work* (New Delhi: Shakti Books, 1985), p. 24 in Ibid., p. 393.
150 Ibid., p. 393. Roy directs us to Naila Kabeer, *Reversed Realities: Gender Hierarchies in Development Thought* (London and New York: Verso, 1994), pp. 175–177 for an elaborate discussion on the subject.
151 Tinni Goswami-Bhatacharya, 'Femininity and Imperialism Women and Raj in Colonial Bengal (1880–1930)', Conference Paper Ecole Normale Superieure Paris, 2011, p. 3. https://caluniv.academia.edu/TinniGoswami/Conference-Presentations (Consulted on 1 February, 2014). Also, see Tinni Goswami, *Sanitising Society Public Health and Sanitation in Colonial Bengal 1880–1947* (Delhi: B. R. Publishing Corporation, 2011).
152 Roy builds on Arjun Appadurai and others' arguments on the subject – for example see, Arjun Appadurai, 'Gastro-politics in Hindu South Asia', *American Ethnologist*, vol. 8, no. 3, 1981, pp. 494–511 in Roy, 'Women, Hunger and Famine', pp. 417–418.
153 Roy, 'Women, Hunger and Famine', p. 392. Utsa Ray highlights that domestic manuals on cookery geared towards making the *bhadramahila* the 'taste makers' of the family and household were closely associated with Bengali gastronomic culture and *bhadralok* notions of 'tastefulness' of different types of food and cuisine which also underscored the importance of cooking as a central role for the ideal 'new woman'. Utsa Ray, *Culinary Culture in Colonial India A Cosmopolitan Platter and the Middle-Class* (Cambridge: Cambridge University Press, 2015), pp. 107, 109–121.
154 Roy, 'Women, Hunger and Famine', p. 392.
155 Ibid., p. 392. Roy points out that for a detailed discussion, see, for example, Martha Alter Chen, *Perpetual Mourning: Widowhood in Rural India* (New Delhi: Oxford University Press, 2000), and Chitrita Banerji, 'What Bengali Widows Cannot Eat', *Granta*, vol. 52, 1995, pp. 163–71.
156 Roy, 'Women, Hunger and Famine', p. 393. Roy also discusses statistical figures of such 'missing women' from Jean Dreze and Amartya Sen, *Hunger and Public Action* (Oxford: Clarendon Press, 1989), pp. 50–54 in Ibid., p. 393.

157 Tanika Sarkar, *Words to Win: The Making of Amar Jiban, A Modern Autobiography* (New Delhi: Kali for Women, 1999), pp. 253–57 in Roy, 'Women, Hunger and Famine', p. 393.
158 Judith Richell, 'Ephemeral lives: the unremitting infant mortality of colonial Burma, 1891–1941', in Valerie Fildes, Lara Marks and Hilary Marland (eds), *Women and Children First International Maternal and Infant Welfare 1870–1945* (New York: Routledge, 1992), p. 138.
159 Ibid., p. 137.
160 Richell, 'Ephemeral lives', p. 137; also see Cho Nwe Oo, 'Nutrition in pregnant and lactating mothers', paper presented at second Orientation Course in Nutrition, 1974, Burma, p. 3 in Richell, 'Ephemeral lives', p. 137.
161 J. Pryer and N. Crook, *Cities of Hunger Urban Malnutrition in Developing Countries* (Oxford: 1988), p. 14 cited in Richell, 'Ephemeral lives', p. 139.
162 R. O. Whyte, Rural Nutrition in Monsoon Asia (Kuala Lumpur and Oxford: 1974), p. 61 in Richell, 'Ephemeral lives', p. 140.
163 Richell, 'Ephemeral lives', p. 141.
164 W. T. Gairdner, 'On infantile death rates in their bearing on sanitary and social science' (N.P., 1861), P. 15. In India Office Library, Pamphlets, PT.2348–57, Secretary of State for India Library, and H. S. Shrycock and J. S. Siegal, The Methods and Materials of Demography, edited by E. G. Stockwell (London: 1976), p. 235; in Richell, 'Ephemeral lives', p. 135.
165 Richell, 'Ephemeral lives', p. 137.
166 Ibid., p. 135.
167 L. T. Ruzicka, 'Mortality in India: past trends and future propects', in T. Dyson and N. Crook (eds), *India's Demography* (New Delhi: 1984) p. 18 in Richell, 'Ephemeral lives', p. 135.
168 Lemuel Lucas Joshi, *The Milk Problem in Indian Cities With Special Reference to Bombay* With a Foreword by John A Turner. (Bombay: D.B. Taraporevala Sons & Co., 1916), p. 108.
169 For a discussion on a hygienic model of motherhood, Judy Whitehead, 'Modernising the Motherhood Archetype: Public Health Models and the Child Marriage Restraint Act of 1929', *Contributions to Indian Sociology*, vol. 29, nos. 1 and 2, 1995, pp. 194–195. for a critical analysis of the 'germ theory of disease' and 'a bacteriological revolution', see Michael Worboys, 'Was there a Bacteriological Revolution in late nineteenth-century medicine?', *Studies in History and Philosophy of Biological and Medical Sciences*, vol. 38, 2007, pp. 21–25.
170 Joshi, *The Milk Problem in Indian Cities*, p. 96.
171 Ibid., pp. 96, 109. Also, Joshi, *The Milk Problem in Indian Cities*, pp. 96, 109 cited in Saha, 'Milk, mothering & meanings', p. 105–106.
172 Joshi, *The Milk Problem in Indian Cities*, p. 99.
173 Ibid., p. 97.
174 Ibid., p. 109. Also, on 'bad milk' and 'slaughter of the innocents', Deborah Valenze, *Milk A Local and Global History* (New Haven: Yale University Press, 2011), pp. 215–216.
175 Joshi, *The Milk Problem in Indian Cities*, p. 109.
176 Ibid., p. 108.
177 Ibid., pp. 108–9.
178 Ibid., p. 104.
179 Ibid., p. 108.
180 It is relevant to note that on the international scene, a little earlier, Major E. D. W. Greig was the Government of India representative at the international Congress to curb infant mortality at Berlin in 1911, see for example, 'Note on the Proceedings of the Third International Congress for the Protection of Infant Life, attended by Major E. D. W. Greig, I.M.S. representing the Government of India',

Deputation of Major E. D. W. Greig, I.M.S., to attend the International Congress on Infant protection, held at Berlin in September 1911, Proceedings 3-4, December 1911, Department of Education, Sanitary A, 1911, NAI.

181 Surgeon-General Sir Charles P. Lukis in *English-Speaking Conference on Infant Mortality Report of the Proceedings of the English-Speaking Conference on Infant Mortality, held at Caxton Hall, Westminster, on August 4 and 5, 1913* (London: National Association for the Prevention of Infant Mortality and for the Welfare of Infancy, 1913), p. 39.

182 Ibid., p. 211.

183 Cecelia Van Hollen, *Birth on the Threshold Childbirth and Modernity in South India* (Berkeley: University of California Press, 2003), pp. 50–51.

184 Lukis in *English-Speaking Conference on Infant Mortality*, pp. 210–211.

185 Ibid., p. 211.

186 Lukis in *English-Speaking Conference on Infant Mortality*, p. 39.

187 Ibid. On tuberculosis, also see Joshi, *The Milk Problem*, pp. 101–104.

188 Lukis in *English-Speaking Conference on Infant Mortality*, p. 210.

189 Rai Bahadur Dr. Chunilal Bose, *The Milk Supply of Calcutta* (Calcutta: H. W. B. Moreno at the Central Press, 1918), p. 18.

190 Charu Gupta, 'The Icon of Mother in Late Colonial North India, "Bharat Mata", "Matri Bhasha" and "Gau Mata"', *Economic and Political Weekly*, vol. 36, no. 45, 2001, pp. 4295–4297; also Saha, 'Milk, mothering & meanings', p. 106.

191 As also mentioned in Chapter 1, p. 66n164, see Utsa Ray, 'Constructing a "Pure" Body: The Discourse of Nutrition in Colonial Bengal', Institute of Development Studies Occasional Paper 40, 2012, p. 15 in Prasad, *Cultural Politics of Hygiene in India, 1890–1940*, p. 32. Also, 'untouched' in the context of general food items like bread, see Ray, *Culinary Culture in colonial India*, pp. 161, 175.

192 Prasad, *Cultural Politics of Hygiene in India*, p. 27, also on effeminacy Ray, *Culinary Culture in colonial India*, pp. 157–158; and Mrinalini Sinha, *Colonial Masculinity The 'Manly Englishman' and the 'Effeminate Bengali' in the Late Nineteenth Century* (Manchester: Manchester University Press, 1995); about how 'dyspepsia served as a catch-all category for a great many disorders' and milk as a possible cure – see Valenze, *Milk*, mainly pp. 202–209.

193 S. B. Ghose, M.B. Chemical Analyst, Municipal Corporation, Calcutta 'Food Adulteration in Calcutta', *Calcutta Medical Journal* (October, 1907) in Kabita Ray, *Public Health in Colonial Calcutta and the Calcutta Corporation 1923–1947* Selections from Journals and Newspapers (Kolkata: Corpus Research Institute, 2010), pp. 119–121.

194 Saurabh Mishra, *Beastly Encounters Livelihoods, Livestock and Veterinary Health in North India* (Manchester: Manchester University Press, 2015), p. 111.

195 Ibid., pp. 111–112. Mark Harrison argues that the colonial state was gradually becoming interested in public health matters by the late nineteenth century. Mark Harrison, *Public Health in British India Anglo-Indian Preventive Medicine, 1859–1914* (Cambidge, Cambridge University Press, 1994), p. 188 in Mishra, *Beastly encounters of the Raj*, p. 111.

196 Mishra, *Beastly Encounters*, pp. 104–8, 114.

197 Sudeshna Banerjee, '"Non-Bengali" Icons of Malevolence', in Banerjee et al. (eds), *Calcutta Mosaic*, p. 235 in Mishra, *Beastly encounters of the Raj*, p. 107.

198 Regarding diet of lactating mothers and infants of easily digestible foods like barley, arrowroot and so on, see Margaret Ida Balfour Pronito (composed), *Bharater desi daider jonno dhatrisikkha* (Calcutta, Printed at the Baptist Mission Press, 1922), p. 28 Title Translation: Midwifery for the Indian indigenous midwives; Suhrawardy, 'The Care of the Expectant Mother and Newborn Infant', p. lxix.; among others; also see Saha, 'Milk, mothering & meanings', p. 106.

4

CHILD-MOTHERS AND *MOTHER INDIA*

This chapter aims to provide a fresh look at the already enormously researched field of child marriage particularly in colonial Bengal.[1] It addresses problematic questions raised about the 'immature' mother's capacity for childbirth and effective lactation and its impact on community, national and/or 'racial' health and manly vigour mainly in the context of Calcutta. In this regard, it will problematise and analyse the largely underexplored medical and medico-legal opinions about the nature of lactation, breast milk and breastfeeding in early motherhood. I argue here that medical and medico-legal debates about age of consent reform tied to ideas about eugenics or 'good in birth',[2] progress and civilisation were also intimately connected with breastfeeding in early motherhood or 'premature maternity'[3] which was mainly supposed to have devitalised community and national health and strength. The 'physical deterioration of the human stock' also implied 'effeminacy, mental imperfection, and moral debility'.[4] The particular time frame of this chapter delimited by the Age of Consent Act (1891) and the Child Marriage Restraint Act (1929) contributes towards situating breastfeeding amidst the broader context of intense discussions on the body, sexuality, conjugality, maternity, nutrition and high infant and maternal mortality rates.

The focus here is on the Hindu Bengali *bhadramahila* as the 'immature' child-mother who was often blamed for the creation of the Bengali-Hindu 'dying race'.[5] By the 1920s, the 'child marriage question' was reframed in order to centre around the proper management of childhood as a universal 'age of life' constituted by broader intersecting issues like the 'management of sexual habits, eugenic procreation, child-rearing, and political-racial futures'.[6] Nationalist representations of the *bhadramahila* as the 'traditional' and 'modern' literate 'new woman' whose main duty was to become a *sugrihini* or 'good' wife, and mother had to tackle with the fact that she was usually the problematic 'girl-child/woman' who lacked girlhood and legal personhood.[7] Writings on child marriage and early maternity often revealed the urgent need to differentiate between the bodily makeup of the girl child and woman to ensure bodily maturity before enduring intercourse, childbirth and childrearing:

 DOI: 10.4324/9781003327837-5

> Is menstruation an evidence and proof of sexual maturity. . . . Taking maturity to mean bodily and mental maturity, are immature mothers more liable to the penalties of child-birth . . . than mature? Are they as good nurses – is their milk equally abundant and rich? . . . [W]hat is the effect of early marriage and maternity on the stamina physical, moral, and mental of the race?[8]
>
> The first appearance of menstruation, even in its natural course; not hastened by hot-house manipulation – child marriage, is merely an indication that the girl is at best on the threshold of womanhood.[9]

Reform was also considered necessary as many saw the child-wife-and-mother's 'emaciated' and 'exhausted' body, instead of its earlier inviolable purity, incapable of sustaining national health and vigour.[10] The validity and authenticity of socio-religious ceremonial beliefs and practices surrounding child marriage were also fiercely debated.[11] This chapter also looks into other problematic factors mainly 'dirty' lying-in rooms, ritual pollution, unhygienic practices, mostly blamed on traditional birth attendants or *dais*, and frequent pregnancies among child-mothers that were believed to have vastly added to the high incidence of maternal and infant malnourishment, morbidity and mortality which gravely affected the 'biological stock of nations'.[12] Concern about the 'welfare and progress of the family and community' often took precedence over 'the mental and physical well-being of the infant girls'.[13] Moreover, colonial '[i]nterventions in issues of domestic indigenous conjugality were deemed doubly dangerous, encroaching on both religion and femininity'.[14] The Revolt of 1857 followed by takeover by the Crown and the Queen's Proclamation in 1858 was supposed to ensure non-interference in such potentially volatile issues. Colonial rule based on political exigencies and the 'orthodox "status quo"' often determined involvement or lack thereof in socio-religious matters.[15]

The age of consent debates had its inception with the controversies around the enactment of the Native Marriage Act of 1872, followed by the Rukhmabai case on the restitution of conjugal rights in the 1880s and finally the Phulmani Dasi case in the 1890s.[16] A flexible and multipronged discourse on degeneration also emerged from the debates on child marriage beginning as early as the 1860s.[17] At the time, motherhood and infant care gradually became 'scientific' and 'modern', medicalised taught activity which required expert knowledge, skills and training. Spreading awareness through print, in English and Bengali, about successful lactation, breastfeeding and artificial feeding of infants was an integral part of the colonial and nationalist quest for knowledge/power by interfering with the everyday lives of individuals, families and communities. It was with the enactment of the Native Marriage Act of 1872 that Brahmo leader Keshub Chunder Sen, at the head of the Indian Reform Association, pushed through the notion that child marriage, a 'potent sign of Indian otherness',[18] was primarily a 'physiological' problem and 'its "religious bearings must be determined by the verdict of physiology".'[19] In this regard, he had invited expert medical opinion from doctors practicing in Bengal stating:

> It seems necessary, therefore, that competent medical authorities should be consulted in the matter, and their judgement made known for the guidance of the Native community. I beg therefore respectfully to request, you will be pleased, after a careful consideration of the facts that have come to your knowledge, and of the climatic and other influences which govern the physical development of women in tropical countries to state what you consider to be the age of puberty of Native girls and their minimum marriageable age.[20]

Sen's request for expert opinion sought to determine child marriage as a 'physiological' problem and the 'earliest marriageable age consistent with the well-being of mother, child and society'[21] by so-called impartial and objective medical men. Neatly dovetailing Manchester surgeon John Roberton's study of women's 'comparative periodicity' across the British empire in 1851, these doctors pointed out that there was no ' "natural" age of menstruation'. They pointed to the existence of 'forced puberty' due to the culture of child marriage and oversexed Bengali households which led to the 'hereditary transmission of early puberty over time'.[22] Child marriage became a biocultural problem. Their main idea was that the female body was primarily shaped by culture, rather than climate or biology alone – thus, there was no excuse to blame the tropical excesses for sexual pathologies which were supposed to be intimately associated with the culture of child marriage itself.[23] A very similar discussion by Assistant-Surgeon and Teacher of Medicine at the Campbell Medical School, Calcutta, Bolye Chunder Sen on child marriage as a 'physiological' problem in 1891 is outlined in detail in the first section of this chapter. Anxieties were voiced about early menstruation, 'precocious sexuality',[24] and 'premature' consummation and maternity which were most often variously associated with the tropical environment and the culture of child marriage – both blamed for the degeneration of the 'Bengali race' and its defencelessness against disease and colonialism.[25]

In the 1890s, the age of consent came to be fiercely debated about as 'a huge outcry rocked the Indian public when Phulmoni Dasi, 11, died of "injuries inflicted on her on her wedding night" by her husband Hari Mohan Maiti, 37'.[26] The 'medicalized idiom in which her death was discussed' led to the case being called 'the "exciting cause" for the passage of the Age of Consent Act of 1891 in Bengal'.[27] The enactment of the Age of Consent Act 1891 was ideally meant to ensure that the consummation of marriage would occur with the *garbhadhan* ceremony (literally 'gift of the womb'[28]) performed at a proper time to prevent girls from 'premature intercourse'.[29] Colonial and nationalist (revivalist and reformist) impassioned exchanges led to the Criminal Law Amendment Act X of 1891 that revised Section 375 of the Indian Penal Code of 1860 to raise the age of consent for married and unmarried girls from 10 to 12 years.[30] Previously, a husband could legally cohabit with a wife who was ten years old whereby the revivalist Bengali-Hindu intelligentsia believed that the new act made a nuisance of the 'fundamental ritual observance in the life cycle of the Hindu householder – that is, the "garbhadhan" ceremony, or the obligatory cohabitation between husband and wife which took place immediately after the wife reaches her puberty'.[31] The compromise upset orthodox Hindu pundits and revivalists who claimed that this interfered with the *garbhadhan* ceremony as menstruation usually occurred before the age of 12 while reformists argued that menstruation often took place in girls over 12 years and puberty did not mean full maturity required for 'safe intercourse'.[32] Revivalist and reformist worldviews often contradicted and overlapped with each other, however. It may be argued that reformists usually preferred legal intervention by the colonial state, whereas revivalists usually sought to revive the community from within. By 1927, with the publication of pro-imperialist American journalist Katherine Mayo's famous book, *Mother India*, which primarily criticised Hindu socio-religious beliefs and practices concerning child marriage – there was a huge uproar that led to a nationalist-feminist consensus about child marriage and early motherhood as a health problem. It, therefore, accelerated the enactment of the Child Marriage Restraint Act (CMRA) in 1929. This chapter is divided into three sections namely: 'Premature Maternity' Criticised; 'Premature Maternity' Defended; and 'Mother India' and Childcare.

'Premature Maternity' Criticised

> With the progress of puberty the organs concerned with copulation develop in the same way as breasts. . . . With undeveloped organs the amount of pain experienced in early connection or attempts at it must be intense, and serious injuries must be inflicted, sometimes proving fatal, as in the case of Phulmani Dassi. Amongst animals 'consent' is apparently necessary for fertile intercourse, as the immature female will not permit the access of the male if the approach produces pain instead of the reverse. In this lies a safeguard which is not allowed to the unfortunate human child-wife. . . . It cannot be conducive to the moral health of any community to practically allow the rape of its female children and their exposure to all the possible horrors of premature maternity.[33]

Surgeon-Major C. H. Joubert lashed out against the 'want of accuracy of the natives of India with regard to age' and 'a national custom' of child marriage as 'rape' of 'female children' which also exposed 'all or most young females to the risks of immature maternity' as incompatible with the 'moral health of any community' in British India. These were supposed to be a crucial marker of racial, moral and civilisational differences between England and India.[34] He also raised questions like whether 'outward signs of perfect puberty or maturity' exist and whether conceptions can occur without menstruation.[35]

As this chapter examines medical advice on the child-mother's capacity for effective lactation and nursing of infants, it coincides with Tanika Sarkar's argument that the 'new nationalist world-view' conceptualised 'the family as a contrast to and critique of alien rule'.[36] However, it attempts to move beyond Sarkar's argument that '[t]he household generally, and conjugality specifically, came to mean the last independent space left to the colonised Hindu'[37] as 'conjugality was constituted as the centre of gravity around which the discursive field on the family organised itself' – that '[a]ll other relations, even the mother-child one (which would come to take up its place as the pivotal point in the later nationalist discourse) remained subordinated to it up to the end of the 19th century'.[38] It is instead argued here that an enormous corpus of advice about early motherhood and nursing of infants also became visible at the time. This, in turn, reflects subject formation of the colonised Hindu Bengali middle class, predominantly male and gradually female, as it strove to leave its mark in history.[39]

As colonial and nationalist debates about child marriage and 'premature maternity' were particularly concerned about the child-wife-and-mother's 'sexual or maternal body'[40] – these also expressed concerns about meticulously differentiating between the figures of the 'girl-child/woman'.[41] Simply put, a far from simple matter however, as Surgeon-Major Norman Chevers, Principal of the Calcutta Medical College stated – '[i]t stands to reason that a wife ought to be a person whom the least observant would declare to be a "woman" and not an immature "child".'[42] Also visible in contemporary Bengali medical works like *A Treatise on the Science and Practice of Midwifery* by allopathic and homeopathic practitioner, Annada Charan Khastagir, a serious attempt was also made at defining female maturity on the basis of both her bodily maturity related to puberty and behavioural modesty such as turning *lajjito* and *banito*, shy and modest, alongside other changes which, he believed, made her keen for marriage and ready for women's great purpose (implying motherhood) *strijati* or womenfolk have been created for.[43]

Myriad socio-religious, medical and medico-legal colonial and nationalist, revivalist and reformist, understandings of child marriage and parenthood, and their impact on community and national health led to different conceptualisations of 'mature' and 'healthy' male and female bodies. Together with 'new disciplines of the body', there was a conscious attempt at indigenous '"self" constitution and a vernacular modernity'.[44] However, colonial and nationalist worldviews also shared a common definition of the age of consent to mean – 'a certain physical capacity when a girl could sustain intercourse without much damage'.[45] Differences of opinion came up, however, over 'subsidiary issues' like: Did menstruation indicate 'full puberty' and 'sexual maturity'? What happens if the girl begins to menstruate before she is 12 years old and thereby she is unable to perform the *garbhadhan* ceremony?[46] This points to the fact that:

> it was her body that signified consent, and it was her body that would enjoy legal immunity till then. The protected person was nothing more than a protected body; personhood for her did not extend to anything beyond sheer physicality.[47]

Moreover, as Mrinalini Sinha points out, 'female consent' was also 'the reproductive capacity of women: the age at which women could be considered physically fit to bear healthy children without injury to themselves or to the future of the race'.[48]

Renowned *daktar* Gangaprasad Mukhopadhyay (B.A., M.B.) pointed out that the three stages or conditions (*abastha*), namely pregnancy/*garbhabastha*, childbirth/*prasababastha* and breastfeeding/*stanndanabastha*, were correlated.[49] He believed in the significance of following a good disciplined life before and after childbirth in order to ensure the mother's well-being and comfort during these stages.[50] He argued that child marriage usually took place around the age of 7 or 8 for girls and 14 or 15 for boys.[51] He emphasised that child maternity caused bodily and mental disorders in the offspring. Child-mothers gave birth to weak bodied children who, in turn, bore children thereby making their bodies prematurely *bhagna* or 'ruined'.[52] About breastfeeding, Mukhopadhyay argued that child maternity often led the infant's body to become *kharbba o shirna*, weakened and atrophied, due to *prochur porimaaney standughdher abhaabey* or excessive scanty lactation in the child-mother.[53] Even if the mother was able to produce milk and breastfed her child, her *sharir* or body became *durbal* or weak in the process of nourishing the infant.[54] He asked that if healthy middle-aged mothers found childbirth and nursing of infants difficult, then how could the child-mother's body tolerate such bodily exertion and mental stress.[55] He also considered male bodily and mental strength compromised as they became entangled in child marriage and domestic affairs prior to full growth and proper education.[56]

Racialised anxieties about Bengali-Hindu manhood in relation to child marriage and early motherhood featured prominently in Bolye Chunder Sen's[57] paper presented at the ninth meeting of the Calcutta Medical Society on September 10, 1890.[58] He argued, in alignment with many European and indigenous medical practitioners, that the culture of child marriage, instead of 'race' or tropical climate alone, led to early menstruation in Bengal. He challenged the notion of 'the early development of everything under the tropics' which, he pointed out, had 'probably got abroad from seeing the luxuriant vegetation that meets the eye of a foreigner from a colder latitude, who fails to observe "that man seems the only growth that dwindles here".'[59] In order to validate his arguments, he cited Norman Chevers' views from *A Manual of Medical Jurisprudence for India* based on Baboo Modhusoodun Gupta's arguments that 'according to Sushruta, the menstrual discharge begins after the twelfth, and ceases after the fiftieth year' and usually 'catamenia appear sooner or later according to the mode of living of the females, and the sexual excitement to which they may be subjected'.[60] Therefore, Sen authoritatively argued, this has been briefly cited as an excerpt around the beginning of this chapter, that:

> As medical men . . . we know full well the time required for the growth and development of the body. It is twenty-five years, and some even believe it to extend to the thirtieth year for its completion. The first appearance of menstruation, even in its natural course; not hastened by hot-house manipulation – child marriage, is merely an indication that the girl is at best on the threshold of womanhood.[61]

Subsequently, Sen deployed the categories of 'race', gender and community in his discussion of the problem of child maternity. He considered child maternity as a 'physiological' problem responsible for the degeneration of the 'Bengalee-Hindoos'.[62] He questioned the desirability of child marriage from 'a physiological point of view, to have a girl subjected to sexual intercourse, and be saddled with conception, parturition and lactation on the first appearance of menstruation'.[63] He blamed child maternity for infantile diseases due to 'inherent weakness in the children' such as 'refusing the breast'.[64] He appealed to his European 'Aryan' brethren to compare their musculoskeletal structure with the degenerate Bengali-Hindu men 'that have sprung from the same stock', but 'imperfect and immature seed' and were 'nursed in ill-developed nestling ground'.[65] Sen was primarily concerned about child maternity resulting in the poor build of Bengali males, specifically the 'diminished size of the population of "weak, unfortunate Bengal", originally a "pure Aryan race" like the Europeans'.[66]

Indira Chowdhury-Sengupta argues that the nationalist argument about a 'common Aryan race' associated with the colonising 'master race', with Bengalis as a 'Hinduised Aryan race', was closely related with Orientalist, Social Darwinist and ethnographic discourses.[67] She discusses 'Aryan womanhood'[68] and highlights that colonial understandings of the 'effeminate' and 'non-martial' Bengali 'race' enormously influenced the 'nationalist construction of the *birmata*, or the brave mother' and her calling to nourish 'fearless sons' at her breast to rescue 'the fallen race of Bengalis'[69]:

> Rise, Oh sisters!
> Oh wives and mothers of the brave!

Instruct your offspring,
As you nurse them at your breast
In legends heroic!
So the blood vibrates with pride as it flows in their veins.[70]

Furthermore, Sen was responding to colonial discourses about child marriage resulting in 'Bengali effeminacy' which was not merely about 'likening the unfitness of native civilians to the unfitness of women' but a set of pseudo-scientific racialised explanations of 'native effeminacy' associated with the 'unnaturalness' inherent in the 'effeminate Bengali's' body and character.[71] It was directly correlated with problematic practices like *purdah* and the confinement of women in the *zenana*,[72] alongside premature consummation, early motherhood and masturbation.[73] This confirmed the supposedly degenerate pathological nature of the Bengalis and justified their disqualification from self-government and continuance of colonial rule. As Pande highlights, liberal racialism (i.e. liberalism and 'race science' combined) provided the framework for 'colonial governmentality' in India.[74]

Ayurvedic practitioners also advocated maturity of the body to enable effective mothering and to ensure that a healthy (strong) infant was born. For example, Ayurvedic and allopathic practitioner Surendranath Goswami's *Arya Dhatribidyas* which collated parallel data from Ayurveda and allopathic medicine on each page throughout the book, pointed out child marriage as being responsible for the 'shattered constitution' of the mother as well as 'less fertile' and 'weak' children.[75] Similarly, Kabiraj Srijukta Girijabhushan Ray Sengupta's article titled '*Sishupalan*' or 'Child-Rearing', advocated a particular mode of childrearing in accordance with 'chikitsasastra' or 'medical science' especially for the education of '*bhadra*' 'Bengali parents who were predominantly underage, frail and malnourished girl-child and boy-child' themselves who, in turn, gave birth to malformed and feeble children.[76]

In the 1920s, premature motherhood was often coupled with the issue of the population problem, for instance, by the Bengali intellectual and prolific author, Chandra Chakraberty in his book *National Problems* published in 1923. He argued that girls are fitted for wifehood and motherhood between the ages of 21–23 and

> The parents should and ought to investigate the character, fitness and heredity of the suitors of a girl. . . . Girls can not be trusted to use good judgement and discretion upon a question which has such a vital bearing on her happiness before she is 21 or 23. . . as civilization advances, more than physical fitness, mental fitness rather becomes the criterion of motherhood for the fulfilment of the complicated task which modern life demands, or the race suffers. Mother is the highest teacher, and home is the best school, and her influence is predominant in forming the character and educative

> materials of the child. With premature motherhood there is race lethargy and retrogation, precocious senility and excessive child-mortality, thus arresting progress at the biotic fountain-head, and leading to racial, physical and mental degeneracy.[77]

His eugenic arguments are evident in his protest against birth control as he argued that the 'saturation point' of earth's population is still far away,[78] and, in India, according to

> [t]he last census . . . in the preceding decennium, the population has hardly increased, and the increment has been gained from the lowest stratum of society, and the middle class, the custodian and the hope of the future is slowly dying.[79]

He believed that the middle class or 'the best elements of the nation' needed to 'increase for the regeneration of the country, if the race is not to sink to the lower level of culture by the rapid multiplication of the under-world'.[80] Between the 1920s and the 1940s, the population problem had become a communalised, civilisational, Malthusian issue of numbers and resources. Unlike the educated upper and middle class and caste Hindus, lower classes and mainly Muslims were often 'castigated for their backward rather than modern controlled reproductive behaviour' due to their supposed lower intellectual capacity and higher fertility resulting from later consummation of marriage, polygamy, and other causes.[81]

By the late 1920s, there was also a gradual consensus that came together around the issue of child marriage and premature motherhood as health problems.[82] Public protests following the publication of Katherine Mayo's *Mother India* in 1927 also expedited the enactment of the Child Marriage Restraint Act (CMRA) in 1929. The Age of Consent Committee, referred to as the Joshi Committee, was established in June 1928 and headed by Sir Moropant Joshi, formerly Home Member of the Central Provinces.[83] It surveyed public opinion about legal intervention by the colonial state to raise the age of consent for sexual intercourse. Jyotirmoyi Ganguli (M.A., 1889–1945) of Calcutta, daughter of Kadambini Ganguli (first female medical practitioner from Bengal), in her written and oral evidence to the Committee favoured state legislation to raise the age of consent for girls because she believed that child marriage was a customary practice not bounded by religious sanction. Her main argument may be summed up as follows:

> Our race has deteriorated physically to a large extent; nervous disorders and a low percentage of calcium in the blood are common and these make us an easy prey to death. This condition is largely due, I think to very young parentage and so an advance in the present law is entirely justified. . . . To me it seems that people are actuated

> more by custom when they practise early consummation of marriage at puberty than by religious injunction, because many of the Slokas of our Shastras advocate marriage of fully-developed girls and men and almost all of them demand of the bride healthy, well-developed, well-formed, brave and mighty children and not the puny ones child-mothers give birth to. . . . When a young girl becomes a mother she has not got the proper development, and she cannot give the child the proper amount of calcium which the child needs.[84]

The Brahmo Samaj and the Arya Samaj were brought together in the figure of Ganguli as she was a Brahmo lady and former principal of both the Brahmo Girl's School in Calcutta, and the Arya Samajist Kanya Maha Vidyalaya in Jullunder.[85] Members of the Brahmo Samaj shared a nationalist, Hinduised and gendered vision of motherhood with a strong desire for patriotic sons to rescue the motherland. Child marriage was also criticised by the Arya Samaj which grew out of Punjab in the 1870s 'for being a deviation from vedic ideals when women ideally did not marry before age 16 and men before age 25, and on the grounds that they produced weak offspring which eventually led to the degeneration of the race'.[86] Despite differences between secular and vedic reformers from the Brahmo Samaj and the Arya Samaj, the 'progress of the Indian nation' was often measured by the 'physical and moral health' of its mothers and children.[87]

The Arya Samaj and the British Eugenics Society also 'bore uncanny resemblances' as both considered that 'only marriages between mature individuals could produce vigorous offspring'.[88] Dayananda Sarasvati's *Satyarth Prakash*, integral to the *Arya Samaj* movement, motherhood was primarily about the 'breeding of Aryans' and reviving Hindu masculinity.[89] It allowed men to attain 'perfect physical strength, perfect wisdom', 'perfect development of good qualities', and their 'reproductive element perfected'. He also suggested various foods like milk, butter and others to improve the 'reproductive element . . . of the highest quality, free from all faults and imperfections' and provided detailed guidelines 'to copulate', as the main function of women was to become 'reproducers' to produce children of a 'superior' order.[90] Anshu Malhotra points out that 'Dayananda may have believed, like many in the nineteenth century, that lactation acted as a natural method of birth control'. Joseph S. Alter 'has shown how in the Vedas, milk is referred to as *vrsnyam payas* or virile "seed-like" milk, with women's milk implied as female seed, the symbolic opposite of male semen'.[91] Thus, it was advised, 'It is best . . . for the mother not to suckle her child. Plasters should be applied to the breast that will soon dry up the milk'[92] and the mother would have 'to hire a wet-nurse for feeding her child' because 'the substance of the infant high caste body' was 'apparently unaffected by the nurturing of a low caste woman'.[93]

In short, this section discussed anxieties about the intimate connections between the 'maturity'/'immaturity' of the female body, her capacity for intercourse and maternity, and their impact on community and national health and manliness. The following section explores problematic medical and medico-legal opinions expressed in support of child marriage and premature motherhood in colonial Bengal.

'Premature Maternity' Defended

'[D]octors who have opposed the Age of Consent Bill' in the Bengali newspaper *Sanjivani* on February 14, 1891 emphasised:

> Susruta says that a child born of a mother under sixteen does not live and is very weak if it lives, and this view is supported by Raghunandan in his *Jyotishtattwa*. According to the Hindu *shastras*, a son is required to offer the *pinda* to his ancestors. But what spiritual good will a Hindu father derive from a son, brought forth prematurely, who will die before him? It is to be regretted that even those who pique themselves upon their education look more to the established practice than to the real spirit and object of the *shastras*. Dr. Jagabandhu Bose's statements cannot be accepted as authoritative, so long as he does not support them by quotations from works on Physiology.[94]

However, based on experiments with pregnant, growing guinea pigs by American embryologist and Harvard Medical School Lecturer, Charles Sedgwick Minot (M.D.), famous Calcutta *daktar* Juggobundhu Bose (M.D.) questioned whether 'there is an inherent opposition between growth and reproduction' as follows:

> The other point for consideration is whether the reproductive process interferes with the natural growth of an organism. . . . It has been asserted by Herbert Spencer . . . that there is an inherent opposition between growth and reproduction, because the assimilative process cannot perform enough to supply material for the growth of mother and offspring both . . . but as Minot has pointed out . . . Spencer's view is erroneous. For growing guinea pigs will bear one-third of their own weight of young while growing, and still reach as full an adult size as those producing no young (Hensen). My own experiments suggest that they become even larger . . . Charles Sedgwick Minot M.D., 'Lecturer on Embryology at the Harvard University. (Hand-Book of Reference of Medical Science, Edited by Marcus Beck.)'. . . . My humble opinion coincides with Minot.[95]
>
> (emphasis added)

Bose added that lack of 'good food', '[w]ant of physical exercise' and '[m]ental work, its effects on the body', instead of child marriage and premature motherhood should be held responsible for the 'physical deterioration in the race'.[96] He also argued that 'native' doctors have confirmed that young girls usually go through childbirth in 'perfect safety'.[97] He pointed out that 'native' doctors were more knowledgeable in the field of childbirth among young girls because European physicians were called only in critical cases.[98] In the Bengali newspaper *Samaya* on March 5, 1891, an article boldly ridiculed Dr. Jagadbandhu Bose's premise, however, by emphasising that whereas Bose

> says that premature cohabitation is not prevalent in this country; but experienced medical men . . . say in one voice that the practice of premature cohabitation widely prevails here. Dr. Jagadbandhu affects to be sleeping though awake. It is impossible to bring him to his senses.[99]

Hindu revivalists were against raising the age of consent to 12 years because they believed the failure to consummate the marriage when menstruation began (the *garbhadhan* ceremony) implied that the girl's father incurred the sin of foeticide as the womb became polluted, future sons would not be able to offer ritual offerings (*pinda*) to ancestral spirits, and women were destined to be widows in many successive births.[100] The age of consent debates also often correlated child marriage with the problems of Bengali effeminacy and racial degeneration. Mrinalini Sinha argues that medical practitioners like Babu Juggobandhu Bose and the entire revivalist nationalist camp's defence against raising the age of consent for sexual intercourse, however, amounted to an empty victorious claim to a 'revitalised Indian masculinity', instead of a 'reversal of the colonial emasculation of the Indian male'. This occurred as the favourite colonial arguments were usually about such 'eugenics-based distinction between child-marriage and premature consummation for the physical and moral development of the race'.[101]

Contradictory medical opinions were also voiced in this regard, sometimes by the same person – as in the case of homeopathic practitioner, Haranath Ray (L.M.S.) in 1887, in his book *Midwife's Vade-Mecum*, that usually in about a year and a half after 'premature menstruation, a girl became *enceinte*, and gave birth to a child in or before the due time'.[102] He argued, '[W]hat wonder that her child should be weak, feeble, and of stunted growth' and the child-wife-and-mother suffered from 'the *sutiká* disease after delivery' and she spent the rest of her life suffering from 'the effects of menstrual and many other diseases'.[103] In his description, child marriage was a modern phenomenon in response to Muslim threats which resulted in physiological problems like scanty lactation in the child-mother, whereby a wet nurse was hired or animal milk procured, in turn, leading to a weak Bengali-Hindu male body.[104] He went on to argue that the general climate of thought was that development of the male body with the help of exercise (*vyam*) and 'manly activities' (*puroshochit kriya*) led to national progress.[105] While the male body became strong and matured fully through *vyam*, Ray questioned whether a weak male body produced by child marriage could undergo these strenuous activities.[106] In contrast, however, is Ray's letter of 1891,[107] from the section 'Medical Opinions on the Alleged Cruelty to Tender Aged Wives by Their Husbands' in the proceedings of the public meeting to protest against the Age of Consent Bill held at the residence of the late Maharajah Kamal Krishna Deb, Bahadur, in Calcutta in January 1891. In the letter, he protested against the Age of Consent Bill, arguing that 'I am no advocate of early marriage, but I cannot subscribe to the statement that the offspring of early marriage are stunted, imperfect, dwarfish and Lilliputian bipeds'. He also added that menstruation depended on 'individual constitution' of girls, therefore 'the Bill is no effective remedy for the evil, and as it interferes with the religious institutions and social usages of the country, it ought to be shelved'.[108]

The Dacca Prákásh argued, using the tropical climate as an excuse, that the 'present Bill owes its origin to a mistaken notion in the mind of the English people. In England, which is a cold country, no girl becomes fit for sexual intercourse before that age'.[109] It was suggested:

> Opinions which have been given by English doctors on this subject are opinions based upon English notions, and . . . [i]t will, therefore, be, in the highest degree, wrong to pass the proposed law on the strength of those opinions.[110]

The Bill was further opposed as it was argued that child-wives did not become 'sickly' due to 'early cohabitation' with their husbands and 'the earlier born are invariably found to be stronger than the later born'.[111] This same line of argument that apparently 'superior children' were born from child-mothers was still being used in the late 1920s, as evident from attorney Charu Chandra Mitra's written submissions in the *Age of Consent Committee Evidence*. On child-mothers' capacity for effective lactation and the superiority of her children to those of adult mothers, and the medical merits of child marriage not just for India, as child marriage was promoted as an antidote to the 'evils of deferring marriage' in Europe and America, Mitra emphasises:

> I should think that a propaganda in favour of early marriage should be carried on in the interest of the girls themselves not only here but in Europe and America. The evils of deferring of marriage and its attendant evils due to long sexual abstinence, such as diseases of menstruation, neurasthenia, hysteria and other nervous diseases, sexual perversions, inversions, unnatural means of satisfying sexual desires, spread of venereal diseases, unhappy marriages, animosity between the sexes, have become so great in Europe that the evils of child marriage, if it is an evil at all, are negligible in comparison . . . Klienwa'chter indeed, found that the younger the mother the bigger

> the child. It is not only physically that the child is superior to those of older mothers, both in conduct and intelligence, provided the fathers are not too old or too young. . . . E. B. Wales of New Jersey has recorded the history (reproduced in Medical Reprints, Sept. 15, 1890) of a coloured girl who became pregnant at the age of 11. . . . Delivery was easy and natural. . . . The child was a fine healthy boy weighing not less than eleven pounds. Mother and child both did well and there was a great flow of milk.[112]

When cross-questioned, however, he answered that he was prepared to reconsider his answers if physiologically 'maternity before 16 was proven injurious' to the mother and child – 'I care for facts and not opinions. Opinions are never admitted as proof in medical science. . . . Physiological objections should outweigh all other objections'.[113] Thus, the age of consent debates between the 1890s and the 1920s was 'steeped in the language of physiology' and 'mapped in terms of the biological criteria of sex and age'.[114]

Medical practitioners like Bidhu Mukhi Bose (M.B.) from Calcutta also expressed that 'she does not consider early marriage harmful to the infant because in Bengal where the practice is prevalent children are born healthy'.[115] Dagmar F. Curjel's MD (Glasgow), of the Women's Medical Service in her paper titled 'The Weight at Birth of Infants in India' (1920–1921) went a step further as she highlighted:

> In 1849 Indian infants the average weight at birth was 6.48 lbs. In 201 European and Anglo-Indian infants born in India, the average weight at birth was 7.64 lbs. The writer considers the Indian birth weight compares favourably with the European birth weight, considering the heavier build of European mothers, and looks on this as evidence that *Indian infants are not unfavourably affected by the earlier marriage age.*
>
> (emphasis added)[116]

In the Age of Consent Evidence, perspectives on child marriage and early motherhood were also complicated by prioritising related issues. Edith Ghosh, representative of the Bengal Presidency Council of Women, a private practitioner among women for seven years and occasionally in-charge of the Corporation Maternity Hospital in northern Calcutta, linked together child marriage, frequent pregnancies and insufficient lactation:

Q. *Is frequent child-birth or early maternity more responsible for the physical deterioration of the girls.*

A. In my opinion *provided child-birth does not frequently come on, early maternity is not so disastrous.* In the case of frequency of child-births the mother does not get any rest to recoup her health.

Mrs Nehru: Do you think that the later children of young mothers are better than the children who are born earlier?

A. What I find is that if there is a frequency of child-births the later children are not so good. Even if they are born fairly good, *the mother is unable to feed them properly.*

Dr. Beadon: Do you find that the girl mothers have sufficient nourishment for the babies?

A. They can manage with the first and second babies. *In our Baby Clinique we very rarely get first and second children. But even these children they cannot feed for more than about 9 months. . .* [emphasis added].[117]

Frequent pregnancies were also blamed by C. I. Remfry (Mrs. Douglas Remfry), 'Acting Honorary Secretary, Bengal Presidency Council of Women', Calcutta as she argued that 'Indian girls', at 'no age', were 'competent to give an intelligent consent but it is impossible to generalise'. She believed that child-mothers spent their lives as a '*baby factory*', which led to insufficient physical and mental development alongside lack of proper childcare.[118] It is pertinent to locate the problem of frequent pregnancies within the wider context of the eugenic debates on population control in colonial India, also briefly discussed in the previous section. Sanjam Ahluwalia points out that birth control was 'not communalized' within women's politics[119] – even though 'some opponents argued that use of contraceptives was against their religion, for the most part, organized women's politics was not divided and fractured along religious lines'.[120] They promoted birth control as a national medical necessity with eugenic health concerns resulting from frequent pregnancies, various traditional beliefs and practices and high maternal and infant mortality figures.[121]

Between 1891 and 1928–1929, several socio-religious, medical and medico-legal worldviews were voiced in support of child marriage and early motherhood. These exchanges pieced together contemporary understandings of the Bengali-Hindu child-mother's bodily capacity for reproduction and infant nursing believed to have been crucial to the rejuvenation of community and national manly vigour.

'Mother India' and Childcare

This final section closes the discussion on early motherhood in the age of consent debates by taking a closer look at the conceptualisation of the nation as mother and mother-goddess, *Bharat Mata* (or Mother India), in the context of colonial Bengal. It is followed by an examination of the problems in nursing of infants related to dirty lying-in rooms, *dais* and unhygienic birthing and infant feeding ritual beliefs and practices as these figured in pro-imperialist American journalist Katherine Mayo's (1867–1940) *Mother India* published in 1927. The controversy following the publication of the book accelerated the age of consent debates primarily involving the Hindu Child Marriage Bill, the nationalist movement, and all-India women's organisations, and the enactment of the Child Marriage Restraint Act (CMRA).[122]

To begin with, representations of India as mother and mother goddess were central to the nationalist 'glorification of motherhood'.[123] Jasodhara Bagchi begins her discussion on the Bengali nationalist conceptualisation of the *Bharat Mata* by asking, '[W]as the choice of the mother merely an accidental one? Or was there something about the culture of the Bengalis that created the requisite precondition for such a choice?'[124] Motherhood was always 'a culturally privileged concept' in Bengal as social interactions in Bengal have been most often permeated by 'the address of mother'.[125] It was not just a form of address used by her children and their spouses and by servants addressing the mistress of the household, but even by strangers to unknown women and girls passing by in the street.[126] Mother India/'[M]other Bengal' gradually became a major source of 'mass contact' spreading the message of cultural and economic *Swadeshi*.[127] The symbol of swadeshi nationalism Bharat Mata painted by Abanindranath Tagore, was 'a blend of Bengali women with her conchshell bangle and the image of Shri, the harvest goddess of prosperity'[128] She was also the 'ideal of Bangalakshmi'.[129] Ramendra Sundar Trivedi also involved Bengali women in the 'anti-partition Swadeshi of 1905 by giving the call of ' "[a]randhan" (no cooking)'.[130] Mothers were considered as central to the project of education of their offspring and the guardian of indigenous values.[131] The nationalist 'mother image' was 'a combination of the affective warmth of a quintessentially Bengali mother and the mother goddess Shakti, known under various names as Durga, Chandi or Kali, who occupies a very important position in mainstream religious practice'.[132] Shakti as a political ideal of swadeshi certainly was specific to Bengali culture, fed by the literary experiments of Bankimchandra and the Kali cult of Ramakrishna, popularised by Swami Vivekananda and Sister Nivedita. Motherhood, therefore, became the basis for the contrast between the East and the West. In the words of Swami Vivekananda –

> In the west, the woman is wife. The idea of womanhood is concentrated there as the wife. To the ordinary man in India the whole force of womanhood is concentrated on motherhood.[133]

Moreover, as Bagchi argues 'Bengal/India, the land itself became the mother'. Worship of the mother goddess coincided with the empowering of the imageries of the mother figure in Bengal.[134] Bagchi traces the trajectory back to an early Sanskrit text of the fifth/sixth centuries which provided references to

> the presiding deity of Bharat well famed as the Bharat-mata (Mother India). To her north is the Himalaya and Kanyakumari in the south is forever present. Prayer to this great Shakti frees men from re-birth. (*Samavidhana Brahman*).[135]

Sumathi Ramaswamy's study on the intermeshing of the map of India and the anthropomorphic Mother India further illustrates that the colonial 'scientific' cartographic form had to be supplemented with the divinity of the mother/goddess *Bharat Mata* (or Mother India) to demand sacrifice for the motherland.[136] However, she emphasises that few illustrations actually visualised Mother India engaged in acts of 'maternality'.[137] The *Bharat Mata* that appeared in the magazine *Intiya* on April 10, 1909, edited by Tamil poet-patriot Subramania Bharati (1882–1921), was unusual as she held four infants in her arms, two of whom were suckling from her 'discreetly exposed breasts'. Ramaswamy argues that this may be characterised as 'patriotic milk kinship'.[138] She clarifies that the partly concealed breasts are not threatening – being involved in a task that reasserts 'the woman's primary identity as child bearer and nurturer'.[139] Attempts at visualising *Bharat Mata* as the 'mortal mother' were usually overshadowed by the multitude of images of her as a divine figure due to the 'dominant habit of divinizing her, with her suprahuman and godly status, revealed by the large halo that rings her head, the multiple arms her body bears, and the abhaya mudra "fear-not" gesture her hand generally assumes'.[140]

Powerful goddesses with minds of their own, such as Durga and Kali, with ferocious and uncontrollable proclivities could have been a 'potential embarrassment in a social climate increasingly governed by norms of bourgeois respectability and sexual propriety'.[141] Therefore, they became 'shakti incarnate' and 'venerable repositories of power' that the patriot needed for his 'new goddess of territory', but she was under the control of her patriotic sons.[142] The 'women's question' was integrally linked to the 'new patriarchy' of the western-educated middle-class Hindu men and the 'new ideology of bourgeois motherhood' that emerged in late colonial India.[143] The nation came to be closely associated with 'home' and 'family' whose well-being depended on the figure of the educated mother who raised 'productive citizens'.[144] Thus, 'while the home is under the custodianship of the woman as mother, the nation as home is presided over by her archetype, Mother India'.[145]

Durga is a warrior Goddess yet she is depicted as 'a smiling, matronly beauty'. Her strength is overlaid with 'a domesticated gentle feminity'. Motherland/*Deshmata*/country 'is abstracted from the people and is then personified as the Mother Goddess' from the Hindu pantheon.[146]

'The people, then, are not the "desh" itself, but are sons of the Mother'.[147] Unlike Sarkar's Motherland-Deshmata as a 'cultural artefact',[148] Sugata Bose points out that for nationalist thinkers like Bipin Chandra Pal, the Motherland

> was in origin 'not a mere idea or fancy, but a distinct personality. The woman who bore them and nursed them, and brought them up with her own life and substance was no more real a personality in their thought and idea than the land which bore and reared, and gave food and shelter to all their race'.[149]

Anti-colonial nationalism was an 'oppositional ideology' fighting British stereotypes of Bengali babu that, unlike the 'manly' 'British public school boy-cum-administrator' or the Indian 'martial races', was an 'effeminate creature'.[150] Moreover, even though imperialism had fashioned its own Mother Goddess in the figure of Queen Victoria[151] – the Bengali-Hindu nationalist conceptualisation of Shakti blended victimhood and triumphant strength in the vocabulary of kinship and home, often based on natural ties rather than self-interest.[152]

Partha Chatterjee argues that the *bhadramahila* as 'new woman' was conceptualised by the nationalist 'new patriarchy' as different from and 'superior' to the 'modern' memsahib, 'ignorant' women of older generations, and those from lower (castes and/or) classes.[153] She belonged to the 'spiritual or the inner sphere as an "uncolonized space" wherein the essence of Indiannness could be located'.[154] Tanika Sarkar argues that nationalist iconography in nineteenth-century Bengali literature in fact connected, what Chatterjee argues were separate inner/spiritual versus the outer/materialist domains, primarily through the powerful imagery of a ' "race of mothers" – "mayerjati" '[155] who would rejuvenate the nation by creating patriotic (Hindu) *sons*.[156] Chatterjee further contends that 'unlike the women's movement in nineteenth and twentieth century Europe or America, the battle for the new idea of womanhood in the era of nationalism [in India] was waged in the home'.[157] By way of contrast, Sinha argues,

> [T]his neglect of women's agency in the outer world of nationalist politics not only underestimates the discourse of Indian feminism in the early women's movement, but it also freezes the gendered logic of Indian nationalism to a single moment supposedly defined by the singular problematic of the assertion of national cultural 'difference' from the West.[158]

The *Mother India* controversy actually challenged the cultural nationalist discourse on the 'modern Indian woman' as a 'signifier of an "essentialized Indianness" for the assertion of cultural difference from the West' as liberal feminism 'refashioned' her as 'agent of, and model for, an abstract nationalist Indian modernity'.[159] Representations of the nation as Mother India and the figure of the Indian woman as the very essence of Indianness allowed new opportunities for women's activism.[160] Like Sarojini Naidu (1879–1949), the 'modern' Indian woman often combined 'westernization' with the traditional, 'glorious ideals of Indian womanhood' in the process of voicing her opinions and becoming the female object and subject in the discourse on 'Indian womanhood'.[161] The 'modern/westernized' Indian woman, Naidu, was sent as the official representative of the All-India Women's Conference (AIWC) at the Pan-Pacific Women's Conference in Honolulu.[162] She aimed 'to educate the American People about the "real" Mother India'.[163] She lectured in the United States on 'The Interpretation of Indian Womanhood' and 'The Political Situation of India'.[164] She aimed to undo the images of the 'unregenerate' Indian nationalism and the 'downtrodden' Indian woman in Mayo's *Mother India.*[165]

Finally, Mayo's *Mother India* specifically criticised Hindu social practices related to precocious sexuality, early marriage, premature motherhood, 'dirty' lying-in rooms, and *dais*, alongside superstitions and 'strange substances' that were used in childbirth and for infant feeding purposes.[166] Mayo provided horrific details of childbirth often presided over by the 'allegedly filthy, louse-infested, unscientific Indian *dai*, or midwife' while listing the 'terrible consequences of child marriage on Indian women and children' which were 'the main contributions of the book.[167] Mayo also touched on superstitions, ritual pollution and caste structure associated with childbirth in the hands of the traditional, low caste *dais* and their assistants as '*narkata*' or 'cord-cutters'.[168] The 'title referred to a central chapter of the book, which depicted in gruesome detail the horrors to which the Indian mother was subject during childbirth', as well as to the hollowness of 'popular nationalist iconography of the nation as Mother India'[169]:

> According to the Hindu code, a woman in child-birth and in convalescence therefrom is ceremonially unclean, contaminating all that she touches. Therefore only those become *dhais* who are themselves of the unclean, 'untouchable' class. . . . If the delivery is at all delayed, the *dhai* is expected to explore for the reason of the delay . . . she makes balls of substances, such as hollyhock roots or dirty string . . . or earth mixed with cloves, butter and marigold flowers . . . any irritant – and thrusts them into the uterus, to hasten the event. In some parts of the country, goat's hair, scorpion stings, monkey skulls, and snake-skins are considered valuable applications . . . the 'cord-cutters' . . . cut the umbilical cord . . . a task so degrading . . . The end of the cut cord, at best is left undressed . . . In . . . less happy cases, it is treated with...substances, including cow-dung . . . As the child is taken from the mother, it is commonly laid on the floor, uncovered and unattended, until the *dhai*

> is ready to take it up. If it be a girl child, many simple rules have been handed down through the ages for discontinuing the unwelcome life then an there . . . the first feedings are likely to be . . . *gutli*, a combination of spices in which have been stewed old rust-encrusted lucky coins and charms written out on scraps of paper. These things, differing somewhat in different regions, castes and communities, differ more in detail than in quality of intelligence displayed . . . the mother . . . is usually kept without any food or drink for from four to seven days from the outset of her confinement . . . the baby is not put to the breast till after the third day – a custom productive of dire results.[170]

In putting together this discussion on childbirth and feeding of infants, Mayo referred to various sources, including briefly quoting from Sub-Assistant Surgeon in Barabanki, Mrs. Chowdhri's graphic account of traditional birthing practices in eastern Bengal. Taking a look in detail at Chowdhri's report reveals that, like many indigenous medical practitioners at the time, she argued that confinement was 'arranged in some place where none of the members of the family are likely to go (she believed it was 'very often where the refuse matters are thrown'). Furthermore, as mentioned earlier, '[a] number of medicines are quoted as being used for child-birth – these include goat's hair, scorpion stings, monkey's skull, snake skin'; '[c]amel's hair is believed to attract a foetus and for this reason is applied in a bunch at the vulva', and a 'cock's head is tied near for the same purpose'. Chowdhri explained: '[m]any other extraordinary methods are practised. It is believed among the women that disease is the manifestation of the advent of a god and that any medical treatment will drive away and offend the god. Hence they prefer supernatural treatment.'[171]

Mayo also referred to Edris Griffin's (Nursing Sister, Health Visitor, Delhi) main argument that infants died within the first week because the mother 'not being fed, naturally has very little milk'.[172] It is relevant to note that Griffin further pointed out that the 'unfortunate baby is given honey, sherbert, a concoction of ghur and spices, bazar milk, in fact anything but its mother's milk'. She described the 'indigenous dai is an institution that, like superstition, will die hard. She is a great power in the land, her methods account for the greater part of the mortality among mothers and babies'. She also recommended educating mothers as '[a]part from teaching the dais, the people themselves must be taught and shown the need for improvement. The mothers and mothers-in-law have their own ideas as to how confinements should be conducted, and they insist on the dai doing it according to their notions.'[173]

She insisted that mothers should be told about the fact that 'the dai should not be allowed to insert her finger into the child's rectum . . . to produce the motion', or 'down its throat', 'to open it', whereby babies were 'unable to take the breast'.[174] Both Chowdhri and Griffin agreed that *dais* needed training, with constant supervision by women doctors, else they would 'very quickly revert to their old methods'.[175]

Sinha explains that *Mother India* was 'primarily a public health document that had revealed the unsanitary and unhygienic practices of Indians to the world'.[176] It put forward 'the moral justification of British imperialism'.[177] This 'limited frame focused only on Indian cultural practices, and thus conveniently ignored any negative impact that colonialism had on the condition of women in India'.[178] Sinha further argues that more blatant was Mayo's 'communal card' in Volume II (1931) which mainly quoted excerpts from the Age of Consent Committee (Joshi Committee) appointed by the colonial government to explore public opinions on the age of consent, and *The Face of Mother India*, 'a pictorial representation of India and of Indian women'.[179] On the other hand, the Indian women's movement, mainly comprised of the three major national women's organisations (the Women's Indian Association, the All-India Women's Conference (AIWC), and the National Council of Women in India), emphasised on their condemnation of *Mother India* together with the need for social reform.[180] The imperialist/nationalist controversy in the wake of the publication of *Mother India* was characterised by a consensus around medical concerns about the health of child-mothers and their children, as also evident in the Joshi Committee evidence.[181] The 'various activities of organized women to garner support from members of the all-male Central Legislative Assembly' included 'the holding of public meetings, the passing of resolutions, the lobbying of leaders of various political parties, the publishing of newspaper and journal articles, and the picketing by women outside the assembly' which 'underscored the significance of the Sarda Bill for the project of nationalist modernity'.[182] The Women's Indian Association (WIA) in its journal, *Stri Dharma*, championed the bill, aligning it with issues related to child and maternal welfare and female education.[183] Sinha argues that due to the 'dilatory tactics'[184] of the colonial state in the age of consent debates, Indian nationalist reformers publicly assumed the mantle of being the instrument of modernity in India.[185]

Finally, whereas Sinha argues that the colonial government 'first tried dilatory tactics to kill' the bill 'prematurely' or opposed it until the eve of its passing in September 1929 – Andrea Major counters Sinha's arguments by highlighting that the 'assumption of homogenous colonial opposition to the measure simplifies the state's position, however'.[186] Judge and Arya Samajist, Rai Bahadur Har Bilas Sarda's Hindu Child Marriage Bill (asking for age of consent to be fixed at 12 for girls and boys at 14 years along with the annulment of child marriages for Hindus) in February 1927 bore little resemblance to the Child Marriage Restraint Act (CMRA) of September 1929. She argues that the redrafting of the Sarda Bill to alter 'invalidation' of child marriage clause to 'penalization' of adults who organised child marriages, circulation of the bill and the Joshi Committee surveys – did not amount to blocking the Bill. She highlights that ultimately the colonial state deployed an entire gamut of strategies from active support to delaying the final Bill in order to curb public agitations and ensure its own survival.[187] The Child Marriage Restraint Act (CMRA) of 1929 provided the definition of a child for females as anyone under 14 and for males under 18.[188]

In conclusion, this chapter focused on the relatively underexplored problem of breastfeeding in early motherhood in relation to the 'maturity'/'immaturity' of the female body as well as her capacity for sexual intercourse and motherhood, as discussed in the age of consent debates (1890s–1920s). It examined the 'women's question' in relation with the nation as mother and mother-goddess, *Bharat Mata* (or Mother India) in the context of colonial Bengal, and concluded with a look at the traditional birthing and infant feeding practices as discussed in Mayo's *Mother India*. Mayo explained that she had 'chosen the title deliberately to awaken the women of India by contrasting the actual treatment of women with their glorification in nationalist discourse'.[189] The chapter also explored the nationalist-feminist consensus on child marriage and premature motherhood as health concerns, which led to the passing of the CMRA in 1929, and thereby the definition of childhood according to age across communities.[190]

Notes

1 See Dagmar Engels, 'The Age of Consent Act of 1891: Colonial Ideology in Bengal', *South Asia Research*, vol. 3, no. 2, 1983, pp. 107–131; Tanika Sarkar, 'Rhetoric against Age of Consent: Resisting Colonial Reason and Death of a Child-Wife', *Economic and Political Weekly*, vol. 28, no. 36, 1993, pp 1869–1878; Tanika Sarkar, 'A Prehistory of Rights: The Age of Consent Debate in Colonial Bengal', *Feminist Studies*, vol. 26, no. 3, 2000, 'Points of Departure: India and the South Asian Diaspora', pp. 601–622; Mrinalini Sinha, *Colonial Masculinity The 'Manly Englishman' and the 'Effeminate Bengali' in the Late Nineteenth Century* (Manchester: Manchester University Press, 1995); and Ishita Pande, *Medicine, Race and Liberalism in British Bengal Symptoms of Empire* (London: Routledge, 2010), among others.

2 Margaret Lock and Vinh-Kim Nguyen, *An Anthropology of Biomedicine* (Chichester: Wiley-Blackwell, 2010), p. 118.

3 From Letter 'Dated Calcutta, the 9th August 1890 From – Surgeon – Major C. H. Joubert, Professor of Midwifery, Medical College, Calcutta, To – The Inspector-General of Civil Hospitals, Bengal', Government of Bengal, Judicial Proceedings, June 1893, West Bengal State Archives, WBSA.

4 'Child-Wives' in 'Extracts from the Indian Medical Gazette for September and October 1890' in Home Department, Judicial Branch, October 1890 Proceeding, File 211 National Archives of India (NAI). Also, see *Pande, Medicine, Race and Liberalism in British Bengal*, p. 163; Sinha, *Colonial Masculinity*, p. 158.

5 David Arnold, '"An ancient race outworn": malaria and race in colonial India, 1860–1930', in Waltraud Ernst and Bernard Harris (eds), *Race, Science and Medicine, 1700–1960* (London: Routledge, 1999), pp. 134–138. Arnold explores the concepts of 'race' and class in relation to the debilitating effects of malaria in colonial Bengal. Also, see Pradip Kumar Datta, '"Dying Hindus": Production of Hindu Communal Common Sense in Early 20th Century Bengal', *Economic and Political Weekly*, vol. 28, no. 25, 1993, pp. 1305–19.

6 Eleanor F. Rathbone, *Child Marriage: The Indian Minotaur. An Object-Lesson from the Past to the Future* (London: George Allen & Unwin, 1934), pp. 73–74 cited in Ishita Pande, *Sex, Law, and the Politics of Age Child Marriage in India, 1891–1937* (Cambridge: Cambridge University Press, 2020), p. 78.

7 On the 'girl-child/woman', Ruby Lal, 'Recasting the Women's Question the Girl-Child/Woman in the Colonial Encounter', *Interventions*, vol. 10, no. 3, 2008, p. 322; on the idea of personhood, including legal personhood, Tanika Sarkar, 'A Prehistory of Rights', pp. 601–622.

8 Dr. Kenneth McLeod, 'Nubile Age of Females in India' in 'Extracts from the *Indian Medical Gazette* for September and October 1890', File 211 in 'The age of consent under section 375 of the Indian Penal Code. Substitution for the word "ten" the word "twelve" in section 375 of the Indian Penal Code', Home Department, Judicial Branch October 1890, Files 210 to 213; National Archives of India (NAI). Also see K. Mcleod, 'Nubile Age of Females in India' cited in 'Transactions of Medical Societies', *Indian Medical Gazette*, vol. 25, no. 9, 1890, p. 279.

9 Bolye Chunder Sen, 'The Nubile Age of Females in India Physiologically Treated', *British Gynaecological Journal*, vol. VI, no. 24, 1891, p. 612. Also, sections of this article cited in 'Transactions of Medical Societies, The Calcutta Medical Society, October 1890' in 'Extracts from the Indian Medical Gazette for September and October 1890', File 211 in 'The age of consent under section 375 of the Indian Penal Code. Substitution for the word "ten" the word "twelve" in section 375 of the Indian Penal Code', Home Department, Judicial Branch, October 1890, Files 210 to 213; NAI. On menstruation and child marriage in Bengali periodicals like *Chikitsa Sammilani*, for example, Shri Pulinchandra Sanyal (M.B.), 'Striloker Mashik Rajahshrab ba Ritu', *Chikitsa Sammilani*, vol. 4, 1294 Bengali year, c. 1887, pp. 53–59, 101–103. Also see Shri Pulinchandra Sanyal (M.B.), 'Bibaha Bichaar', *Chikitsa Sammilani*, 1294 Bengali year, c. 1887, pp. 193–197, 261–270, 344–348. For a discussion about *daktar* Sanyal's, editor of *Chikitsa Sammilani* from 1887–1890, contradictory arguments on child marriage, see Swapna M. Banerjee, *Fathers in a Motherland Imagining Fatherhood in Colonial India* (New Delhi, Oxford University Press, 2022), pp. 118–119. Banerjee translates 'Bibaha Bichaar' as 'Scrutinizing Marriage Practices'. Moreover, it is interesting to note that in early twentieth century Bengal, menstruation continued to figure in medical writings in connection with anxieties about conception, gender, and even the morality of the child, see brief article S. P. Dutt, 'Susantaner Asha', *Chikitsak Bandhab*, vol 1, no 3, Chaitra 1330 (1924), pp. 9–10. Translation mine.

10 Sarkar, 'A Prehistory of Rights', pp. 608, 612.

11 In the 1890s, the age of consent debates were primarily between men, however, women's voices were also heard – see Government of Bengal, Judicial Proceedings, June 1893, WBSA; and in petitions, for example, 'Memorial from certain "women living in India" praying that the Age of Consent may

be raised to 14 years', Home Department, Judicial Branch, February 1891, Files 155 to 159, NAI; Padma Anagol-McGinn, 'The Age of Consent 1891 Reconsidered Women's Perspectives and Participation in in the Child-Marriage Controversy in India', *South Asia Research*, vol. 12 no. 2, 1992, pp. 100–118. By the 1920s, participation of women activists and women's organisations in India meant that the Child Marriage Restraint Act could not be publicised as merely an act of benevolence of colonialism, colonial officials, and indigenous male reformers – see Pande, *Medicine, Race and Liberalism in British Bengal*, especially p. 232n97; see also Mrinalini Sinha, 'Introduction', in Mrinalini Sinha (ed), *Mother India* by Katherine Mayo. Edited with an Introduction by Mrinalini Sinha (Ann Arbor, MI: University of Michigan Press, 2000, 1998), pp. 1–62; and Mrinalini Sinha, 'Refashioning Mother India: Feminism and Nationalism in Late-Colonial India', *Feminist Studies, Points of Departure: India and the South Asian Diaspora*, vol. 26, no. 3, 2000, pp. 623–644.

12 Lock and Nguyen, *An Anthropology of Biomedicine*, p. 119.

13 Sekhar Bandopadhyay, *Caste, Culture and Hegemony Social Dominance in Colonial Bengal* (New Delhi: Sage Publications, 2004), p. 167.

14 Andrea Major, 'Mediating Modernity: Colonial State, Indian Nationalism, and the Renegotiation of the 'Civilizing Mission' in the Indian Child Marriage Debate of 1927–1932', in Carey A. Watt and Michael Mann (eds), *Civilizing Missions in Colonial and Postcolonial South Asia* (Delhi: Anthem Press, 2012), p. 166

15 Ibid., pp. 166–167.

16 For details see Sarkar, 'Rhetoric Against Age of Consent', p. 1870. On the Rukhmabai case, see Sudhir Chandra, 'Rukhmabai: Debate over Woman's Right to Her Person' *Economic and Political Weekly*, vol. 31, no. 44, 1996, pp. 2937–2947; Antoinette Burton, 'From Child Bride to "Hindoo Lady": Rukhmabai and the Debate on Sexual Respectability in Imperial Britain', *The American Historical Review*, vol. 103, no. 4, 1998, pp. 1119–1146; and Kanika Sharma, Laura Lammasniemi, and Tanika Sarkar, 'Dadaji Bhikajiv Rukhmabai (1886) ILR 10 Bom 301: Rewriting Consent and Conjugal Relations in Colonial India', *Indian Law Review*, vol. 5, no. 3, 2021, pp. 265–287, among others.

17 Pande, *Medicine, Race and Liberalism in British Bengal*, p. 157. On the nature of 'degeneration', ibid., pp. 155–156.

18 Ibid., p. 157.

19 Mahendralal Sarkar, "Babu Keshub Chunder Sen's Circular Letter Addressed to Certain Medical Gentlemen of Calcutta and Their Replies Thereto," *Calcutta Journal of Medicine: A Monthly Record of the Medical and Auxiliary Sciences*, vol. 4, no. 7, 1871, p. 251 cited in Ibid., p. 157. His name has also been spelt as Mahendra Lal Sircar. On the Native Marriage Act of 1872, see Pande, *Medicine, Race and Liberalism in British Bengal*, p. 227n37.

20 Keshub Chunder Sen, 'Marriageable Age of Native Girls', *Calcutta Journal of Medicine: A Monthly Record of the Medical and Auxiliary Sciences*, vol. 4, no. 7, 1871, p. 258.

21 Sarkar, 'Babu Keshub Chunder Sen's Circular Letter', p. 251 cited in Pande, *Medicine, Race and Liberalism*, p. 157.

22 Pande, *Medicine, Race and Liberalism in British Bengal*, p. 158.

23 Ibid., p. 155.

24 Ibid., p. 148; also on 'early menarche' and 'sexual precocity' see Supriya Guha, 'The Nature of Woman: Medical Ideas in Colonial Bengal', *Indian Journal of Gender Studies*, vol. 3, no. 1, 1996, pp. 27, 32.

25 See mainly Sinha, *Colonial Masculinity*, pp. 138–180; and Pande, *Medicine, Race and Liberalism in British Bengal*, pp. 151–176.
26 Pande, *Medicine, Race and Liberalism in British Bengal*, p. 160.
27 Ibid.
28 Anagol-McGinn, 'The Age of Consent 1891 Reconsidered', p. 107.
29 Sarkar, 'A Prehistory of Rights', p. 607.
30 Sarkar, 'Rhetoric Against Age of Consent', p. 1870. Also, for a discussion on the subject, see 'The age of consent under section 375 of the Indian Penal Code. Substitution for the word "ten" the word "twelve" in section 375 of the Indian Penal Code', Home Department, Judicial Branch, October 1890, File Nos 210–213, (including 'Notes', pp. 1–24), NAI. On child marriage and the history of emotions, see Ishita Pande, 'Feeling Like a Child: Narratives of Development and the Indian Child/Wife', in Stephanie Olsen (ed), *Childhood, Youth and Emotions in Modern History: National, Colonial and Global Perspectives* (Basingstoke, Hampshire: Palgrave Macmillan, 2015), pp. 35–55.
31 Sarkar, 'Rhetoric Against Age of Consent', p. 1870.
32 Sarkar, 'A Prehistory of Rights', p. 607. Also, on whether meanings of 'puberty' and 'maturity' were interchangeable – see for example, Letter 'Dated Calcutta, the 1st September 1890 From – W. J. Simmons, EsQ., Honorary Secy. Public Health Society of Calcutta To – The Chief Secretary to the Government of Bengal, Judicial Proceedings, Government of Bengal, June 1893, Progs Nos 105–106 File No. J C/17 2, WBSA. On extension of the period of 'childhood', by delaying marriage and the problem of 'precocious sexuality', as an indication of civilisational progress and a higher position on the evolutionary ladder, see discussion in Pande, *Medicine, Race and Liberalism in British Bengal*, p. 167; on childhood, adulthood and sexuality see Pande, 'Feeling Like a Child'.
33 See Letter 'Dated Calcutta, the 9th August 1890 From – Surgeon – Major C. H. Joubert, Professor of Midwifery, Medical College, Calcutta, To – The Inspector-General of Civil Hospitals, Bengal', Government of Bengal, Judicial Proceedings, June 1893, WBSA. Sections of this excerpt have also been cited in Pande, *Medicine, Race and Liberalism in British Bengal*, p. 166. On the heated debates on the problem of marital rape, see Sinha, *Colonial Masculinity*, pp. 160–166; also on age, body and child rape in medico-legal debates on 'difference/indifference', with a specific focus on Norman Chevers' racialised arguments on rape as a 'cultural crime' in colonial India, see Ishita Pande, 'Phulmoni's Body: The Autopsy, the Inquest and the Humanitarian Narrative on Child Rape in India', *South Asian History and Culture*, vol. 4, no. 1, 2013, pp. 9–30, mainly pp. 5–7, 15n6, 16n22.
34 Letter 'Dated Calcutta, the 9th August 1890 From – Surgeon – Major C. H. Joubert, Professor of Midwifery, Medical College, Calcutta, To – The Inspector-General of Civil Hospitals, Bengal', Government of Bengal, Judicial Proceedings, June 1893, WBSA.
35 Excerpt from paragraphs 3 to 8 in Ibid. Also for a discussion of the climatic, socio-cultural and physiological causes of menstruation by Joubert and others, see for instance, Ishita Pande, *Medicine, Race and Liberalism in British Bengal*, 148, 151–174, 183–84.
36 Sarkar, 'Rhetoric Against Age of Consent', p. 1870. Also, see Partha Chatterjee, 'The Nationalist Resolution of the Women's Question', in Kumkum Sangari and Sudesh Vaid (eds), *Recasting Women. Essays in Colonial History* (New Delhi: Kali for Women, 1989), pp. 233–253.

37 Sarkar, 'Rhetoric Against Age of Consent', pp. 1870–1871.
38 Ibid., p. 1870.
39 See Srirupa Prasad's argument on the middle class writing itself in history, Srirupa Prasad, *Cultural Politics of Hygiene in India 1890–1940 Contagions of Feeling* (New York: Palgrave Macmillan, 2015), p. 17.
40 Sarkar, 'A Prehistory of Rights', p. 612.
41 Lal, 'Recasting the Women's Question', p. 322.
42 Letter from Norman Chevers, Dated Medical College, 8 April, 1870 cited in Sen, 'Marriageable Age of Native Girls', p. 260.
43 Paraphrased from Annada Charan Khastagir, *A Treatise on the Science and Practice of Midwifery with Diseases of Children and Women Manab-Jatna Tattva, Dhatribidya, Nabaprasuto Sishu o Stri Jatir Byadhi-Sangraha* (Calcutta: Author, 1878 second ed., first ed. 1868), p. 31. Also see, Bipradas Mukhopadhyay, *Jubati Stri-Jibaner Aadorsho* (Calcutta: Sanyal and Brothers, Bengali year 1296). Title Translation: Young Woman The Purpose of a Woman's Life. Khastagir's work has been also cited in Ranjana Saha, 'Infant Feeding: Child Marriage and "Immature Maternity" in Colonial Bengal, 1890s–1920s', *Proceedings of the Indian History Congress* Platinum Jubilee (75th) Session 2014, 2015, p. 709. It is of particular relevance to note that he also discusses the problem of female masturbation, see Meredith Borthwick, *The Changing Role of Women in Bengal, 1849–1905* (Princeton: Princeton University Press, 1984), pp. 135–136. On ' "scientific" marriage manuals' on the rise at the time – Ibid., p. 134. Secondary sources on masculinity, *brahmacharya*, wrestling and milking of cows as similar activities due to amount of bodily strength required, milk (as semen of the god of fire, Agni) and its androgynous qualities and the importance of types of food for diet and disposition in Ayurveda, see Joseph S. Alter, *The Wrestler's Body Identity and Ideology in North India* (Berkeley: University of California Press, 1992), pp. 100–128, also on diet and masculinity, see Parama Roy, *Alimentary Tracts Appetites, Aversions, and the Postcolonial* (Durham: Duke University Press, 2010), pp. 75–114. Khastagir's arguments on female modesty and motherhood also ties up neatly with discussion on female modesty in Chatterjee, 'The Nationalist Resolution of the Women's Question', p. 242. On the nationalist 'glorification of motherhood' and significance of the 'motherhood archetype' see Jasodhara Bagchi, 'Representing Nationalism: Ideology of Motherhood in Colonial Bengal', *Economic and Political Weekly*, vol. 25, no. 42/43, 1990, pp. WS65–WS71; and Judy Whitehead, 'Modernising the motherhood archetype: Public health models and the Child Marriage Restraint Act of 1929', *Contributions to Indian sociology*, vol. 29, nos. 1 & 2, 1995, pp. 187–209.
44 Pande, *Medicine, Race and Liberalism in British Bengal*, pp. 157, 174.
45 Sarkar, 'A Prehistory of Rights', p. 615. Also, similar discussion in Engels, 'The Age of Consent Act of 1891', pp. 111, 116; Pande, *Medicine, Race and Liberalism in British Bengal*, 162–173, among others.
46 On questions about the 'subsidiary issues', see Sarkar, 'A Prehistory of Rights', p. 615.
47 Ibid.
48 Sinha, *Colonial Masculinity*, pp. 170–171.
49 Gangaprasad Mukhopadhyay, *Matrisiksha Arthat Garbhabasthay o Sutikagrihey Matar ebong Ballabastha Porjonto Santaner Sasthyarakkha Bishayak Upodesh* (Calcutta: United Press, second ed. 1902), p. 3. Title Translation: Educating the Mother Meaning Healthcare Advice During Pregnancy and in

the Lying-Room for the Mother and the Infant till Childhood. *Santan and ballabastha* mean child and childhood, for definitions see Shri Sailedra Biswas, *Samsad Bengali-English Dictionary* Revised by Sri Subodhchadra Sengupta (Calcutta: Sahitya Samsad, 1968), pp. 895, 1174–1175. However, it has to be borne in mind that the legal definition of a child was based on the age of consent at the time of this edition which was 12).

50 Mukhopadhyay, *Matrisiksha*, pp. 2–3.
51 Ibid., p. 234.
52 Ibid., p. 241.
53 Ibid., p. 236.
54 Ibid.
55 Ibid.
56 Ibid., p. 238; also see Ranjana Saha, 'Milk, mothering & meanings: Infant feeding in colonial Bengal', *Women's Studies International Forum*, vol. 60, 2017, p. 100.
57 He was a member of the Calcutta Medical Society, Licentiate in Medicine and Surgery (L.M.S.), Assistant-Surgeon and Teacher of Medicine at the Campbell Medical School, Calcutta.
58 Bolye Chunder Sen, 'The Nubile Age of Females in India Physiologically Treated', *British Gynaecological Journal*, vol. VI, no. 24, 1891, p. 610. Also, sections of this article cited in 'Transactions of Medical Societies, The Calcutta Medical Society, October 1890' in 'Extracts from the Indian Medical Gazette for September and October 1890', File 211 in 'The age of consent under section 375 of the Indian Penal Code. Substitution for the word "ten" the word "twelve" in section 375 of the Indian Penal Code', Home Department, Judicial Branch, October 1890, Files 210 to 213; NAI.
59 Ibid., p. 610. Also, 'Indian pathologies' especially early menstruation and 'pathological' sexuality were often associated with the 'culture of child marriage', see mainly Pande, *Medicine, Race and Liberalism in British Bengal*, pp. 155, 158, 227n32.
60 Sen, 'The Nubile Age of Females in India Physiologically Treated', p. 608.
61 Ibid., 612.
62 A very similar discussion by Keshub Chunder Sen on the age of consent issue in relation with the idea of racial degeneration along 'true physiological grounds' by apparently impartial and objective 'medical men' was cited by Mahendralal Sarkar in the *Calcutta Journal of Medicine* in 1871. Sarkar, 'Babu Keshub Chunder Sen's Circular Letter', p. 252, in Ishita Pande, *Medicine, Race and Liberalism in British Bengal*, p. 158. In this discussion Pande includes Mahendralal Sircar, 'The Earliest Marriageable Age', *Calcutta Journal of Medicine*, vol. IV, no. 7, 1871, pp. 251–256; and also Letters by Keshub Chunder Sen and others titled 'Marriageable Age of Native Girls', *Calcutta Journal of Medicine*, vol. IV, no. 7, 1871, pp 258–273. Discussion on 'physiology' and child marriage also in Letter 'Dated Baidyanath, the 4th March 1891 From – Dr. Mahendra Lal Sircar To – The Chief Secretary to the Government of Bengal', Proceeding no. 213 File J 7-A/2 91, Government of Bengal, Judicial Proceedings, June 1893. See Pande, *Medicine, Race and Liberalism in British Bengal*, pp. 157–159.
63 Sen, 'The Nubile Age of Females in India Physiologically Treated', p. 612.
64 Ibid., p. 615. B. C. Sen understood refusal of the breast as resulting from weakness in infants from early motherhood. Refusing the breast was earlier associated with the customary practices of 'exposure of infants' in a basket hung up on a tree due to fears of malignant spirits – already discussed in Chapter 3.

65 Ibid., p. 616.
66 Guha, 'The Nature of Woman', p. 32.
67 Indira Chowdhury-Sengupta 'The Effeminate and the Masculine: Nationalism and the Concept of Race in Colonial Bengal', in Peter Robb (ed), *The Concept of Race in South Asia* (New Delhi: Oxford University Press, 1995), pp. 284–286.
68 Uma Chakravarti, 'Whatever Happened to the Vedic Dasi? Orientalism, Nationalism and a Script for the Past' in Sangari and Vaid, *Recasting Women*, pp. 27–87 in Chowdhury-Sengupta 'The Effeminate and the Masculine', p. 292.
69 Chowdhury-Sengupta 'The Effeminate and the Masculine', p. 292.
70 Yogindranath Sarkar, *Bande Mataram* (Calcutta: n.p., 1908, sixth ed.), p. 136 in Chowdhury-Sengupta 'The Effeminate and the Masculine', pp. 292–293.
71 Sinha, *Colonial Masculinity*, p. 41
72 Ibid., p. 44.
73 Ibid., pp. 19–20.
74 Pande, *Medicine, Race and Liberalism in British Bengal*, pp. 22–23, 69.
75 Surendranath Goswami, *Arya Dhatribidya. A Treatise on the Ayurvedic System of Midwifery. With Sanskrit text and English translation. Part I.* (Kumarkhali: Author., 1899), p. 24.
76 Kabiraj Srijukta Girijabhushan Ray Sengupta, 'Sishu-Palan' ('Child-Rearing'), *Janmabhumi*, Ashar or Monsoon season, Bengali Year 1317 or c.e. 1910 in Pradip Basu (ed), *Samayiki Purano Samayik Patrer Prabondho Sankalan, Ditiyo Khanda: Griha and Paribar* (Kolkata: Ananda Publishers Private Limited, 2009), mainly pp. 713–715. Title Translation: *Journal on Current Topics Collection of Old Essays from Periodicals* Second Volume: Home and Family.
77 Chandra Chakraberty, *National Problems* (Calcutta: Ram Chandra Chakraberty, 1923), p. 75. On timely breastfeeding and charts on composition of breast milk and various kinds of animal milk, see Chandra Chakraberty, *Infant Feeding and Hygiene* (Calcutta, Ramchandra Chakraberty, MA, 1923), pp. 4, 6, 8.
78 Ibid., p. 96.
79 Ibid., p. 99.
80 Ibid.
81 Sanjam Ahluwalia, *Reproductive Restraints Birth Control in India 1877–1947* (Ranikhet: Permanent Black, 2008), pp. 37–40; and on feminist challenges to the nationalist glorification of motherhood, Ibid., pp. 102–105.
82 On the new nationalist consensus on the 'women's question' and the discourse of liberal Indian feminism', see Sinha, 'Refashioning Mother India', pp. 623–44.
83 For details see Whitehead, 'Modernising the motherhood archetype', p. 201.
84 "Written Statement of Miss Jyotirmoyi Ganguli, M.A., 6, Guru Prosad Chaudhuri Lane, Calcutta" and "Oral Evidence of Miss Jyotirmoyi Ganguli, M.A., 6, Guru Prosad Chaudhuri Lane, Calcutta (*Calcutta 18th December 1928.*)," in *Age of Consent Committee Evidence 1928–1929* Volume VI *Oral Evidence and Written Statements of Witnesses from Bengal Presidency* (Calcutta: Government of India Central Publication Branch, 1929), pp. 11, 14. She also highlighted that her argument about calcium deficiency was sound, based on contemporary ongoing research on the subject conducted by Dr. Charu Chandra Roy, Dr. N. C. Bhattacharji, and Dr. Ananda Kumar Sen. Also, Ganguli's mother provided her information about cases of child maternity under 15 with difficult delivery where physical damage occurred to the mother and the children who survived were 'always weak'. Ibid., pp. 14–15. Also, the fact that

'very weak' children were born from child mothers belonging to 'Bhadralog' families mostly of ages 14–17 usually as a general problem among patients who visited the Chittaranjan Seva Sadan maternity hospital in South Calcutta, founded in 1926, has been confirmed by Mrs. Latika Basu, Secretary of Chittaranjan Seva Sadan. 'Oral Evidence of Mrs. Latika Basu, Chittaranjan Seva Sadan, 148, Russa Road (South Calcutta). (*Calcutta 19th December 1928*)', *Age of Consent Committee Evidence* Volume VI, p. 68. Jyotirmoyee Ganguly (her name has been spelt like this as well) also chaired a Youth Conference in Jessore where papers on *sateetva* or women's chastity were discussed. *Ananda Bazar Patrika* editorial and report, 19 June 1929 on the Youth Conference, Kalia, Jessore in Sabyasachi Bhattacharya, *The Defining Moments in Bengal 1920–1947* (New Delhi: Oxford University Press, 2014), pp. 47–48. On *sateetva* as part of moral rhetoric in manuals for educating housewives among other issues, see mainly Ibid., pp. 49–52.

85 Saha, 'Milk, Mothering and Meanings', p. 100.

86 Whitehead, 'Modernising the motherhood archetype', p. 199.

87 Ibid., pp. 187–190.

88 Ibid.

89 Anshu Malhotra, 'The Body as a Metaphor for the Nation Caste, Masculinity, and Femininity in the *Satyarth Prakash* of Swami Dayananda Sarasvati', in Avril A. Powell and Siobhan Lambert-Hurley (eds), *Rhetoric and Reality Gender and the Colonial Experience in South Asia* (Oxford: Oxford University Press, 2006), pp. 122, 143–145. On Amar Nath Dutt's, President of the Arya Samaj, Burdwan, communalised anxieties regarding the wellbeing of the Bengali-Hindu 'race' especially in relation to conditions in eastern Bengal which had a Muslim majority and the idea of *Swaraj*, see 'Written Statement of Mr. Amar Nath Datt, B.A., B.L., M.L.A., Advocate, High Court, dated 13th August 1928', and 'Oral evidence of Mr. Amar Nath Dutt, M.L.A., Advocate, High Court (Delhi, 11th October 1928)' in *Age of Consent Committee Evidence 1928–1929 Volume VI*, pp. 1–11.

90 Malhotra, 'The Body as a Metaphor for the Nation', pp. 131–137.

91 For details see Alter, *The Wrestler's Body*, p. 148 in Ibid., p. 145.

92 Dayananda Sarasvati, *Light of Truth*, (or an English Translation of the *Satyarth Prakash* by Dr. Charanjiva Bharadwaja), (United Provinces of Agra and Oudh: Arya Pratinidhi Sabha, second ed. 1915), pp. 21–22, 108, cited in Ibid., p. 144.

93 Malhotra, 'The Body as a Metaphor for the Nation', pp. 122, 143–145.

94 *Sanjivani*, 14 February, 1891 in Report on Native Papers for the week ending the 21st February 1891, No. 8 of 1891, *Report on Native Newspapers Bengal, January – June, 1891*, NAI.

95 Letter 'Dated Calcutta, the 9th March 1891. From – Babu Juggobundhu Bose, M.D., To The Secretary, British Indian Association', Bengal Judicial Proceedings, June 1893, WBSA; and 'Appendix B Note by Dr. Juggobandhu Bose, M. D. on the "Age of Consent Bill" Showing that it is uncalled for even on physiological grounds', in *An Appeal to England to Save India from the Wrong and the Shame of the "Age of Consent" Act* (Published by Báli Sádharáni Sabhá, 25th April, 1891), p. 11.

96 For details see discussion on child maternity see 'Dr. Juggobundhu Bose's Opinion on the Age of Consent Bill', Order No. 217 File J 7-A/2 95, Government of Bengal, Judicial Proceedings, June 1893. Also, Letter 'Dated Calcutta, the 9th March 1891. From – Babu Juggobundhu Bose, M.D., To The Secretary, British

Indian Association', Bengal Judicial Proceedings, June 1893. Also, see 'Appendix B Note by Dr. Juggobandhu Bose', p. ii. His name has been spelt differently in both cases.

97 Letter 'Dated Calcutta, the 9th March 1891. From – Babu Juggobundhu Bose, M.D., To The Secretary, British Indian Association', Bengal Judicial Proceedings, June 1893, WBSA. Also, see 'Appendix B Note by Dr. Juggobandhu Bose', p. 12.

98 Letter 'Dated Calcutta, the 9th March 1891. From – Babu Juggobundhu Bose, M.D., To The Secretary, British Indian Association', Bengal Judicial Proceedings, June 1893, WBSA; and 'Appendix B Note by Dr. Juggobandhu Bose', p. 11.

99 *Samaya* March 5th 1891 in 'Report on Native Newspapers for the Week ending the 14th March 1891', No 11 of 1891 in *Report on Native Newspapers Bengal, January – June, 1891*, NAI.

100 For details, see Pande, *Medicine, Race and Liberalism in British Bengal*, p. 164.

101 Sinha, *Colonial Masculinity*, p. 159.

102 Paraphrased from Haranath Ray, *Midwife's Vade-Mecum*, p. 354 in *Sanjivani* (14 February 1891), cited in 'Report on Native Papers for the Week Ending the 21st February 1891', No. 8 of 1891 in *Report on Native Newspapers Bengal, January – June 1891*, NAI. About the book, see Haranath Ray, *Midwife's Vade-Mecum. Dhatrisikkha Sangraha Ba Garbha Chikitsa Bishaya Pancha Bingshoti batsarer pariksha o adhayaner fal Chikitsak, chatra, dhatri, sikkhita strilok o grihaswamidiger nimitto sangrihito o o birochito* (Calcutta: Shri Binod Kishore Ray, 1887). [His name was spelt as Haranath Ray in his book]. Title Translation: Midwife's Vade-Mecum an Anthology on Midwifery Or Obstetrics A Result of Twenty-Five Years of Examination and Deep Study About Obstetrics. Compiled and Composed for the Doctor, Student, Midwife, Educated Women and Married Men.

103 Ibid.

104 Ray, *Midwife's Vade-Mecum*, p. 355. On related arguments about 'Hindu wombs' and the threat of 'Muslim progeny', see Charu Gupta, 'Hindu Wombs, Muslim Progeny: The Numbers Game and Shifting Debates on Widow Remarriage in Uttar Pradesh, 1890s–1930s', in Sarah Hodges (eds), *Reproductive Health in India. History, Politics, Controversies* (Hyderabad: Orient Longman, 2006), pp. 167–198.

105 On the role of *vyam* to prevent diseases as a motto popular among *daktars* including Sundari Mohan Das in late nineteenth and early twentieth century Bengal, see Mukharji, *Nationalizing the Body*, pp. 119–124.

106 Ray, *Midwife's Vade-Mecum*, p. 352. Translation mine.

107 Hurro Nath Raya, Letter '5, Sukeas Street, February 1891', in the section 'Homeopathic Practitioners' (Appendix B) 'Medical Opinions on the Alleged Cruelty to Tender Aged Wives by Their Husbands'. Appended to the Full Proceedings of a Public Meeting held on 22 January 1891 at the Residence of the late Maharajah Kamal Krishna Deb, Bahadur, Sabhabazar Rajbati, Calcutta, to protest against the Age of Consent Bill. (Calcutta: The Sabhabazar Standing Committee, 1891), p. 48.

108 The contradictory nature of his statements is pointed out in the newspaper *Sanjivani* (14 February 1891), cited in 'Report on Native Papers for the Week Ending the 21st February 1891', No. 8 of 1891 in *Report on Native Newspapers Bengal, January – June 1891*, NAI. In 1928–29, on the opposite argument of child marriage and premature maternity making 'a nation of weaklings and

dwarfs, ailing and effeminate' and the 'inability' of the child-mother to 'supply her baby with milk'– see Dr. Jadavji Hansraj (D.O.M.S., England) of Bombay, 'Written Statement, dated 12th August 1928, of Dr. Jadavji Hansraj, D.O.M.S., (Eng.), J.P. President, and Mr. Premji Chaturbhuj, Honororary Secretary of the Bhatia Mitra Mandal, 203–5, Horby Road, Fort, Bombay' in *Age of Consent Committee Evidence*, Volume III Oral Evidence and Written Statements of Witnesses from the Bombay Presidency (Continued – Bombay and Poona) and the Central Provinces and Berar (Calcutta: Government of India Central Publication Branch, 1929), p. 150; also cited in Katherine Mayo, *Volume II* (London: Jonathan Cape Ltd., 1931), pp. 140–141.

109 *The Dacca Prákásh*', of the 15th February 1891 in Report on Native Papers for the week ending the 21st February 1891, No. 8 of 1891, *Report on Native Newspapers Bengal, January – June, 1891*, NAI.

110 Ibid.

111 Ibid.

112 'Written Statement of Mr. Charu Chandra Mitra, Attorney-at-law, 5 Hastings Street, Calcutta' in *Age of Consent Committee Evidence 1928–1929 Volume VI*, pp. 21–22. Excerpt on Klienwa'chter and E. B. Wales have been cited from Havelock Ellis' *Psychology of Sex*, Vol. VI, Chapter XII cited in Ibid., pp. 21–22. It is cited in the section on his oral evidence that Mr. Charu Chandra Mitra, Attorney-at-law, Calcutta had been practising for 32 years by 1928 and he had objected to age of consent being raised in 1891, 1925 and again in 1928–1929 respectively. Mitra provided examples of, what he considered, successful child maternity from his own family and reasons why Hindu child marriage was a valid practice in contemporary Bengal alongside recommendations of different types of education for boys and girls as girls needed education primarily to become 'good mothers', see 'Oral evidence of Mr. Charu Chandra Mitra, Attorney-at-law, Calcutta (*Calcutta 18th December, 1928*)' in *Age of Consent Committee Evidence 1928–1929* Volume VI, pp. 23, 30, 36.

113 'Oral evidence of Mr. Charu Chandra Mitra', p. 27.

114 Pande, *Medicine, Race and Liberalism in British Bengal*, p. 165.

115 Dr. Bidhu Mukhi Bose cited in 'Chapter VIII. – Extracts From Papers Written by Qualified Doctors and Nurses', in *Improvements of the Conditions of Childbirth in India Including a Special Report on the Work of the Victoria Memorial Scholarships Fund during the past Fifteen Years and Papers Written by Medical Women and qualified Midwives* (Calcutta: Superintendent Government Printing, India, 1918), pp. 150–151.

116 Dagmar F. Curjel M.D. (Glas), W.M.S., 'The Weight at Birth of Infants in India', *Indian Journal of Medical Research*, 1920–21, cited in Margaret Ida Balfour and Ruth Young, *The Work of Medical Women in India* With a foreword by Dame Mary Scharlieb (London: Humphrey Milford Oxford University Press, 1929), pp. 174–175.

117 'Oral Evidence of Dr. (Mrs) Edith Ghosh representative of Bengal Presidency Council of Women (*Calcutta 19 December 1928*)', in *Age of Consent Committee Evidence 1928–1929* Volume VI, pp. 41–42.

118 'Written Statement, dated 11th August 1928, of C. I. Remfry (Mrs. Doglas Remfry), Acting Honorary Secretary, Bengal Presidency Council of Women, for and on behalf of the Committee, 2, Victoria Terrace, Calcutta', in *Age of Consent Committee Evidence* Volume VI, pp. 37–38.

119 Ahluwalia, *Reproductive Restraints*, p. 94.

120 Ibid.

121 Ibid.
122 Major, 'Mediating Modernity', pp. 165–189, and Sinha 'Refashioning Mother India'.
123 Bagchi, 'Representing Nationalism', p. WS68.
124 Ibid., p. WS65.
125 Ibid., pp. WS65–WS66.
126 Ibid., p. WS66.
127 Ibid., p. WS68–WS69.
128 Ibid., p. WS70.
129 Ibid.
130 Ibid.
131 Ibid., p. WS66.
132 Ibid. 'It is the *Markandeya Puranas* that provides the glorification of the goddess (*Devi mahatmya*) in the form of Durga or Chandi. This is the form in which she is supposed to protect her devotees from all troubles (*durgatinashini*)'. See Ibid., p. WS67. 'Shakti is also manifested in the form of Mahakali, since she embodies the eternal time (*kala*) in her. It is as kala that she not only destroys but creates. From her flow the vibrating dance of creation. It is this all destructive Shakti that controls the creative powers in the cult of Kali worship'. See Ibid.
133 Swami Vivekananda, *Complete Works*, vol. 8 (Advaita Ashram, Mayavati; tenth ed, 1978, 1951), p. 57 in Ibid., p. WS68.
134 Bagchi, 'Representing Nationalism', p. WS66.
135 Ibid., p. WS69. For a discussion on Indo-Asian cosmosophy with its many gods and goddesses encompassing ancient religions, iconography and architecture across Asia, see Anupa Pande and Parul Pandya Dhar (eds), *Cultural Interface of India with Asia Religion, Art and Architecture* (New Delhi: D. K. Printworld (P) Ltd and National Museum Institute, 2004). Also, see Upinder Singh and Parul Pandey Dhar (eds), *Asian Encounters Exploring Connected Histories* (Delhi: Oxford University Press, 2014).
136 See details in Sumathi Ramaswamy, *The Goddess and the Nation Mapping Mother India* (Durham: Duke University Press, 2010), pp. 52–53.
137 Ibid., p. 22.
138 For a detailed discussion, see Ibid., pp. 22–24.
139 Ibid., pp. 22–23.
140 Ibid., p. 70.
141 Ibid., p. 112.
142 Ibid., pp. 112–13.
143 Ibid., p. 113.
144 Ibid.
145 Ibid.
146 Tanika Sarkar, 'Nationalist Iconography: Image of Women in 19th Century Bengali Literature', *Economic & Political Weekly*, vol. 22, no. 47, 1987, pp. 2011–2012.
147 Ibid., p. 2011.
148 Ibid.
149 Sugata Bose, *The Nation as Mother and Other Visions of Nationhood* (Gurgaon, Haryana: Penguin Viking, An imprint of Penguin Random House, 2017), p. 6. For details of this discussion, see Bipin Chandra Pal, *The Soul of India: A Constructive Study of Indian Thoughts and Ideals* (Calcutta: Yugayatri Prakashak, 4th edition, 1958), pp. 102–05, 108–09 cited in Bose, *The Nation as Mother and Other Visions*, p. 6. On nationalist iconography emphasising the

'divinity' of *Bharat Mata* by deliberately ignoring the 'mortal mother' image – see Ramaswamy's arguments discussed earlier in this section – 'Mother India' and Childcare.

150 Sarkar, 'Nationalist Iconography', p. 2011.
151 Ibid.
152 Ibid.
153 Chatterjee, 'The Nationalist Resolution of the Women's Question', p. 248.
154 Mrinalini Sinha, 'Gender in the Critiques of Colonialism and Nationalism Locating the "Indian Woman"', in Sumit Sarkar and Tanika Sarkar (eds), *Women and Social Reform in Modern India* Volume Two (Ranikhet: Permanent Black, 2007), p. 217.
155 Sarkar, 'Nationalist Iconography', p. 2012.
156 Ibid., 2012.
157 Sinha, 'Refashioning Mother India', p. 625.
158 Ibid.
159 Ibid., p. 626.
160 Sinha, 'Gender in the Critiques of Colonialism and Nationalism', p. 225.
161 Ibid., 224–226. On idea of women's place in the home combined with suffrage demands by Naidu, see Anupama Roy, *Gendered Citizenship Historical and Conceptual Explorations* (Hyderabad: Orient Longman Private Limited, 2005), pp. 164–165.
162 Sinha, 'Gender in the Critiques of Colonialism and Nationalism', p. 225.
163 Ibid., p. 226.
164 Ibid.
165 Ibid. Also, it needs to be noted that Naidu was actually an unconventional and adventurous figure who contributed enormously to the Indian National Movement. She participated in the freedom struggle, travelled both as a spokesperson for the Indian National Congress and as an outstanding extempore orator and poet herself across India and abroad. She participated in the Civil Disobedience, Non-cooperation, Salt Satyagraha, and Quit India movements. In post-Independence India, she also became the first Governor of the United Provinces (now Uttar Pradesh). For details, see Makarand R. Paranjape, *Making India: Colonialism, National Culture and the Afterlife of Indian English Authority* (London: Springer, 2013), pp. 163–193.
166 Mrinalini Sinha (ed), *Mother India* by Katherine Mayo. Edited with an Introduction by Mrinalini Sinha (Ann Arbor: The University of Michigan Press, 2000, 1998), pp. 137–151.
167 Sinha, *Mother India* by Katherine Mayo, p. 25.
168 Ibid., pp. 138, 141. Also, see Supriya Guha, 'A History of the Medicalisation of Childbirth in Bengal in the Late Nineteenth and Twentieth Centuries', Unpublished PhD Thesis, 1996, University of Calcutta, pp. 26, 114–115; and Supriya Guha, 'Midwifery in Colonial India The Role of Traditional Birth Attendants in Colonial India', *Wellcome History*, no. 28, Spring, 2–3, 2005, Wellcome Trust, pp. 2–3.
169 Sinha, 'Refashioning Mother India', p. 623.
170 Sinha, *Mother India* by Katherine Mayo, pp. 138, 140–143.
171 Chowdhri highlighted that such an experience of confinement and childbirth could be improved by ensuring:

    1 That legislation should forbid the practice of untrained dais.
    2 That centres should be opened for the training of indigenous dais.
    3 Appointment of trained dais by municipalities.

4 Supervision of these by women doctors. See Mrs. Chowdhri, Sub-Assistant Surgeon, Barabanki cited in 'Chapter VIII. – Extracts From Papers Written by Qualified Doctors and Nurses', in *Improvements of the conditions of childbirth in India including a special report on the Work of the Victoria memorial scholarships fund during the past fifteen years and papers written by medical women and qualified midwives*, Calcutta: Superintendent Government Printing, India, 1918), pp. 151–152.

172 Edris Griffin, Nursing Sister, Health Visitor, Delhi, Chapter VII. – Papers Written by qualified midwives – Miss Patch, Miss Griffin, Mrs. Vonwein in *Improvements of the conditions of childbirth in India including a special report on the Work of the Victoria memorial scholarships fund during the past fifteen years and papers written by medical women and qualified midwives* (Calcutta: Superintendent Government Printing, India, 1918), p. 143; also see Edris Griffin in *National Health*, Oct. 1925, p. 124 cited in Sinha (ed), *Mother India* by Katherine Mayo, pp. 142–143.
173 Griffin, 'Chapter VII. – Papers Written by qualified midwives', p. 143.
174 Ibid., p. 144.
175 Griffin, 'Chapter VII. – Papers Written by qualified midwives', p. 145; also see Ibid., p. 145 cited in Saha, 'Milk, mothering & meanings', p. 99.
176 Sinha, *Mother India* by Katherine Mayo, p. 24.
177 Ibid., p. 29.
178 Ibid.
179 Ibid., p. 27. Also, for a discussion on early marriage in Hinduism see primarily, Mayo, *Volume II*, chapter 'Babies Preferred', pp. 38–48.
180 Sinha, 'Refashioning Mother India', pp. 623–24, 628.
181 Sinha, 'Refashioning Mother India', p. 2, also on 'consensus issue' see Geraldine Forbes, *Women in Modern India* (Cambridge: Cambridge University Press, 1996), pp. 89–90.
182 Sinha, 'Refashioning Mother India', p. 631.
183 Major, 'Mediating Modernity', p. 175.
184 Sinha, 'Refashioning Mother India', p. 630. See for example, Alexander Muddiman, the Home Member of the Government of India, who had announced in 1925 that 'the policy of the government of India was to block the passage of social reform legislations in the assembly'. See note by A. P. Muddiman, 11 July 1927, Home Department, Judicial Proceedings, 382/27, 1927, NAI in Sinha, 'Refashioning Mother India', p. 642n34.
185 Mrinalini Sinha, 'The Lineage of the Indian Modern: Rhetoric, Agency and the Sarda Act in Late Colonial India', in Antoinette Burton (ed), *Gender, Sexuality and Colonial Modernities* (London: Routledge, 1999), p. 207 in Major, 'Mediating Modernity', p. 172.
186 Major, Mediating Modernity', p. 167.
187 See Major, 'Mediating Modernity', pp. 177–185. Also, numerous excerpts have been cited from Legislative Assembly Debates 1927–1929 supporting and criticising raising the age of consent – see Major, 'Mediating Modernity'.
188 Ishita Pande, 'Sorting Boys and Men: Unlawful Intercourse, Boy-Protection and the Child Marriage Restraint Act in Colonial India', *The Journal of the History of Childhood and Youth*, vol. 6, no. 2, 2013, p. 332; and Ishita Pande, *Medicine, Race and Liberalism in British Bengal Symptoms of Empire* (London: Routledge, 2010), p. 232n97.
189 Sinha, 'Refashioning Mother India', p. 623.

190 Sumita Mukherjee, 'Using Legislative Assembly for Social Reform: The Sarda Act of 1929', *South Asia Research*, vol. 26, no. 3, 2006, pp. 219–33; Ishita Pande, 'Coming of Age: Law, Sex and Childhood in Late Colonial India', *Gender & History*, vol. 24, no. 1, 2012, pp. 205–30; and Pande, 'Sorting Boys and Men', pp. 332–58; Sinha, 'Refashioning Mother India', pp. 623–44; and Sinha, *Mother India* by Katherine Mayo, among others.

5

THE CHILD WELFARE EXHIBITION, 1920*

Introduction: Exhibition, Knowledge and Power

This chapter focuses on an in-depth study of the Health and Child Welfare Exhibition held in colonial Calcutta in 1920. Despite a few scholarly references, however, there has been no detailed study till date. The vicereines of India launched child welfare exhibitions motivated by the transnational exhibitory baby health week propaganda initiative to curb infant mortality. These exhibitions were also locally organised and collaborative in nature with an urgent nationalist appeal. The study critically engages with select Exhibition lectures about so-called 'clean' midwifery and 'scientific' motherhood given by famous Bengali medical practitioners and other prominent professionals, predominantly men and a few women. These drew intimate sociobiological connections between the problems of 'dirty' midwifery, ritual pollution, improper confinement, insanitary childbirth, insufficient lactation, and the excessive maternal and infant deaths in Calcutta. The central argument is that these public lectures primarily focused on the very making of the 'ideal' Indian nursing mother, often imagined as the traditional yet modern *bhadramahila* mother figure, for rejuvenating community and national health and vigour. Correspondingly, it highlights the transnational resonance of famous New Zealand physician Frederic Truby King's 'mothercraft' popularised as childcare by the clock. The chapter is, therefore, guided by the twin purposes of filling the gap in our knowledge about child welfare exhibitions in colonial India and illuminating extant scholarship on the global infant welfare movement:

An Appeal on Behalf of the Children of Bengal

Do you know that IGNORANCE is destroying innumerable lives in Bengal?

Do you know that every year over a million people die from preventable causes?

DOI: 10.4324/9781003327837-6

Do you know that of these unnecessary deaths more than half a million occur among children under 10 years of age?
Do you know that each day on the average at least 600 baby lives are needlessly sacrificed?
Do you know that if the infant death-rate of Calcutta was as low as that of New Zealand only 825 babies would have died in the city in 1919 instead of 5,928?
What are you prepared to do to help dispel the ignorance that is destroying the children of the land of your birth or your adoption?
Funds are urgently needed for the purpose.
What will you subscribe?[1]

An exploration of why and how these exhibitions were conceived and carried out reveals that these were primarily based on an emulation of the National Baby Week in London in 1917.[2] This first British baby week set in motion week-long baby health exhibitions, lectures and competitive baby shows.[3] This was a part of the global infant welfare movement which may also be traced back to anxieties of British authorities about the problem of poor fitness of the British soldiers in the Boer War (1899–1902) in South Africa, followed by the strains of the First World War and the recuperating interwar period, which turned motherhood and infant health into national and imperial concerns. 'Mothercraft' and healthy mothering to eliminate 'germs of disease'[4] and high infant mortality to improve community, 'racial' or national health gradually developed in alignment with the main tenets of the worldwide infant welfare movement.

This chapter highlights that many of the Calcutta Exhibition lectures centred on the 'women's question' as crucial to colonial 'civilising missions', nationalism and community-building, and even preservation of the imperial race in India. As mentioned earlier in this book, this, in turn, is intimately connected with the fact that maternal and child welfare propaganda was taken up by quasi-governmental organisations set up by the vicereines of India. These organisations mainly included the National Association for Supplying Female Medical Aid to the Women of India founded by Lady Dufferin in 1885 (also known as the Dufferin Fund), alongside the Victoria Memorial Scholarships Fund (V.M.S.F) established in 1903 by Lady Curzon, The Lady Chelmsford All-India League for Maternity and Child Welfare in 1920 by Lady Chelmsford, and the All-India Baby Weeks by Lady Reading from 1924. These actively encouraged medical training of female doctors, health visitors and midwives; the establishment of female hospitals and baby clinics, and organisation of child welfare exhibitions and propaganda literature. The colonial state mostly left medical care of Indian women to quasi-governmental organisations which were supposed to function as 'saviours of Indian womanhood'.[5] This study highlights that European and indigenous elite men and women were able to share power/

knowledge as they actively propagated and participated in maternal and child welfare initiatives, particularly through these quasi-governmental organisations on a pan-Indian scale.

It is pertinent to note that municipal maternal and infant welfare work in Delhi had already commenced earlier in 1915 and the first infant welfare centre was opened in May 1918.[6] In 1918, the Dufferin Fund Office, with the support of Henry Sharp, Secretary of the Education Department, Government of India, also formed the Association for the Provision of Health Visitors and Maternity Supervisors.[7] One of the main aims of the Association was to 'improve the knowledge and the work of dais'.[8] It was assisted by a government grant of 6,000 rupees and, thereafter, it opened a health school in Delhi in 1918.[9] Around the same time, Vicereine Lady Chelmsford, President of the Central Committee of the Countess of Dufferin's Fund between 1916 and 1921,[10] interested herself in maternal and child welfare work. In 1918, in order to spread awareness about childcare to 'Indian school girls', prizes were distributed at schools at a pan-Indian scale for the best essays on 'The Care of the Baby':

> At the suggestion of Her Excellency Lady Chelmsford a number of prizes were offered for competition among Indian school girls for essays on 'The Care of the Baby'. Essays have been received from about 68 different schools. It is evident that the competition has aroused considerable interest, and both teachers and scholars have taken much pains to give and acquire the necessary information. It is equally evident however from the fact that certain mistakes are constantly repeated in the essays from individual schools that many school mistresses have acquired their information at second or third hand or from text books imperfectly understood or imperfectly translated. Now that Infant Mortality and Infant Welfare are beginning to arouse general interest in India, it would be well if some vigorous effort could be made to supply at least the girls of the country with the most recent and proved knowledge of the subject in simple and practical form. Otherwise we shall have the babies, who, as recommended in some of these papers, are to be fed on mutton bones at six months old, have tea and coffee as articles of diet in their first year, fed with four patent foods simultaneously when symptoms of delicacy appear, and have their feet swathed in flannel binders, regretting the good old days when they were allowed to grow up as they pleased. Twenty-two prizes were awarded for very excellent essays.[11]

Moreover, a public appeal for funds was launched in 1919 and the Lady Chelmsford All-India League for Maternity and Child Welfare was established in 1920.[12] Following the first year, the funds raised for the Lady

Chelmsford League were operated through the Dufferin Office, and the Health Visitors Association also became merged with it.[13] The main objectives of the Lady Chelmsford League included the promotion of maternal and child welfare in India, training of Health Visitors and Maternity Supervisors, propaganda, and the formation and establishment of Branches of the League, and the affiliation of the League with other bodies having similar objects.[14] The League also published a quarterly journal, alongside medical manuals on 'mothercraft' and antenatal care with clocks, regularity and discipline as leading themes. In 1931, the League eventually united with the Red Cross Society to form the All India Bureau of Maternity and Child Welfare. Ruth Young (W.M.S.) was appointed as the first Director of the Bureau.[15]

From the start, the League was involved, with the help of the Red Cross Society and various organisations, in spreading public awareness about maternal and child welfare through exhibitions, baby weeks, lectures and propaganda literature throughout colonial India. Sehrawat points out that the Association of Medical Women in India (AMWI, 1908 onwards) had advocated the improvement of medical services for 'Indian women' with the replacement of the Dufferin Fund and non-medical vicereines as 'incorporated wives' by medical experts and the Women's Medical Service (WMS) in India.[16] Renowned medical practitioner Margaret Ida Balfour eventually reconciled these differences by serving as joint-secretary to the Dufferin Fund (1916–1924) and chief medical officer of the WMS in 1920. Sehrawat emphasises: '[S]he brought to the forefront issues related to infant and maternal mortality, "scientific medical research" on Indian women's health, the need for further training of members of the WMS, as well as female sub-assistant surgeons'. The Dufferin Fund and the Lady Chelmsford All-India League for Maternity and Child Welfare by Lady Chelmsford 'closely reflected Balfour's ideas for a travelling exhibition'.[17]

In March 1919, Balfour pointed out that the suggestion to organise an exhibition resembling the one held in England in 1917 had come from the Association of Medical Women in India as they believed that spreading 'elementary knowledge of maternity and infant welfare among Indian women, would have an excellent effect in improving the conditions of childbirth, and reducing the high infant mortality in India'.[18] Balfour believed that 'to ensure success an effort must be made by all the educated classes of the community. Certain lines on which the exhibition might be organised were suggested'.[19] The organising work of the Maternity and Infant Welfare Exhibition in Delhi 'was done in the Dufferin Fund Office and involved immense amount of labour'.[20] Sir Henry Sharp, Secretary of the Education Department, and the first Chairman of the Lady Chelmsford League, also became the Chairman of the Exhibition Committee.[21] His efforts were crucial to the organisation of the Exhibition and he managed to secure a government grant of Rs. 5000.[22] A local committee was also in place to look over matters and make the Exhibition a successful one.[23] The promotional pamphlet highlighted the overall objectives and organisational structure of the Delhi Maternity and Infant Welfare Exhibition in 1920 as follows:

> [A] knowledge of modern methods of treatment of childbirth and of the rearing of young children should be brought home to the parents of India, men and women both not only in order that countless lives may be spared, but in order that the young of the nation may grow up strong and vigorous.
>
> With this object in view a Committee consisting both of Indian and European ladies and gentlemen has been formed in Delhi to organise an Exhibition in Maternity and Infant Welfare work.
>
> The Exhibition will be held in the Purdah Garden and the ground immediately outside it, during February 1920. It will be reserved for women on certain days but will be open to men at other times. The proper care of mothers and babies will be shown by means of models, exhibits, leaflets, lectures, pictures, magic lantern slides, etc., etc., etc. The Exhibition will be arranged in the following sections:-
>
> 1 Pre-maternity.
> 2 Maternity.
> 3 Infant Welfare.
> 4 Childhood.
> 5 Domestic Hygiene and Sanitation.
> 6 First Aid.
> 7 Home Nursing.
>
> A baby show will also be held.
>
> The whole will be under the kind patronage of Her Excellency Lady Chelmsford.[24]

The 'Infant Welfare' exhibit, which had several sub-sections, also had a subsection on 'Milk' to address key issues like:

> *Milk*. Importance of *Breast Feeding;* Comparison by charts, of mothers, cows, goats, and buffaloes' milk.
>
> Advantages of Breast Feeding. Photos of Breast and Bottle fed infants of the same age. Dangers of Bottle feeding.
>
> How milk is contaminated from the cow, gwala, vessels, flies, bottles or other receptacles (Charts or photos)
>
> If bottle feeding absolutely necessary, care of bottles; care of milk; preparation of diluted milk.
>
> *Weaning* suitable foods to begin with. Explain by diagram alteration in child's digestive processes.

Dangers to mother & child of not weaning. Rickets (with special reference to subsequent child-bearing in girls).
Times of feeding from infancy onward. Diagram of capacity of child's stomach. Show bad results on mother and child of constant feeding. 'Fly' exhibit.[25]

Around this time, on March 27, 1920, the Health and Child Welfare Exhibition was inaugurated at the Town Hall, Calcutta, by the Governor Lord Ronaldshay and Lady Ronaldshay, supported by Sir Bijay Chand Mahatab Bahadur, the Maharaja of Burdwan and Dr. Charles A. Bentley, the Sanitary Commissioner, along with other members of the executive committee set up for the organisation and collection of funds for the Exhibition.[26] It is relevant to note that the Exhibition included a large number of exhibits, many of which were either on loan from the Delhi Maternity and Infant Welfare Exhibition or organised locally, and about twenty-eight different sections representing nearly every aspect of child welfare and public health.[27] Of relevance here, the 'Maternity, Prematernity and Infancy sections' of the exhibits, in particular, were 'grouped together in a "compound" on the first floor' and equipped with model rooms exhibited in Delhi and common in the United Provinces. The Dufferin Hospital also showed a labour ward fitted up ready for a patient and 'a baby-feeding section with local-made Soxhlet sterilizers. All these were a personal loan by famous medical practitioner Ruth Young of Delhi'.[28]

Originally, it was intended to close the Calcutta Exhibition on April 4, 1920 but in response to the persistent demands of the increasing numbers of visitors, the committee members were compelled to extend the period for an additional three days.[29] This Exhibition was a huge event attended by over 25,000 people in total from different parts of Bengal and all over India. Among them about 10,000 people purchased tickets while ladies had free entry on 'ladies' days'[30] or 'pardah days'[31] while thousands of people including college and school students also entered for free.[32] The audience was offered information about their private, ritualistic, and affective world of childrearing practices through a public display of expert 'scientific' and medical advice in the forms of exhibits, lectures, lantern lectures, lantern slides, models, demonstrations and films at the Exhibition, which itself was on display at the majestic location of the Town Hall. In total, at the Calcutta Exhibition, the exhibits comprised nearly 150 different models and about 1,500 charts, posters, pictures and photographs, approximately 1,500 demonstrations, about 600 lantern slides, and 'some 200 pathological and microscopic specimens, insects, samples of food, etc.'[33] There were also a wide variety of exhibitors from the Calcutta Corporation Health Department to companies like the Nestlé and Anglo-Swiss Milk Co. The report, in fact, specially thanked Messrs. Glaxo & Co. for the generous gift of two cases of Glaxo food for sale on behalf of the Exhibition.[34] The Exhibition as child welfare propaganda comes to life here through an exploration of the colonial archive, the official report published in 1921. The front cover of the report had a sketch of a traditional Bengali mother holding her infant and looking apprehensive. After having already undertaken an educative journey through the Exhibition, on the back-cover, she was presentable and neatly attired in a blouse and a *sari* conveniently worn possibly with a pet-ticoat underneath, which was absent in the front cover, confidently playing with not just one, but two healthy children (Figures 5.1 and 5.2).

Before we move forward with a discussion on the Calcutta Exhibition in 1920, it is relevant to note here that the All-India Baby Week initiative was started from 1924 onwards by the Countess of Lady Reading (President of the Countess of Dufferin's Fund between 1921 and 1926). The Lady Chelmsford League and the Indian Red Cross Society together organised the

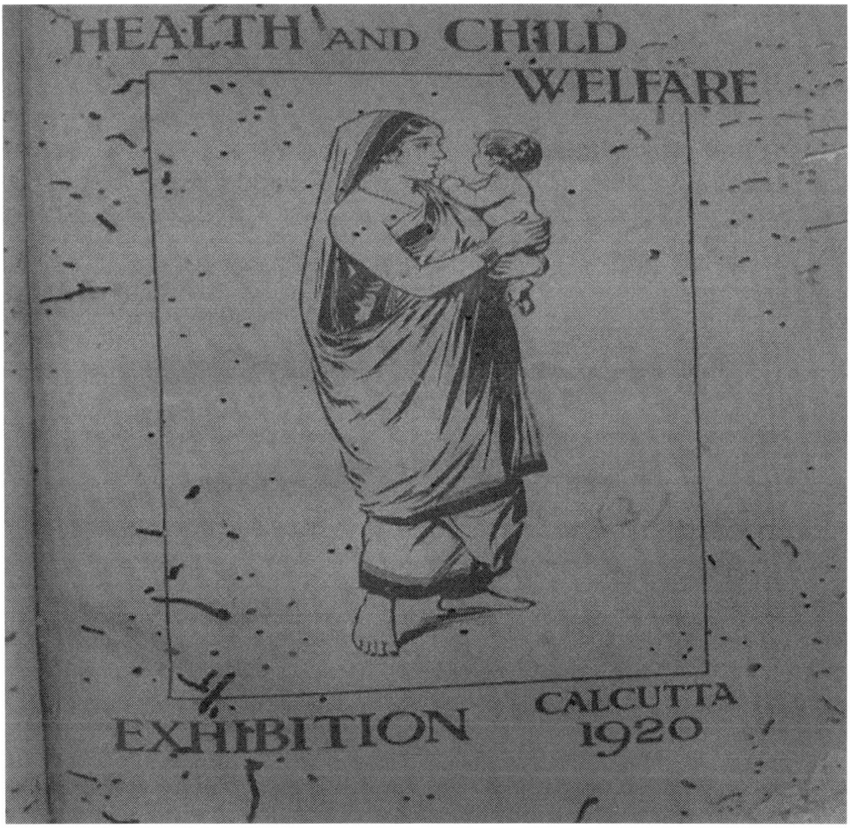

Figure 5.1 Front Cover.

Source: *Health and Child Welfare Exhibition, Calcutta, 1920* [with permission from the National Library, Kolkata].

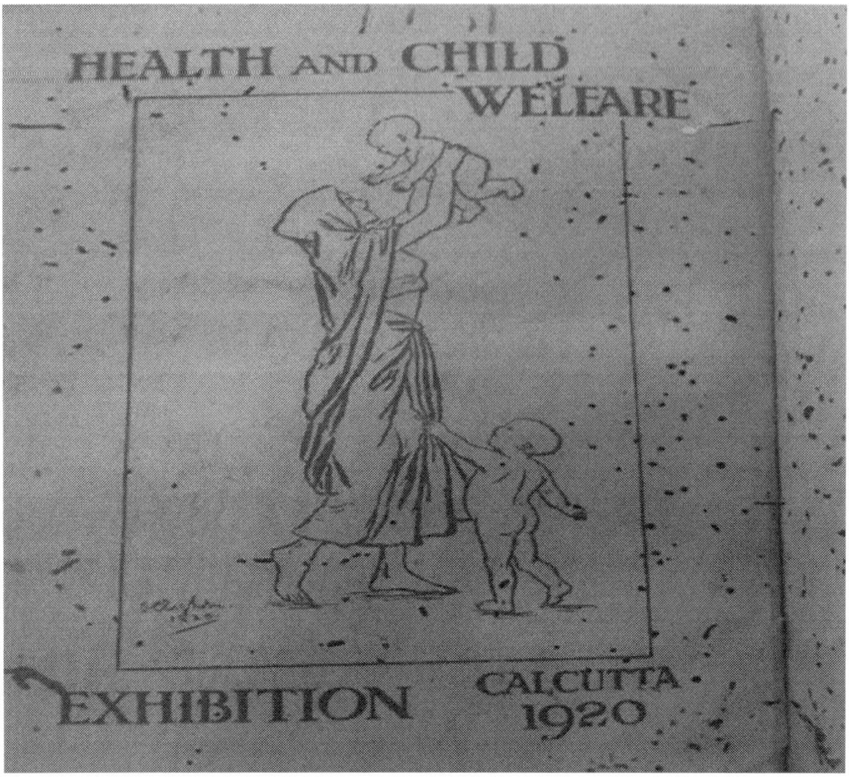

Figure 5.2 Back cover.

Source: *Health and Child Welfare Exhibition, Calcutta, 1920* [with permission from the National Library, Kolkata].

first Baby Week and, at its conclusion, a National Baby Week Council was formed with the League Secretary serving as a secretary in both these organisations. Later on, the Council became merged with the League and Baby Week became one of the activities of the League. In addition, the League possessed a travelling exhibition which could be sent on request to any part of India. The Baby Week movement emerged as a significant contribution to maternal and child welfare across India.[35] It is pertinent to note that Yvonne Fitzroy, Lady Reading's private secretary, in her diary indicates that Lady Reading was interested in child welfare from the time of her arrival in India. In a particular diary entry in Calcutta from December 19, 1921, she wrote that Lady Reading visited two baby clinics in Calcutta, one for Indians and another for Eurasians. It also provides a glimpse of Fitzroy's ideas about Eurasians (which coincided with contemporary stereotypes of Anglo-Indians as they were called from 1911)[36]:

> Wednesday evening Her Ex. Visited two Baby Clinics, one for Eurasians and one for Indians. The latter was very fairly prosperous and supported by the Municipality and all respectable Calcutta, the other flung on the charity of the St. John's Ambulance Nursing Sisters, who are doing wonderful work with little encouragement. The 'domiciled community' as the Eurasians are called, are certainly one of the saddest problems of poor India. Outcaste from every community, hated by European and Indian alike, and fated in every succeeding generation to sink lower in the scale.[37]

Following is an excerpt and illustration about the 'Baby Show'. It promoted breastfeeding and also indicated that the 'average European baby' was the standard frame of reference. It also argued that Anglo-Indian, Indian, and European babies shared a similar average weight up to one year of age irrespective of 'race' (e.g. Figure 5.3):

> In all cases prize babies proved to be breast fed. These babies were far in advance of the ones brought up on artificial food. This was

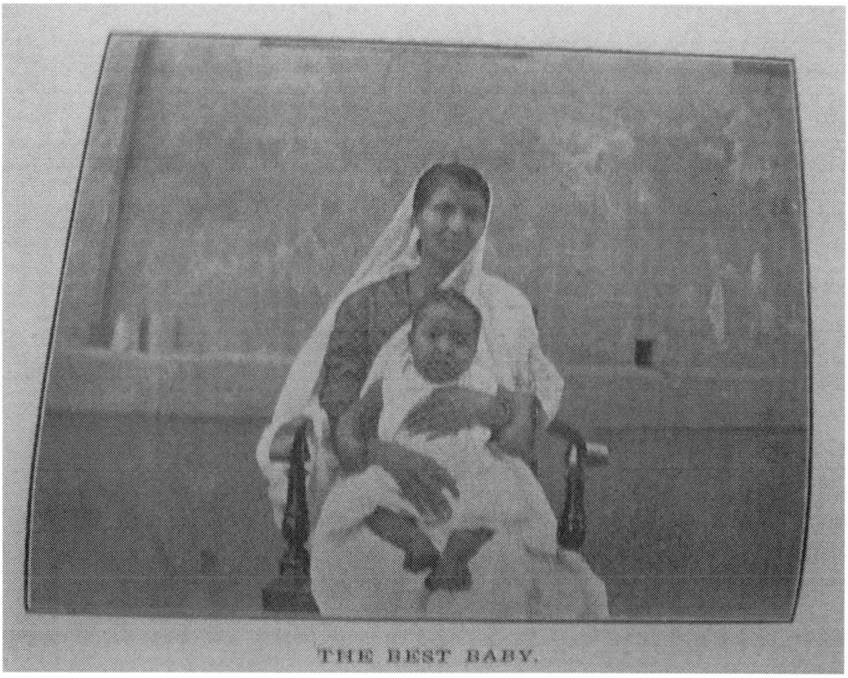

Figure 5.3 'The Best Baby'.

Source: 'Baby Week in the Districts of Bengal' in *Bengal Baby Week 1924* [with permission from the British Library].

> the case in each class of babies examined – European, Anglo-Indian, and Indian. The average of the Indian and Anglo-Indian equalled that of the European baby up to the age of one year, but after this age, the others showed a marked falling off, from the average European baby.[38]

The official report of the *Bengal Baby Week 1924* (Figures 5.4–5.6) claimed that baby week exhibitions and baby shows organised at an all-India level aimed 'to open the gates of learning to Indian mothers; to give to them the knowledge and experience that has been accumulated for the last twenty-five years in Great Britain'.[39] It was further pointed out that the 'Indian mother' particularly needed 'more knowledge of hygiene and what is suitable food for babies'. Therefore,

> everyone who reads this little book should feel that the work they did for Baby Week 1924 was work which was starting a new campaign in India, which will have far-reaching effects in the Home, the Country and the Empire.[40]

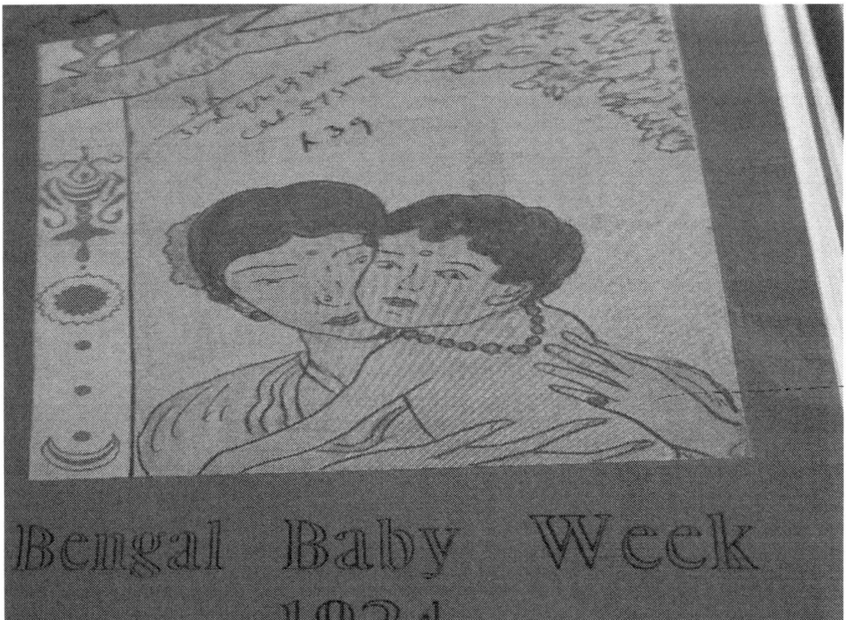

Figure 5.4 Front Cover.

Source: Bengal Baby Week 1924 [with permission from the British Library].

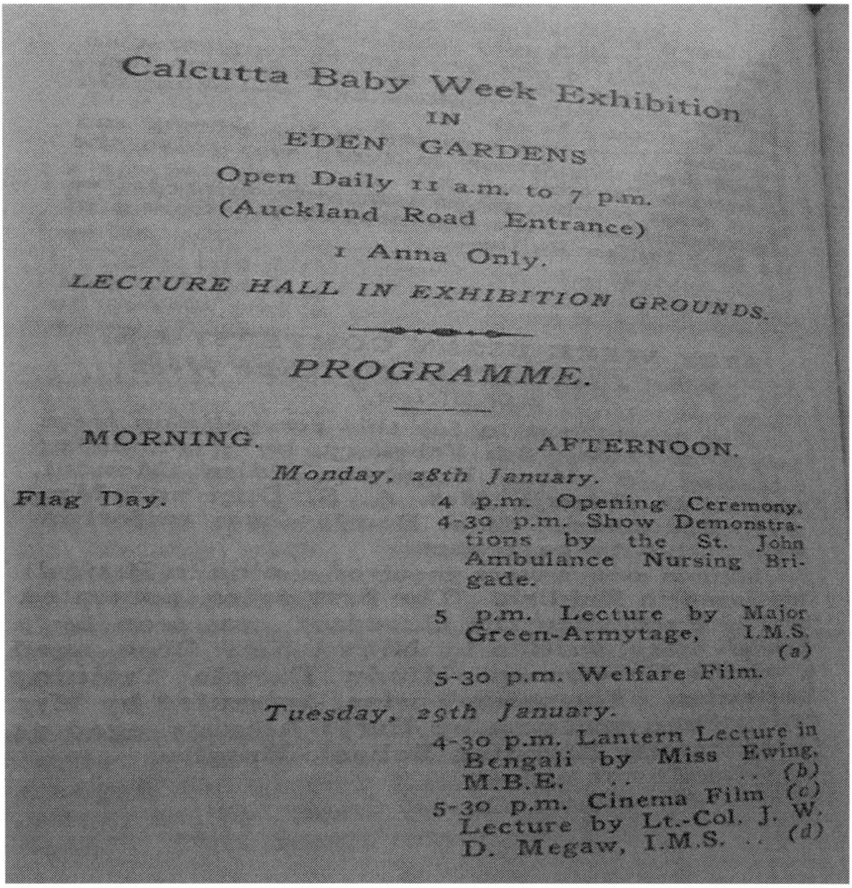

Calcutta Baby Week Exhibition
IN
EDEN GARDENS
Open Daily 11 a.m. to 7 p.m.
(Auckland Road Entrance)
1 Anna Only.
LECTURE HALL IN EXHIBITION GROUNDS.

PROGRAMME.

MORNING.	AFTERNOON.
Monday, 28th January.	
Flag Day.	4 p.m. Opening Ceremony.
	4-30 p.m. Show Demonstrations by the St. John Ambulance Nursing Brigade.
	5 p.m. Lecture by Major Green-Armytage, I.M.S. (a)
	5-30 p.m. Welfare Film.
Tuesday, 29th January.	
	4-30 p.m. Lantern Lecture in Bengali by Miss Ewing, M.B.E. .. .. (b)
	5-30 p.m. Cinema Film (c) Lecture by Lt.-Col. J. W. D. Megaw, I.M.S. .. (d)

Figure 5.5 Calcutta Baby Week Exhibition Programme.

Source: Bengal Baby Week 1924, p. 22 [with permission from the British Library].

Like the Health and Child Welfare Exhibition in Calcutta in 1920, the Calcutta Baby Week Exhibition in 1924 also featured lectures by many famous Bengali medical men like Sundari Mohan Das and B. D. Mookerjee (Figure 5.6).

Child welfare propaganda frequently deployed the widely pervasive 'doctrine of maternal ignorance'[41] to demand education of 'ignorant' mothers often blamed as the 'house of illness'.[42] As in the metropolis, the ideology of 'scientific motherhood'[43] singled out mothers for the task of childrearing. Yet they were considered ignorant and requiring proper instruction. Working-class mothers, however hardworking, were never the model housewife.[44] In colonial India, 'modernizing maternity' involved bringing the mother and

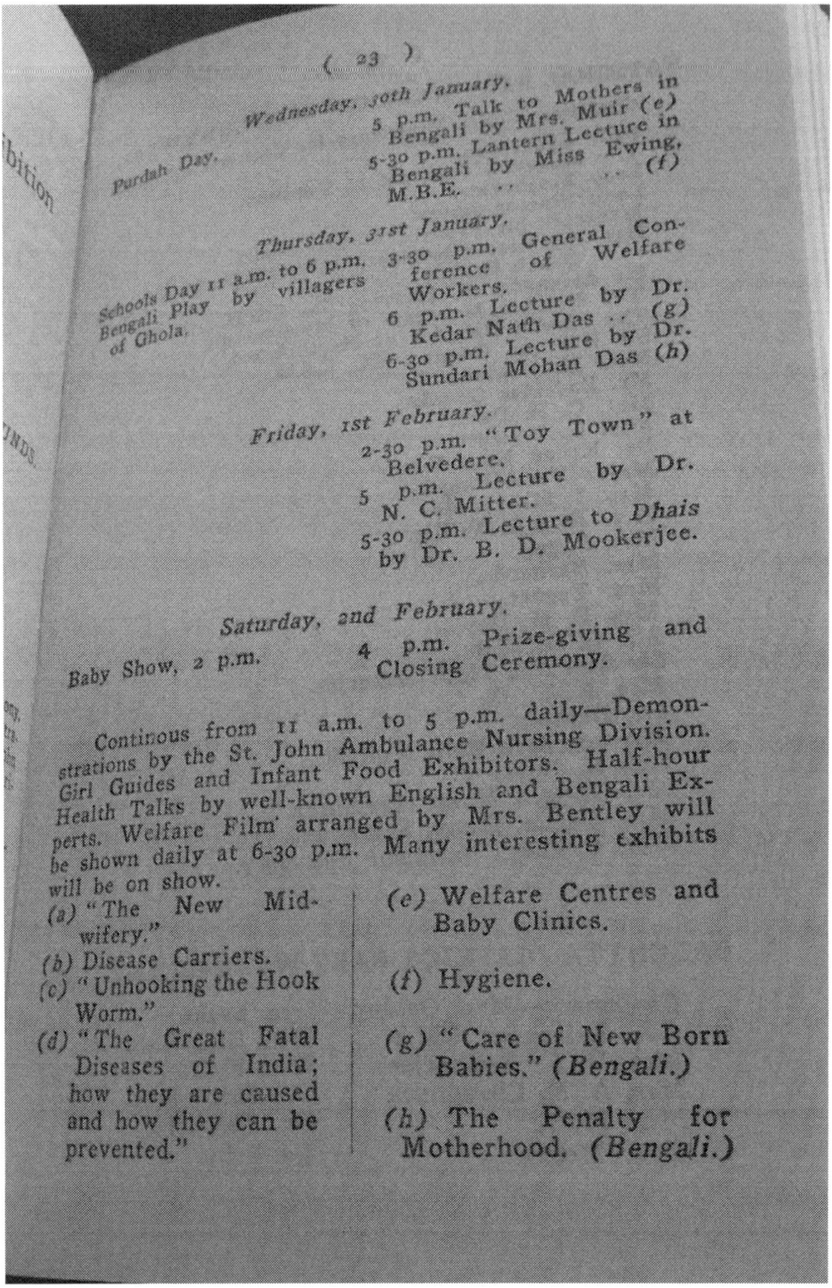

(23)

Wednesday, 30th January.

Purdah Day. — 5 p.m. Talk to Mothers in Bengali by Mrs. Muir (e)
5-30 p.m. Lantern Lecture in Bengali by Miss Ewing, M.B.E. .. .. (f)

Thursday, 31st January.

Schools Day 11 a.m. to 6 p.m. Bengali Play by villagers of Ghola. — 3-30 p.m. General Conference of Welfare Workers.
6 p.m. Lecture by Dr. Kedar Nath Das .. (g)
6-30 p.m. Lecture by Dr. Sundari Mohan Das (h)

Friday, 1st February.

2-30 p.m. "Toy Town" at Belvedere.
5 p.m. Lecture by Dr. N. C. Mitter.
5-30 p.m. Lecture to *Dhais* by Dr. B. D. Mookerjee.

Saturday, 2nd February.

Baby Show, 2 p.m. — 4 p.m. Prize-giving and Closing Ceremony.

Continous from 11 a.m. to 5 p.m. daily—Demonstrations by the St. John Ambulance Nursing Division. Girl Guides and Infant Food Exhibitors. Half-hour Health Talks by well-known English and Bengali Experts. Welfare Film' arranged by Mrs. Bentley will be shown daily at 6-30 p.m. Many interesting exhibits will be on show.

(a) "The New Midwifery."
(b) Disease Carriers.
(c) "Unhooking the Hook Worm."
(d) "The Great Fatal Diseases of India; how they are caused and how they can be prevented."
(e) Welfare Centres and Baby Clinics.
(f) Hygiene.
(g) "Care of New Born Babies." *(Bengali.)*
(h) The Penalty for Motherhood. *(Bengali.)*

Figure 5.6 Calcutta Baby Week Exhibition Programme (Continued).
Source: Bengal Baby Week 1924, p. 23 [with permission from the British Library].

child under medical surveillance often by those separated by both 'race' and 'class'.[45] In a colonial setting, the concept of baby health care was, first and foremost, racialised and amalgamated with the idea of the 'civilising mission' and the uplift of the benighted Indian mother. Indigenous '[m]aternal love was adjudged deficient – being portrayed as variously insufficient, too dispersed or too indulgent'.[46] This study emphasises the salient fact that European and indigenous elite men and women managed to share power/knowledge as they actively promoted maternal and child welfare measures, often through quasi-governmental measures, on a pan-Indian scale. It highlights that these very exhibitions were also locally organised and collaborative in nature with an urgent nationalist appeal to recognise childrearing as a public health concern. Child welfare propaganda was also a '"self-civilizing mission" in the service of a predominantly upper class/caste and male dominated Indian nationalism'.[47] Moreover, as social reformist and nationalist medicalised prescriptions and proscriptions on the 'proper' nurturing of infants were about creating a 'traditional' and 'modern', 'scientific' and 'respectable' domesticity and motherhood – it depended on the subject formation of the colonised elite, usually the upper-caste and middle-class men and gradually women, 'to write itself into history'[48] by discoursing on modernity and bodily hygiene to improve individual, community and national health and vigour. The design of the poster

> arranged for by Her Excellency the Countess of Lytton to be used in perpetuity for "Baby Week" . . . *was a gift from Mr. Tagore and was drawn by one of his pupils*; it is on the cover of this book in a reduced size.
>
> (emphasis added, see Figure 5.4)[49]

The official report, *Bengal Baby Week 1924*, also claimed that mothers 'showed their zeal in exhibiting their babies and hearing lectures on maternity and child welfare'.[50] The brief section on 'Chittagong' in the *Bengal Baby Week 1924*, for instance, pointed out that although it was feared that 'the prejudice and conservative tendency of the people will stand in the way of sending the females and babies to the Show and have them examined by the Doctors'[51] – due to the 'co-operation of all, the active advertisement of the daily "Jyoti" and the untiring energy of Mr. S. C. Mazumdar, the attendance was unexpectedly large'.[52] The report showcases the event as follows:

> 16th of February is a very momentous day . . . The spacious lawn in front of Dr. Khastagir's Girls' School was covered with *shamiannas* and tent and women of the poorer classes with their babies began to pour in from 11am. By 2pm the yard was full, and carriages and motors thronged the Jamal Khan Road in front of the school . . . In all about 500 babies attended with not less than

> 1,000 females. Examination and distribution of prizes commenced and lady judges, with Dr. Denham White and Dr. B. M. Das, carefully distributed the prizes to the most deserving, and consolation prizes to many. All the babies under 3 years were given *jamas*. Of course the mothers of the well-to-do classes did not accept any. Oranges, lozenges and sweets were given to all . . . The delivery of lectures by eminent doctors and Sanitary Inspector and magic lantern show by Health Officer and Sanitary Inspector continued up to 9pm., after which females with babies dispersed. All possible arrangements were made to send them home and there was no complaint of any sort . . . The programme of the 17th was also very successfully carried out, and Dr. N. L. Dutt and Captain Kiron Sen were the lectures of the day. To satisfy the wishes of the mothers there was another magic lantern lecture in the Exhibition ground on the 19th, after which the Baby Week for the year 1924 closed.[53]

Unlike this overenthusiastic report, however, Shudha Mazumdar, wife of aforementioned Satish Chandra Mazumdar of the Bengal Civil Service, narrated a more personalised but pessimistic view of the baby shows and, most importantly, her role in organising them. She pointed out that after moving to Chittagong, she had joined a mahila samiti (women's organisation). 'The District Magistrate's wife, a large and friendly Englishwoman, was the President. A baby show had been proposed by her and I was called to interpret this to the members since she did not know any Bengali'. The response was 'not favourable' primarily due to fear of the 'evil eye'.[54] She pointed out, however, that finally it was agreed upon that 'the uninhibited ones should come forward' whereby 'My small son was then a plump two years and I was asked to set an example by exhibiting him. Wives of other officials were also requested to help in this manner'.[55] The *Amrita Bazar Patrika* went as far as portraying baby shows as 'an insult to Indian motherhood, while the real need was for alleviating malnutrition and providing pure and nutritious milk'.[56] However, the nationalist press had also reconsidered health exhibitions as a 'very good medium of propaganda'.[57] Such exhibitions became widespread and came to be periodically organised by Bengali women's organisations as well as municipalities and district boards in Bengal.[58]

As also mentioned in the Introduction of this book, this fits in with David Arnold's main argument about the significance of the body as the main site of contestation between the coloniser and colonised – the 'corporality of colonialism in India'.[59] Extending beyond Arnold's focus on state medicine, epidemics, western medicine and public health, the emphasis here is on a 'Said-inflected Foucauldian approach' towards western medicine as a discursive practice which allowed the identity formation of the colonised.[60] Decoding of knowledge/power and meanings occurs from the location of a particular subject amidst specific discourses and more crucially, the differentiation between the normal and the pathological most often took place in medical discourses and initiatives.[61] In colonial Calcutta, the emergent discursive landscape of expert knowledge included distinct yet overlapping disciplines like medicine, Home Science, nutrition, sexology, only to name a few. Global bourgeois notions of discipline, domesticity and diet in childcare advice were regulated by clock time. Some of such conduct manuals were written by Bengali *daktars* and other professionals present at the Calcutta Exhibition in 1920. The Calcutta Exhibition is analysed here as an attempt at propaganda to curb infant mortality through the 'provincialization' and 'vernacularization' of western medicine in their local contexts, mainly by *daktars*.[62] For instance, renowned *daktar* Kartik Chandra Bose, author of manuals on nutrition as well as sexual and personal hygiene, set up an exhibit 'Child-Food' at the Calcutta Exhibition in 1920 as a member of the Bengal Social Service League.[63] The League also exhibited charts on child welfare and mortality, food infection, and bacteriology alongside a life-size papier mâché model of the human body with detachable organs; and jar specimens of cow and goat milk with breakup of their relative nutritive ingredients.[64] Moreover, Projit Bihari Mukharji's critical insights into *daktar* Sundari Mohan Das' (who also presented 'Ravages of Putana' paper at the Calcutta Exhibition 1920) *Munisipal Darpan* is particularly relevant in this context. *Munisipal Darpan* is a simply written, quasi-governmental, fictional and dramatised, operational and ethnographic, propaganda text. Mukharji's analysis of the text is reminiscent of Michel Foucault's take on 'modern state power' and 'mechanism of discipline'.[65] Dispersed and discursive colonial state power was 'embedded in social contexts' and embodied in 'the culturally coded bodies'[66] of 'petty officials' like Rameshbabu and '[r]eal-life medical officers' like Das himself.[67] It is relevant here to note that even though they criticised their 'unsanitary habits'[68] and stood 'above the lower caste, working poor of the city'[69] – *Munispal Darpan* also allowed the 'subaltern citizens' to be 'historically capable agents',[70] however limited in scope. Mukharji also draws attention to the glaring silence, which speaks volumes, in the text about demographically significant 'non-Hindu Calcuttans', mainly Muslims.[71] In colonial Calcutta, as Mukharji argues, at the basic day-to-day operational level, the modern '[c]olonial State's visible form is unquestionably that of a Hindu Bengali *Bhadralok*'.[72]

This study critically engages with select Exhibition lectures on so-called 'clean' midwifery and 'scientific' motherhood given by famous Bengali *daktars* and other prominent professionals, predominantly men but also a few women. Many of these were lantern lectures with the help of lantern slides.[73] These lectures focused on the making of the 'ideal' Indian nursing mother, most often imagined as the traditional yet modern *bhadramahila* mother figure. Gender, 'race', class, caste, community and age emerge as fluid and 'pure'/'polluting' biocultural traits associated with blood and milk. The first section interrogates the widely prevalent so-called *bhadra* or 'respectable', often upper caste and middle-class contempt towards the *dai*.[74] This was palpable in the Bengali medical advice on midwifery, childbirth and childcare offered at the Calcutta Exhibition. The second section critically analyses Bengali instruction offered at the Exhibition about the making of the 'ideal' *bhadramahila* mother figure. As also discussed in the previous chapter, the nationalist 'new patriarchy' constructed the *bhadramahila* as the 'new woman', different from and 'superior' to the 'modern' memsahib, the 'ignorant' women of older generations, and those from lower classes.[75] I am interested in the 'women's question' as it related primarily to the conceptualisation particularly of the Hindu Bengali *bhadramahila* in colonial Calcutta. In the process, it also problematises the quotidian, almost commonsensical, usage of the very term *bhadramahila*. The third section discusses crisscrossing imperial intellectual and institutional networks with Britain and the British empire. It draws transnational discursive connections between the very popular King's 'mothercraft' ideas and aforementioned famous Calcutta *daktar* Sundari Mohan Das' childcare advice. Das' deification of the *bhadramahila* as the quintessence of the Indian mother figure as '*Ma Lakkhi*' or the Goddess Lakshmi (Hindu goddess of wealth and prosperity) and her concomitant pathologisation as *Putana*[76] (Hindu mythological demoness) were based on her habit of always breastfeeding which had to be replaced by the modern clock and timely feeds.

From 'Dirty Midwifery'[77] to 'Clean Midwifery'[78]

This brief section problematises and analyses the so-called *bhadra* or 'respectable', often upper caste and middle-class, worldviews mainly disdain towards the *dai* perceptible in the midwifery, childbirth and childcare advice offered at the Calcutta Exhibition.

As discussed earlier in Chapter 2, in her *Antenatal Work in India*, Ruth Young advised that the *dai* should be treated as a 'colleague'.[79] The *dai*, however, was rarely considered a 'colleague' and instead she was most often seen as a major obstacle to doctors and trained midwives' efforts in providing antenatal and postnatal care across colonial India. The dark and insanitary lying-in room set aside for confinement of the parturient *bhadramahila* represented fears of physical and ritual impurity associated with childbirth which together with so-called primitive and unhygienic traditional midwifery practices were most often blamed for the prevalent high maternal and infant morbidity and mortality rates in colonial Bengal.[80] On April 2, 1920 ('ladies' or 'pardah day'), famous Bengali obstetrician Dr. B. D. Mukharji's Exhibition lecture 'Child Welfare and Indigenous Dais' addressed to the *bhadramahilagan* pointed out that the life and death of the mother and child entirely depended on the '*dhatri*' (or *dai*).[81] In Mukharji's description, in ancient times, the 'upper castes performed midwifery work' while, in contemporary India, *dais* were most often women from the '*neechajati*' or lower castes like the '*hadi, muchi, dom*, etc.' due to ritual pollution associated with childbirth.[82] He advocated that instead 'uccho Hindu o Musalman jati', that is upper caste and/or class Hindus and Muslims need to opt for midwifery training.[83] He also expressed his horror about the dirt carried by *dais*' uncut nails, unwashed hands and clothes alongside their use of sharpened bamboo edges for delivery.[84] According to the Calcutta Census of 1911, high infant mortality was mainly due to

> [t]he practice of cutting the umbilical cord with dirty instruments (e.g. a piece of split bamboo, or a conch shell) and of applying cow-dung ashes to the freshly cut end commonly results in tetanus neonatorum and causes a very large number of deaths among healthy infants every year.[85]

On April 3, 1920, famous Bengali medical man Hasan Suhrawardy, already discussed in detail in Chapter 3 of this book, in his lantern lecture 'The Care of the Expectant Mother and Newborn Infant' at the Calcutta Exhibition also expressed his horror that instead of

> a clean accoucher or a midwife, a dirty low class woman, with long and filthy nails and fingers crammed with dirty rings made of base metals, recruited from the untouchable caste of the *Chamar* or the *Dosad* is requisitioned to usher into life the infant who is the hope and future of the country.[86]

He criticised the fact that the '*parda* or *gosha* system necessitates confinement of women within the narrow walls of the courtyards of their houses, indeed many live within the four walls of their rooms only'.[87] Suhrawardy's lecture also displayed 'the web of nationalist and communal issues that had come by 1920, to colour questions of reproductive health in colonial Bengal'.[88] He was mainly anxious about the higher rate of infant mortality among Muslims than Hindus. He believed that the 'chooth or the theory of pollution by touch' and the 'institution of atoor' or confinement during childbirth, were 'all foreign to Islam'.[89] Moreover, his own caste-related prejudices are evident from the fact that while pointing to the need for personal hygiene, he commented that '[a] high caste Bengali Hindu hardly needs this advice'. He lamented that unlike the earlier 'presence of a large number of public hot and cold baths called "*Hamams*" in every Muslim town' and Muslim awareness and 'propaganda of personal cleanliness which their religion preached and which they practised' – 'to-day I am sorry to see that some of the Musalmans are the greatest sinners in this respect'. He appealed that 'unfortunately the Muslims are losing ground everywhere' while 'those who infected them' were 'now free', 'making rapid marches towards progress' having broken the 'shackles of custom and fetters of caste prejudice'.[90] As also discussed in Chapter 3, Suhrawardy believed that child welfare propaganda was 'the best Swadeshi and Nationalist movement'.[91] In his description, he witnessed the slums of East End of London and Edinburgh as well as the tenement house of the back streets of 'Dirty Dublin' but 'nowhere have I come across anything so repugnant' as the insanitary lying-in rooms where both Hindu and Muslim parturient women among 'the well-to-do *bhadralog* Indians' were incarcerated, particularly due to 'ritual impurity' and fears of 'the evil eye, the *dain* or village witch and the evil spirits' for a period of three weeks to 40 days.[92]

The *Bhadramahila* Ideal

This second section examines Bengali instruction offered at the Exhibition about the 'women's question' as it primarily related to the conceptualisation of the 'ideal' *bhadramahila*, particularly of the Hindu Bengali *bhadramahila*, in colonial Calcutta. In the process, it problematises the quotidian, almost commonsensical, usage of the very term *bhadramahila* and the themes of 'science' and discipline which underscored everyday lives.

The main purpose of the Calcutta Exhibition was to attempt health education propaganda in order to create educated mothers and healthy children. Yet this appeal was sometimes *only* addressed to the 'several cultured Hindu ladies of high classes' present at the Exhibition 'to explain to their less educated and ignorant sisters the prime necessity of a supply of fresh air in abundance not only for their own health but for the sake of the health of their babies' – as in District Health Officer of the Calcutta Corporation, J. Chakravarti's lecture 'The Need of Fresh Air'. He pointed out that 'Calcutta has been described by some as a matricidal city and rightly so; amongst other causes, vitiated air plays no unimportant part in producing this' He asked, '[I]f you will please go through the vital statistics of Calcutta, you will find that comparatively more females die amongst Hindus and Muhammadans. Why?' He explained that too much 'expired air' in the overcrowded houses in Calcutta resulted in 'still-born children or children who die within three or four days of their birth from debilitated condition'. If they survived the initial days, they suffered from malnutrition unless they could get 'plenty of mother's milk' and a 'sickly mother can never give sufficient quantity of milk necessary for the proper healthy growth of the child'. His list of causes also problematised pardah lifestyle particularly among Muslims as follows – 'I have often seen small windows provided in many houses of Calcutta above a man's height. This I noticed especially in quarters intended to be occupied by parda women amongst the Muhammadan community'.[93]

In the lecture 'Impure Air and Infant Mortality' at the Exhibition on March 29, 1920, Rai Bahadur Chunilal Bose, Chemical Examiner, Calcutta, argued that confinement figured prominently among the main causes responsible for the 'abnormally high death-rate among infants' and maternal mortality in early twentieth-century Calcutta – insanitary living conditions, malnutrition due to poverty, premature motherhood, 'seclusion of women, ignorance, superstition, bad midwifery, want of proper care, of the mother before confinement, inexperience of young mothers to take proper care of themselves, and their babies, impure and inadequate milk-supply, etc.' He emphasised that insanitary lying-in rooms 'considerably adds to this increased death-rate among new-born babies'. He pointed out that '[o]n thousand seven hundred and ninety-one infants died in this city in 1918 before they were a week old, i.e. while they were still confined within the four walls of the dungeon known as *atoor ghar* in Indian houses'.[94] He also echoed the governing assumption that there was a 'higher death-rate among Muhammadan women and children'[95] because they were usually confined for a longer duration than among Hindus which contributed to a 'longer process of simmering in a foetic atmosphere'.[96]

'Purdah as Pathology' often meant that Muslim women were perceived as 'the most disadvantaged'.[97] Purdah was even sometimes labelled as an essentially Muslim practice stemming from Mughal rule and divested from 'Indian identity'.[98] It was also gradually becoming common for medical reports to allocate their findings on women's morbidity and mortality by religious community whereby the 'health status of women became an issue related to that of the relative "backwardness" of communities'.[99] The census statistics offered a comparative 'tally sheet for registering the progress or decline of each religious community'.[100] It is relevant to note that around the time of the Calcutta Exhibition – in numbers, 'Muhammadans form the most important religious community in Bengal'. However, Hindus outnumbered Muslims in 'the six districts of Western Bengal, the 24-Parganas, Calcutta, Khulna, Jalpaiguri, Darjeeling, and the Chittagong Hill Tracts'.[101] There was also an anxiety-ridden narrative about the perceived decline of the Hindus as 'a dying race' connected with a popular network of tropes and stereotypes fuelling the growing 'discursive power of Hindu communalism' in colonial Calcutta.[102]

The leading notion was that ideally 'educated mothers would improve the physical health and mental vigor of future generations of Bengali *bhadralok*'.[103] *Bhadramahila* most often implied 'the mothers, wives, and daughters of the many school-masters, lawyers, doctors, and government servants who made up the English-educated professional Bengali "middle class" or *bhadralok*'.[104] It is also significant here to draw attention to the fact, as Sonia Nishat Amin argues, that although the term *bhadramahila* predominantly implied 'respectable' Brahmo and Hindu Bengali women, the self-expression of a number of Bengali Muslim women, especially writers and educationists as *bhadramahila* also dates from as early as the 1870s.[105] However, like Amin, Mahua Sarkar questions the widespread and unambiguous usage of the term *bhadramahila* for and by Muslim women. Brahmo and Hindu Bengali women also sometimes basked in a 'feeling of relative well-being' and expressed disdain for Bengali Muslim women as 'mute, backward' and not '*bhadra* in similar ways'.[106] Even renowned Bengali writer, social reformer and educationist, Rokeya Sakhawat Hossein's call for women's self-sufficiency and her 'denouncement of women's collusion in perpetuating their own exploitation' was labelled as 'a kind of rabid reaction stemming from the extreme exploitation of Muslim women within "Muslim society" '.[107] These reveal 'the [bhadramahila's] construction of images of power and freedom' and 'their complicity in communal identity formation'.[108] Begum Rokeya's essay 'Dhangsher Pathe Bangiya Muslim' (which translates as Bengali Muslim on the Road to Destruction) compared the Muslim *bhadramahila* with the more advanced Brahmo women.[109] In her lecture 'Care of Babies' at the Calcutta Child Welfare Exhibition on April 6, 1920 ('ladies day'), she addressed the 'Ladies present' or 'Upasthit bhadramahilagan' as inclusive of Hindu and Muslim Bengali women. She quoted medical opinion of Dr. Bharat Chandra to make her main argument, in alignment with the worldwide mothercraft movement, that the 'duties of a mother' simply had to be learned.[110] Here I draw attention to her emphasis on lessons about infant mortality taken at the global scale by European countries from the Anglo-South African Boer War and the First World War.[111] She began her lecture by quoting infant mortality statistics particularly in Calcutta. She then pointed out that '[a] lot of infants die in the confinement room in consequence of dirty habits and conditions; they are not properly washed and bathed'.[112] Even the 'cups and pots in which milk is prepared for those children, who do not get mother's milk, are not properly cleaned'.[113] She lamented that '[i]t often happens that a fly falls in the milk; it is simply taken out and the milk is given to the child. There are lots of such irregularities – how many instances am I to cite?'[114] Similarly, the very harmful effects of flies sitting on food in the kitchen has been elaborated on by Miss H. Bose, Special Assistant, Inspectress of Schools, Calcutta, in her lecture 'Flies' at the Calcutta Exhibition.[115] Begum Rokeya also believed that '[o]ne of the chief causes of so much infant mortality in Calcutta proper is that, owing to the poor health of the mother, the baby does not get sufficient nourishment from the mother's breast'.[116] She blamed the practice of child marriage and early motherhood in India. In addition to delaying marriage, she encouraged female education and physical exercise, alongside 'proper nourishment of females', instead of them being 'starved, because a lot of money has to be spent on their marriage. They are the future mistresses and they are the mothers of the future progeny'.[117]

As already discussed in detail in the previous chapter, child marriage and early motherhood were supposed to have led to 'physical deterioration of the human stock'.[118] Racialised anxieties particularly about Bengali Hindu manhood in relation to child marriage and early motherhood also became visible, for example, *daktar* Bolye Chunder Sen[119] pointed out that child maternity was a 'physiological' problem which was a major cause for the degeneration of the 'Bengalee-Hindoos'.[120] By the late 1920s, pro-imperialist American journalist Katherine Mayo's famous book, *Mother India*, a 'public health document'[121] which specifically criticised Hindu social practices related to precocious sexuality, child marriage and early motherhood; and sparked imperialist-nationalist controversies intensifying the age of consent debates which involved the 'dilatory tactics' of the colonial state alongside various voices of the nationalist movement and all-India women's organisations right until the enactment of the Child Marriage Restraint Act in 1929.[122] Here I highlight, as Durba Mitra argues, that the very shaping of modern social thought by the colonial state and the Bengali elite involved 'a common language of the control of female sexuality in "an exchange of mutual self-representation" '.[123] As the age of consent laws were debated on an international stage, puberty and maturity also became sexological problems discussed on a global scale. As Ishita Pande points out, 'sexual practices appeared as an index of development of nations'.[124] In particular, Hindu sexology aimed to turn the 'colonial charge of allochronism – of inhabiting another time – into a bald claim of having always been modern'.[125] While challenging their colonial claims, therefore, westernised bourgeois notions of 'respectability' and temporality were incorporated into emergent distinct nationalist and reformist, social scientific texts. Popular North Indian nationalist and reformist 'global/Hindu sexology', which combined global and Hindu 'modernist' sensibilities about sexual and marital hygiene and routine, also brought clock time into a domestic setting, primarily governed by women's 'biological clock'.[126] It claimed to be a 'modern science' with a standardised 'time for sex' for 'disciplining of productive bodies'[127] – as captured in Kaviraj Harnam Das' (1929) analogical imagery of the woman as a watch – '[w]omen too must be wound up after regular intervals of time'.[128]

Child's Cries to Ticking Clocks

'Mothercraft' advice is unpacked here as consisting primarily of clock-regulated infant care, mainly regular breastfeeding, under medical supervision. With a focus on famous Brahmo and nationalist *daktar* Sundari Mohan Das' childcare advice, this section demonstrates the transnational resonance of famous Truby King's mothercraft advice circulating in colonial Calcutta. In the process, it also discusses the unexplored role of the Calcutta Exhibition in the preservation of the image of European invincibility in India.

New Zealand physician Frederic Truby King demanded that the mother only follows regular feeding by the mechanised ticking of the clock. The global mothercraft movement was enormously influenced by King, along with the popular concept of the 'King Baby' raised on his childcare methods.[129] Mothercraft was 'defined by the medical profession – doctors, nurses, trained midwives and trained health visitors'.[130] Motherhood under medical supervision popularised as 'mothercraft' primarily implied expert knowledge and training required by 'ignorant' mothers in childcare, usually 'feeding by the clock' and especially of newborn babies.[131] The modern clock was indispensable to the mothercraft movement. Childcare by the clock meant that mothers had to learn to ignore the child's cries. As also mentioned in the Introduction of this book, from Indo-European 'ma', which is 'imitative, deriving from the child's cry for the breast, as *The American Heritage Dictionary* explains', is 'a linguistic universal', and 'a speaking voice' in current 'baby-led' or 'demand feeding', as opposed to earlier clocked feeding.[132] Bengali advice literature was steeped in the 'transnational, hegemonic discourse' of an apparently 'natural', 'modern' and 'civilised' 'global domesticity', which saw science, system, order and efficiency as essentials for 'daily home life'.[133]

As you might recall from our discussion in Chapter 3, in her popular manual, *Maternity and Infant Welfare*, renowned medical practitioner Ruth Young pointed out that she was influenced by the famous Dr. King's *The Expectant Mother* and *Feeding and Care of Baby*.[134] Her main argument was that clocks and routine were central to the medical instruction of 'Indian mothers' about their ways of nursing their (male) child:

> The value, or rather the necessity, of regularity has been emphasised particularly in regard to feeding, but it is no less important in the other functions of life, *e.g.*, sleep, exercise, action of the bowels, etc. It should be remembered that training can and should begin immediately after birth. The baby *can* be trained in good habits. If *he* is not, bad ones will develop, and it is far more trouble to eradicate these than to take pains in the beginning. . . . It means training the child to be the minimum amount of trouble to himself and to others, to control his own impulses, and later to guide them into right channels. *Such training is for the child's good, and therefore shows truer love than indulgence which harms him.* It demands self-denial and self-control on the part of the mothers who is constantly tempted to yield to the child's cries . . . *the Health Visitor must be careful to explain in simple language, but as fully as possible, the reasons for such action, and lay stress on its advantages both to mother and child.*
>
> (emphasis added)[135]

Young's writings reflect the general climate of European and indigenous medical opinion which aimed to pathologise and medicalise Indian motherhood, and preferred to address the male child for childcare reforms. This, in turn, is related to the broader context of imperial and nationalist panic about national and 'racial' health and manly vigour beginning with the revelation of the unfitness of British soldiers in the Boer War. In this regard, King believed that '[t]he military power of the Empire clearly depended upon a population of healthy boys who would become fit young soldiers and on healthy girls who would be capable mothers'.[136] King 'had become determined to teach proper care and, especially, the practice of breast-feeding for the development of a worthy imperial race'.[137]

'Feeding by the clock' was popularised by many contemporary medical practitioners; however, its leading advocate was King whose visit to London in 1917 was followed by the establishment of the Mothercraft School at Highgate, London.[138] In fact, it was following the success of the 'New Zealand exhibit' at the first British baby week in 1917,[139] that 'mothercraft' expert King secured his position on the Baby Week Council, and thereafter, enormously influenced the founding of the Mothercraft Training Society (Babies of the Empire) in London in 1918.[140] Their manual was also heavily influenced by King as follows:

> *The Mothercraft Manual* was based on Truby King's *Feeding and Care of Baby*, first published in 1913 and reprinted in Britain four times over the next 5 years. Early editions exploited press coverage of infant mortality and the declining birthrate, and appealed directly to mothers of all social classes to recognize childrearing as a matter of national rather than personal concern. Indicative was the cover of the 1925 revised edition which bore a badge inscribed 'To help the mothers and save the babies' and advertized 'The Mothercraft Training Society (Babies of the Empire)'. In the text itself, copious illustrations of starving and subsequently healthy infants demonstrated the success of Truby King's methods of meeting infant needs, basic requirements including an abundance of cool air, clean water, absolute regularity and, above all, the baby's birthright, mother's milk, 'the only perfect food'.[141]

'Extracts From Letters' in an issue of the *Mothercraft Training Society Magazine* provides a detailed discussion of a successful case of Truby King methods applied by memsahibs in the rearing of their infants in the tropical environment of India.[142] The magazine also reveals that Truby King methods or 'T.K. methods' were also applied in case of Indian mothers as such ideas journeyed to Ludhiana, Punjab.[143] The problem of prolonged lactation or breastfeeding beyond the weaning period alongside the general disinterest of most Indian mothers in regular feeding and the domineering presence of older women of the household were considered the main problems faced at this child welfare clinic.[144] In colonial Calcutta, in his childcare manual *Saral Dhatri-Sikkha*, Das acknowledged that he was influenced by the famous Truby King, besides other authors of canonical western medical and Ayurvedic texts.[145]

Based on Sundari Mohan Das' medical writings on maternal and infant welfare, this section argues that breastfeeding became a significant site for the *bhadramahila*'s propitious transfiguration into *Ma Lakkhi*. In this regard, it aims to build on and extend Dipesh Chakrabarty's arguments about the Bengali 'modernity of tradition' and education tied to the *Lakshmi/Alakshmi* and the '*grihalakshmi*/memsahib' debates.[146] In the process, it highlights that medical knowledge systems were often combined and hybridised in their application in anti-colonial nation-building. It also emphasises, as Sumathi Ramaswamy points out, that visual patriotism often resulted from a combination of the visual and the textual together.[147]

Dipesh Chakrabarty arguments about the Bengali 'modernity of tradition' with the literate *bhadramahila* as the ideal wife and mother/*sugrihini* were tied to the opposition between the '*grihalakshmi*/memsahib'. Unpacking Chakrabarty's arguments further about 'Bengali modernity' and 'the modern yet fully national Bengali woman' reveals that it was an 'ideal' based on both dharmic and civilising discourses, often centred around the 'Hindu goddess Lakshmi' and built on fears about 'Alakshmis (anti-Lakshmis)' from 'uneducated'/ '(over)-educated' women.[148] Chakrabarty's arguments are also intimately related to Maneesha Lal's citation of Das' 'Mātā kā Navjīvan' ('New Life for Mother'). It was published in *Stri Darpan* after being translated from Das' original article 'Resurrection of Motherhood and Fatherhood'.[149] The Hindi women's magazine *Stri Darpan* ('The Mirror of Women') had a nationalist feminist approach and focused on nationalist medical (on both western medicine and Ayurveda) writings about motherhood and childcare. It was edited by Rameshwari Nehru[150] and published in Allahabad from 1909. As already mentioned earlier in the chapter, it aimed to educate 'ignorant' mothers who were frequently considered to have been a 'house of illness'.[151] Lal highlights that, in his article, Das praised the *Shastras* for Indian mothers' eagerness for motherhood while he criticised birth control from the West.[152] He argued that motherhood was 'the highest function of female life. So much so that God has been represented as having taken birth as a human babe to taste a mother's love'.[153] Das also drew transnational comparisons to encourage female education to reduce the prevalent high infant mortality rates in Bengal.[154] My analysis of this medicalised and Hinduised nationalist idealisation of Indian motherhood aims to move beyond Lal and Chakrabarty's arguments by emphasising that the medicalised deification of the Indian mother as *Ma Lakkhi* was based on educating the 'ignorant' mother alongside a naturalisation of her habit to always breastfeed whenever the child cried.[155] She became the symbolic 'mother of her people'[156] – akin to Mother India, a 'nurturing mother figure who gave birth to the millions' and 'nourished them on her milk'.[157] Her breasts were desexualised and sacralised through 'maternality', alongside her breast milk being likened to *amrita* or heavenly ambrosia.[158]

Saral Dhatri-Sikkha begins with an illustration of a Bengali-Hindu *bhadramahila* wife and mother in the traditional white sari with a red

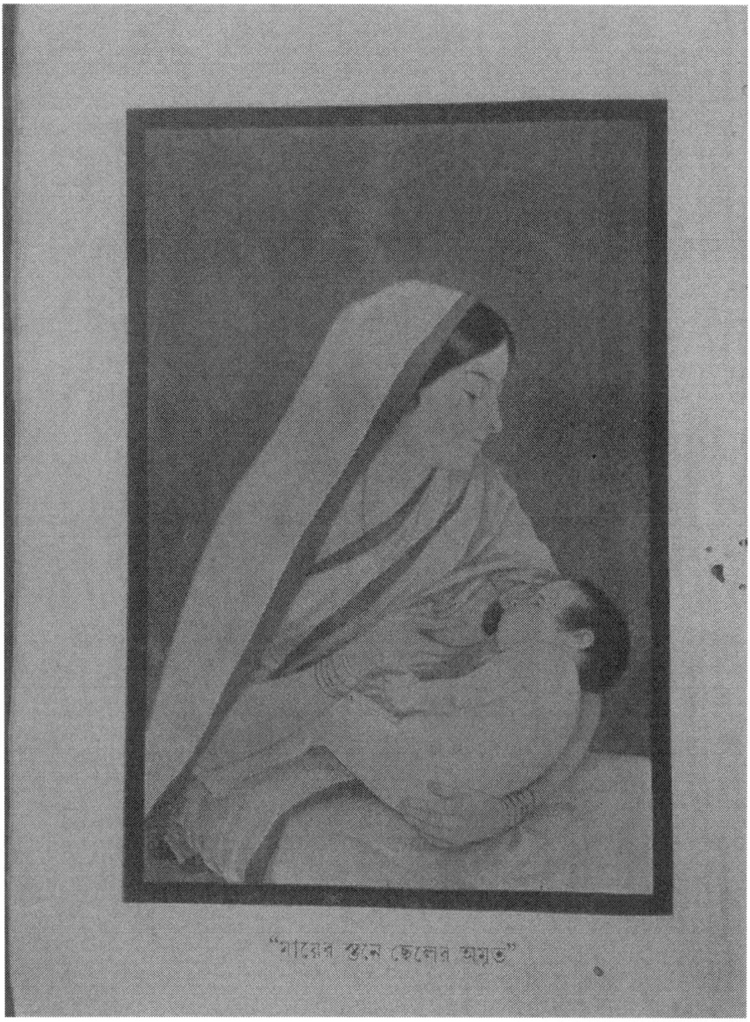

Figure 5.7 *Bhadramahila* Breastfeeding Her Boy Child with Bengali Caption 'Mother's Breasts Have Ambrosia for the Male Child'.

Source: Das, *Saral Dhatri-Shikkha Kumar-Tantra O Stri-Rog* [with permission from the National Library, Kolkata].

border covering her head and with one bare breast nursing her boy child with the caption – '*mayer staney cheler amrita*', that is, 'mothers' breasts have ambrosia for the male child' (Figure 5.7).[159] In alignment with 'the Bengali stereotype' of the non-breastfeeding memsahib,[160] Das considered Indian women to have been *Ma Lakkhi*, because of their habit to always breastfeed.[161] This particular illustration also elucidates,

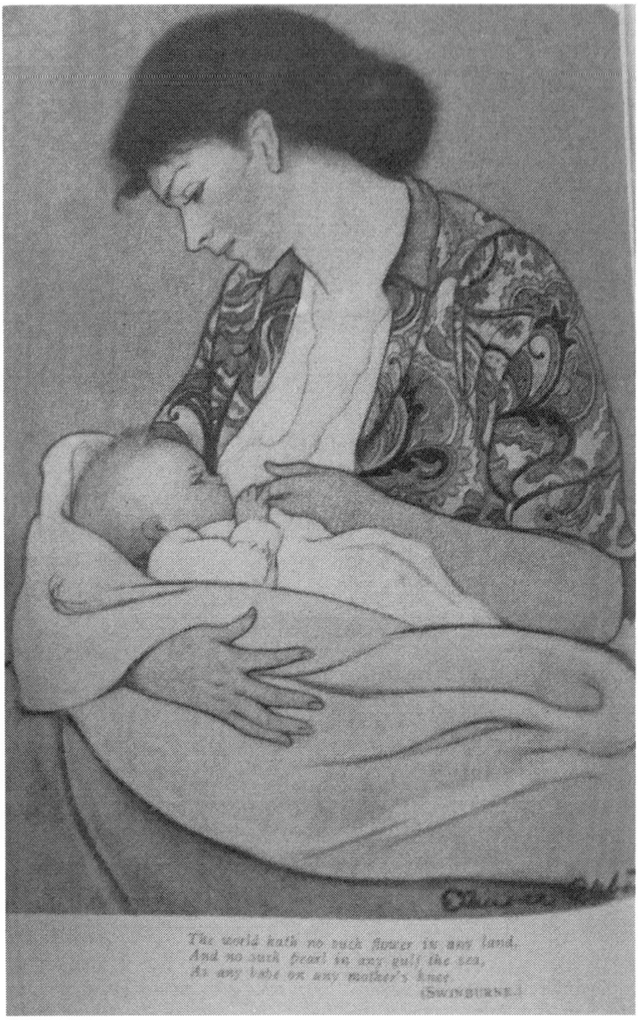

Figure 5.8 Mother Breastfeeding Her Child.

Source: F. Truby King, *Natural Feeding of Infants.*, n.p. [with permission from the British Library].

as Sumathi Ramaswamy argues, that visual patriotism is often a result of suturing the visual and the textual together which occurred frequently as neither is 'dispensable or adequate in and of themselves for patriotic mobilizations'.[162] As Jacques Derrida's 'double logic' of the 'process of supplementarity' illustrates – 'the supplement adds and substitutes at the same time'.[163] It is a 'plenitude enriching another plenitude, the *fullest measure* of presence'.[164] In this regard, Ramaswamy also deploys Kajri Jain's argument to highlight another side to this problem – it could also be that 'the image is potentially treacherous, that it cannot be trusted to do the job on its own'.[165]

In 1918, the popular medical manual *Natural Feeding of Infants* began with a picture of a 'white' mother breastfeeding her child with her blouse partially open at the front.[166] Famous English poet Algernon Charles Swinburne's words read as the caption – 'The world hath no such flower . . . as any babe on any mother's knee' (Figure 5.21).[167] Petrina Brown also quoted Swinburne to express the plight of physicians striving to achieve the ideal of maternal breastfeeding after childbirth by fighting puerperal fever and the soaring maternal mortality rates in nineteenth-century Europe.[168] In colonial Calcutta, medical practitioners also voiced their anxieties about confinement, childbirth and childrearing, including associated ailments like puerperal fever. Licentiate *daktar* Rames Chandra Ray published an article 'Duties toward Parturient Women' which appeared in the monthly medical magazine *Bhishak-Darpan*.[169] In his description, childbirth was 'a *natural* function' which, unless there were any mistakes or obstacles, should not have caused any ailments in parturient women.[170] He attributed multiple causes to the 'occasional severe puerperal fever' including the use of discarded clothes and an unsuitable location within the house as a lying-in room.[171] In order to fight puerperal fever, he stressed on the responsibilities of the doctor and midwife which included 'surgically' clean hands during delivery to securing an 'aseptic' environment with adequate sunshine and fresh air.[172] He further brought out an elaborate series on 'Child Welfare'. In 'Child Welfare VIII (B) Mothercraft and Housewifery' (May 1, 1919), he emphasised:

> [E]very girl and every prospective mother and housewife should know her exact duties. True, the lower animals do not require to be schooled into dutiful mothers or expert housewives; but women do . . . at present, a girl is taught a large quantity of some dead language, a still larger quantity of mathematics but is left to pick up shaky knowledge about her functions child-bearing, child-nurture and housewifery from her ignorant mother. She has no knowledge of the immense importance of breast-feeding of the delicate mechanisms of the child's body and of the intricate functions of her own sex organs. That is why in this country our girls foolishly bathe in cold water on the fourth day of the 'period' and hereby court painful and lasting diseases of the womb. This dense ignorance is responsible for the horrors of the Indian natal chamber as well as for all the evils wrought by the quack midwife in the name of self-advertised experience and efficiency. The feeding of the child is one

> series of blunders in several cases. In a word the price paid for ignorance in mothercraft and housewifery is immense.
>
> It is ignorance alone that makes women forget that maternity is one of their normal or physiological duties – in fact their chief duty in life. . . . Women who would not leave the purdah should nevertheless receive proper education in anatomy, physiology and hygiene as well as in mother craft. But for those who can go into public schools or colleges for women. What is the incredible stupidity of cramming grammar and logic and all that rubbish into the brains of girls for? . . . The studies essential to women are physiology and sanitation. The diploma of graduation for women in public schools should be that of a trained nurse. Properly, grounded in the fundamental principles, the graduate of women's college should be fully qualified, after a post graduate course of one year in a maternity hospital to take to Red cross work. Thus equipped, she is fit for her maternal duties . . . in all public schools for girls, practical instruction in these should be made compulsory:- physiology, hygiene, first aid, infant care, home nursing (specially in regard to – washing the body, weighing it, dressing it, preparing its food and feeding it and putting it to sleep, the importance to breast-feeding the value of the different milk and foods. . . . For the teaching of mother craft, practical instructions should be given. . . . My object is not to exhaust the list nor to formulate schemes but to open the eyes of my countrymen to what others are doing abroad and to what we can and ought to do.[173]

Ray's opinions have been elaborately quoted here to give a sense of what he believed to be 'ideal' ways to overcome the horrors of the Indian natal chamber and quack midwifery alongside his faith in the benefits of emulating the transnational mothercraft movement.

In *Feeding and Care of Baby*, issued by the Royal New Zealand Society for the Health of Women and Children (Incorporated) and followed by the Mothercraft Training Society (Babies of the Empire) in London, King insisted on clocked feeding under medical guidance.[174] It is fascinating to note that, in order to do so, the famous Truby King pointed to the various types of child's cries and their different remedies. For instance, in its most simplified form, he primarily outlined the 'Three Main varieties of Crying in Babyhood' namely: '[p]rimary, painless, reflex crying, needed for expansion of lungs and exercise', '[c]rying due to bodily discomfort, or to being "out of sorts", ill, or in actual pain' and '[c]rying without pain, merely to gain attention. This is the cry of the "spoiled" infant, and needs firmness, not further attention and yielding'.[175]

The elaborate 'Clock Faces'[176] were vital to his main argument – to 'never resort to feeding as a mere means of stopping crying – never feed except at feeding times'.[177] Das' clocks for feeding 'weak'[178] and 'strong'[179] babies alongside his tables for clocked feeding in several ways closely resemble King's 'Clock Faces' and infant feeding tables.[180] Artificial infant feeding, to supplement or replace breastfeeding, was also routinised and had a quantifiable nutritive value.[181]

Since the maternal and child welfare movement was a transnational phenomenon, King's childcare methods spread throughout the British Empire. For example, in 1920, an advertisement publicising the first baby week in New South Wales, Australia used the catchphrase 'Long Live King Baby!' because 'the hope of Australia lies in healthy living babies, fewer dead babies, stronger children, and a fitter race'.[182] At the same time, at the Calcutta Exhibition, Das' lecture 'Ravages of Putana' pointed out that *Indian mothers know that mother's milk is baby's life*.[183] The use of the gender-neutral term 'baby' illustrates that the predominant focus on the boy child in his other childcare writings did not mean different childcare methods for girl and boy children.[184] He was a *Brahmo* and nationalist supporter of *Swadeshi* and female education with a Hinduised view of glorious

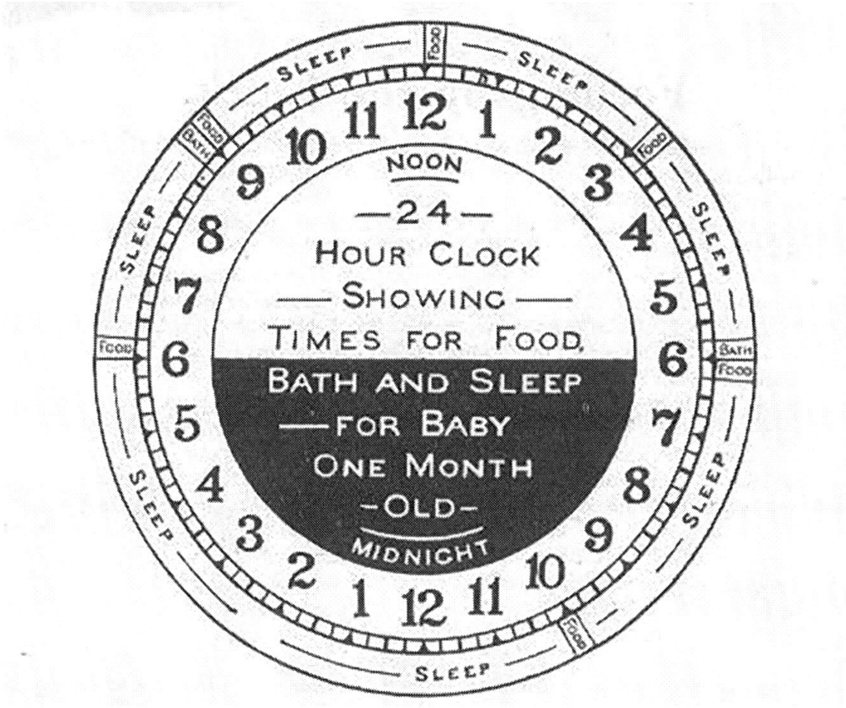

Figure 5.9 'Clock Face'.

Source: Frederic Truby King, *Feeding and Care of the Baby*, p. 35 [with permission from the Wellcome Library]

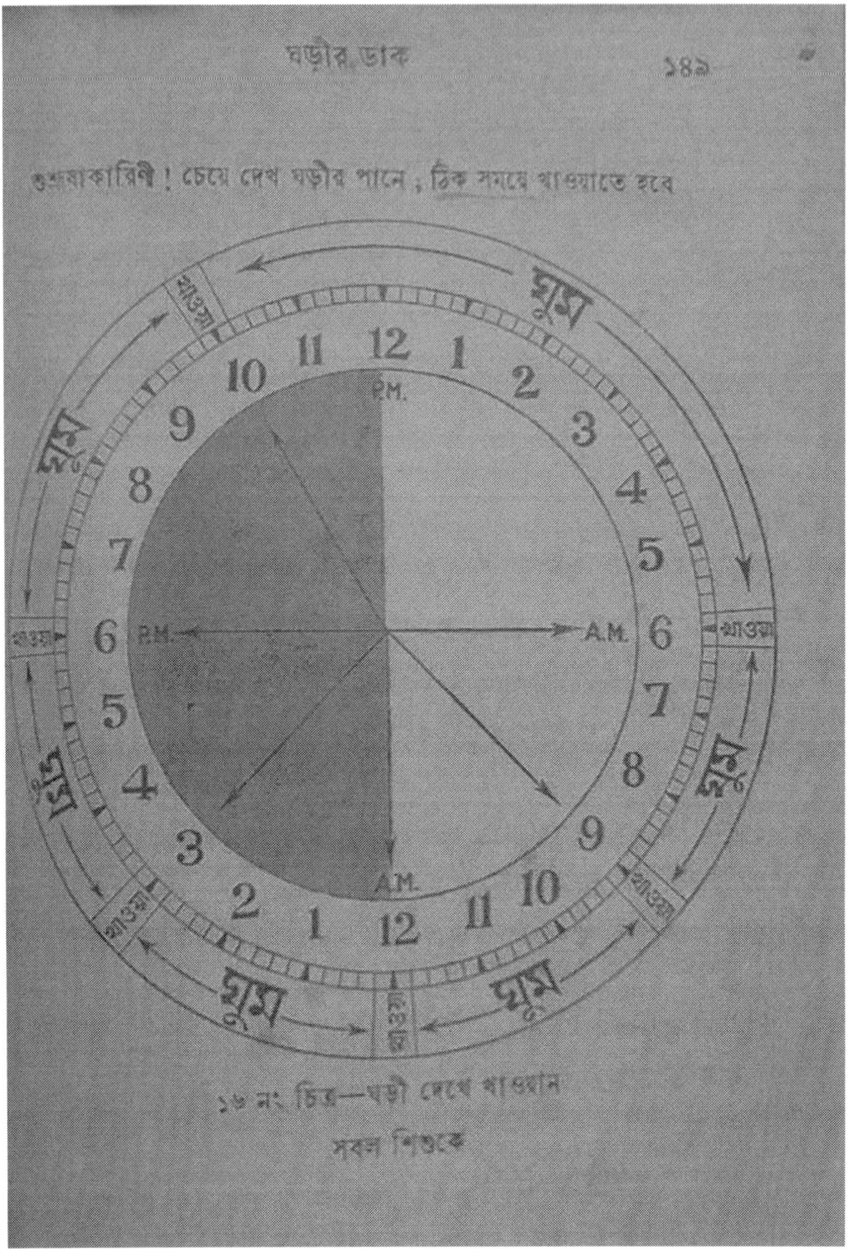

Figure 5.10 Feeding by the Clock of the *Sabal Sishu* or *Strong Infant*.

Source: Sundari Mohan Das, *Saral Dhatrisikkha*, p. 149 [with permission from the National Library, Kolkata]

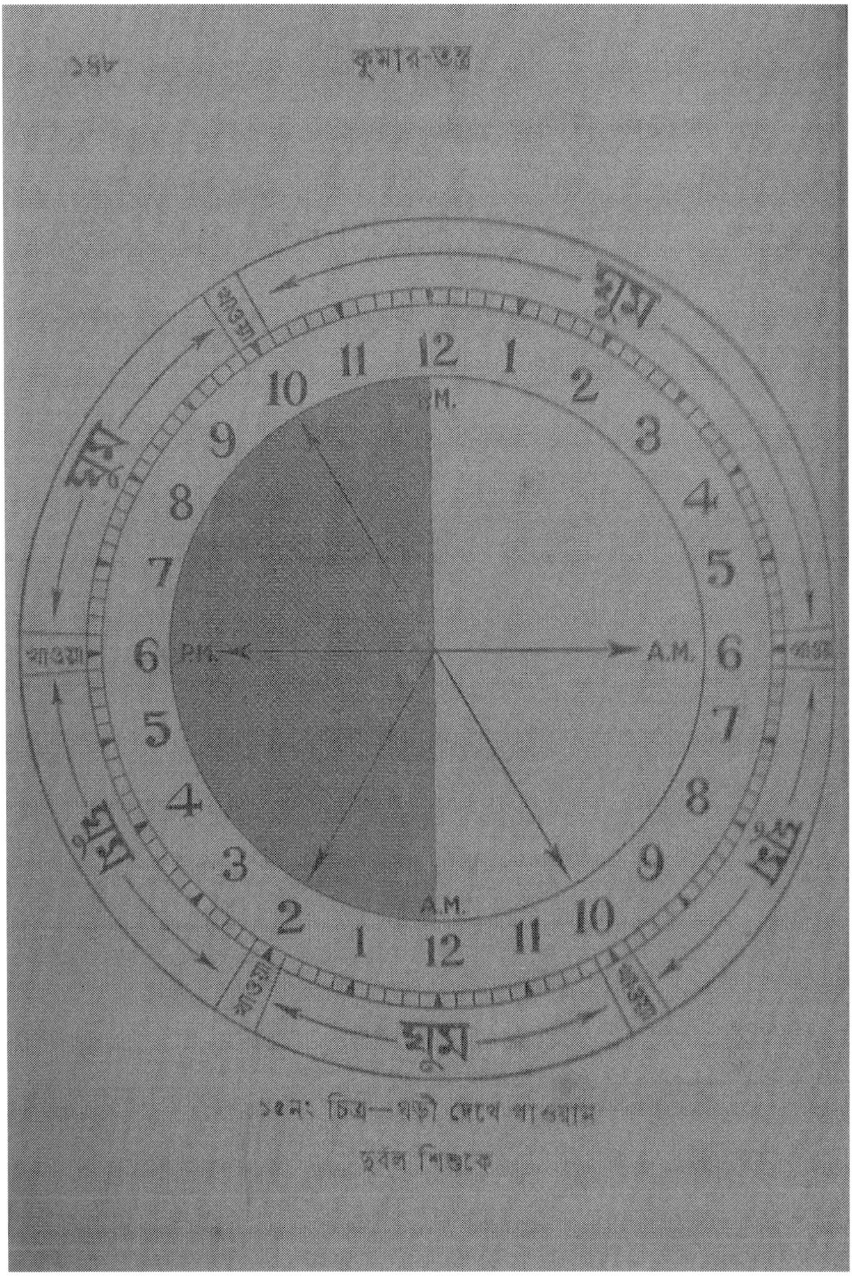

Figure 5.11 Feeding by the clock of the *durbal sishu* or weak infant.

Source: Sundari Mohan Das, *Saral Dhatrisikkha*, p. 148 [with permission from the National Library, Kolkata].

motherhood comprised of goddess-like mothers and producing patriotic sons for anti-colonial nation-building.[185] Despite the Brahmo emphasis on the Christian fatherhood of God, 'the pervasiveness of the Mother Goddess cult in Bengal' meant that the 'idea of divine maternity was integrated with the Brahmo view of women'.[186]

> *Putana*, according to the Ayurveda, is a group of infantile diseases which prove rapidly fatal. One of these diseases is identical with *tetanus of the new-born*. . . . The midwife with her dirty hands and instruments is also a *Putana*, killing mothers in numbers and by poisoning them with various microbes. . . . Even if the mother survives, the milk is suppressed and the babies die of diarrhoea and other sequelae of bad feeding. Those who without rhyme or reason refuse to nurse their babies are so many *Putanas*. In England the rate of infant mortality from diarrhoea is 12.6, in Calcutta about 6, i.e. less than half. Why? *Indian mothers know that mother's milk is baby's life*. Bad food, bad dress, late hours, intemperate habits exposure to infection, irritable temper, all these deteriorate breast milk in quantity and quality. Mothers who do not avoid these, fall under the category of that hideous demoness. Those Indian mothers who suckle their babies at all hours without any regularity or continue to do so even during the weaning period which is generally 9 to 12 months, are so many infanticides. . . . Mothers who unconsciously infect their children with their own poison are so many *Putanas*. . . . Tuberculosis mothers transmit to their children consumption. . . . Syphilitic mothers transmit their poison to their own children by suckling. . . . We, who do not try to prevent preventable diseases like Malaria and Small-pox, which kill a large number of mothers and babes, can be identified with *Putana*.
>
> (emphasis added)[187]

Das used *Putana* to primarily describe mothers particularly inattentive towards regular breastfeeding of their babies.[188] Thus, the deification of the Hinduised *bhadramahila* as the quintessence of the Indian mother figure as '*Ma Lakkhi*' and her concomitant pathologisation as *Putana* (Hindu mythological demoness) were both based on her *natural* habit of always breastfeeding which, Das believed, had to be replaced by regular feeding of infants. In his description, the Hindu mythological demoness Putana, in Ayurveda was a metaphor for tetanus and other infantile disease. Putana had attempted to kill baby-god Krishna by applying poison on her breast. Krishna, however, killed Putana by sucking her milk and life out of her. Das also argued that from a story in the Hindu scriptures it is shown 'how resurrection of motherhood meant resurrection of fatherhood' to give 'an impetus to the child-welfare movement. A strong appeal was made to the ladies to bestir themselves and stir up the gentlemen on behalf of the movement'.[189] Das emphasised, '[I]n New Zealand, child-welfare movement . . . has brought down infant mortality to 50 per 1,000'.[190] Das' clocks for feeding 'strong'[191] and 'weak'[192] babies alongside his tables for clocked feeding in several ways closely resemble King's 'Clock Faces' and infant feeding tables.[193]

King's mothercraft mainly promoted 'ideal' childcare as regular 'breast-feeding for the development of a worthy imperial race'.[194] It is relevant to note that although he was an 'international infant welfare expert', he was a psychiatrist, and not a paediatrician, who had also worked among those deemed 'unfit' and his underlying concern was, therefore, with 'racial degeneration'.[195] Cathy Urwin and Elaine Sharland point out that in King's works 'lack of regularity in babyhood was held responsible, not only for hysteria, epilepsy and imbecility, but also for other forms of degeneracy or conduct disorder in adults'.[196] It is relevant to note that, in 1912, as part of the Baby Week in Cape Town, South Africa, an exhibition was organised by the Society for the Protection of Child Life (SPCL).[197] It was a part of South Africa's infant welfare movement and mothercraft propaganda which gradually developed following the Anglo-South African Boer War period of nation-building. One of the exhibits at this exhibition organised by the SPCL in 1912, drew attention to the 'gendered quality' of the danger posed by the 'feeble-minded' by which he meant that feeble-minded girls were considered to lack self-control, be sexually precocious and prone to prostitution.[198]

Similarly, in 1920, the Calcutta Exhibition lecture 'Feeble-Mindedness in India' by Miss de la Place, Lady Superintendent, Children's House, Kurseong, Bengal revealed that the 'feeble-minded' woman posed a great threat to the well-being of the European community and 'preservation of the race' in India.[199] In her description, the feeble-minded woman was supposed to be 'insensitive to moral restraints . . . who live the life of shame'.[200] She complained that such 'children are usually of a worse type of degeneracy than their parents, and if both parents happen to be affected the results are indeed terrible'.[201] This discussion neatly dovetails with Luzia Savary's most recent study which paid attention to 'feeble-mindedness' connected to the 'para-scientific' and 'para-eugenic' notions in *santati śāstra* or 'science of the progeny' on the hereditary influence of 'mental force' in conjugal love in India.[202] The Children's House claimed to arrest the problem of 'mental deficiency' among Europeans in India with the help of the 'latest scientific methods'.[203] '[T]hough the beginning has been small, the end in view is a very large one, so large that it proposes to embrace in time all the deficient children of the communities classed as European, in India'.[204] Bejoyketu Bose clarifies, however, that the Children's House was an institution for the feeble-minded which admitted European and Anglo-Indian children with accommodation facilities only for 20 pupils.[205] The Bengal Government had made 'a capital grant of Rs. 30,000 for the purchase of a site' and also gave a 'small monthly grant-in aid'.[206] Earlier scholarly works have mainly traced the spread of the global mental hygiene movement to India with the establishment of the Indian Association for Mental Hygiene as late as in 1928 mainly through the efforts of Berkeley Hill as its first President.[207] However, these have ignored the role of the Calcutta Exhibition in spreading eugenicist notions of mental hygiene in India as early as in 1920. By 1931, in the official report of the Calcutta District Health Welfare Exhibition, right next to the section about *Mothercraft and Care of the Mother*, however, Bengali *daktars* had already taken centre stage at the 'mental hygiene' section to demonstrate how the mental make-up of an individual could be determined by a series of tests as 'knowledge of mental as well as physical health is necessary for intelligent men and women who wish to keep themselves *normal* and to bring up their children *normally*' (emphasis added).[208]

In conclusion, this chapter with the spotlight on the Calcutta Exhibition aimed to contribute to the existing scholarship on the social history of health and medicine in colonial India by putting forward three critical insights. These public lectures focused on the very making of the 'ideal' Indian nursing mother, often imagined as the traditional yet modern *bhadramahila* mother figure. Exhibition lectures about so-called 'clean' midwifery and 'scientific' motherhood drew intimate connections between the problems of 'dirty' midwifery, improper confinement and birthing practices, insufficient lactation and breastfeeding, and the very high maternal and infant mortality rates in colonial Calcutta. The study emphasised the intersectionalities of the analytical categories of gender, 'race', class, caste and community, which were also in the making and far from a prefabricated analytic. As a huge public health propaganda effort primarily to curb infant mortality, the Exhibition played a key role by displaying 'ideal' motherhood to rejuvenate the family, community, nation and empire. In the process, the study revealed the complex ties of the Exhibition lectures to multiple agendas of colonial 'civilising mission', anti-colonial nationalism and community-building, and even the preservation of the image of European invincibility in India.

Notes

* This is a revised version of my article published in the IESHR: 'Motherhood on Display: The Child Welfare Exhibition in Colonial Calcutta', *The Indian Economic and Social History Review*, vol. 58, no. 2, 2021, pp. 249–277.

1 'An Appeal on Behalf of the Children of Bengal', in *Health and Child Welfare Exhibition, Calcutta, 1920* (Calcutta: Bengal Secretariat Book Depot, 1921), np. This booklet was sold at 'Price Re.1–4' at the time. For a detailed discussion on infant mortality in colonial Calcutta at the time, see discussion in the second section of Chapter 3 of this book.

2 For a detailed study of the National Baby Week in London, see Linda Bryder, 'Mobilising Mothers: The 1917 National Baby Week', *Medical History*, vol. 63, no. 1, 2019, pp. 2–23.

3 Anna Davin, 'Imperialism and Motherhood', *History Workshop*, vol. 5, no. 1, 1978, p. 43. The first British Baby Week was celebrated in 1917. Baby shows

were popular especially in London districts like Islington. Linda Bryder, 'Mobilising Mothers', p. 8.

4 Hasan Suhrawardy, 'The Care of the Expectant Mother and Newborn Infant', in *Health and Child Welfare Exhibition, Calcutta, 1920* (Calcutta: Bengal Secretariat Book Depot, 1921), p. lxvii.

5 Samiksha Sehrawat, *Colonial Medical Care in North India Gender, State and Society c. 1840–1920* (New Delhi: Oxford University Press, 2013), p. 185; see also The Countess of Dufferin's Fund, *Fifty Years' Retrospect India 1885–1935* (London: The Women's Printing Society Ltd., 1935), pp. 11–13.

6 Review on Maternity and Child Welfare work at Delhi for the year 1928, Chief Commissioner Series, File 5(56) 1929, Delhi State Archives (DSA), New Delhi.

7 Central Advisory Board of Health, *Report on Maternity and Child Welfare Work in India* by Special Committee (1938), (Simla: n.p., 1940, First Reprint), p. 2; P/V/1128, British Library.

8 NAI, Foreign and Political Department, General Branch, September 1920, Part B in Guha, *Colonial Modernities*, p. 119.

9 Central Advisory Board of Health, *Report on Maternity and Child Welfare Work in India* by Special Committee (1938), (Simla: n.p., 1940, First Reprint), p. 2; P/V/1128, British Library. A similar health school was also opened in Calcutta in the 1920s but without much success. See Guha, *Colonial Modernities*, p. 119. On the other hand, a more positive opinion is found in the words of Dr. Y. Sen, F.R.F.P. & S. (Glasgow), Women's Medical Service, Raj Dufferin Hospital, Bettiah, as she argued that 'Baby Clinics' might not have been a success in Calcutta but health visitors' visiting of homes were. She also gives some suggestions to improve maternal and child welfare work in Calcutta see Dr. Y. Sen, F.R.F.P. & S. (Glas.), in 'Chapter VI. – Papers Continued: Drs. G. J. Campbell, Wallace. Sen, George', in *Improvements of the Conditions of Childbirth in India Including a Special Report on the Work of the Victoria Memorial Scholarships Fund During the Past Fifteen Years and Papers Written by Medical Women and Qualified Midwives* (Calcutta: Superintendent Government Printing, 1918), pp. 129–131; also on the League, health visitors, and child welfare see Magaret Ida Balfour and Ruth Young, *The Work of Medical Women in India* With a foreword by Dame Mary Scharlieb (London: Humphrey Milford Oxford University Press, 1929), pp. 144, 148, 149; and Ruth Young, *Antenatal Work in India A Handbook for Nurses, Midwives, and Health Visitors* [Indian Red Cross Society Maternity and Child Welfare Bureau (Incorporating the Lady Chelmsford All-India League for Maternity and Child Welfare, and the Victoria Memorial Scholarships Fund), 1930].

10 *The Countess of Dufferin's Fund 1885–1935 Fifty Years' Retrospect India 1885–1935* (London: The Women's Printing Society, 1935), Appendix, p. 18. In the Foreword by Lady Dufferin, she mentions that M. I. Balfour and Agnes Scott co-authored this particular report. Hariot Dufferin & Ava, 'Foreword', *The Countess of Dufferin's Fund 1885–1935*, n.p. File PP/MIB/C/4 Countess of Dufferin's Fund, Wellcome Library.

11 H. Austen Smith, Lieutenant-Colonel and M. I. Balfour M.B., W.M.S. Joint Secretary, 'Annual Report of the Central Committee for the Year 1918', in *Thirty-Fourth Annual Report of the National Association for Supplying Female Medical Aid to the Women of India for the year 1918 Including the Fifth Annual Report of the Women's Medical Service for India* (Delhi, Superintendent Government Printing, 1919), p. 6.

12 *Report on Maternity and Child Welfare Work in India* by Special Committee (1938), p. 2. Also, see Balfour and Young, *The Medical Women of India*, p. 145.

13 *The Countess of Dufferin's Fund 1885–1935 Fifty Years' Retrospect India 1885–1935* (London: The Women's Printing Society, 1935), pp. 14–15.
14 'Subject: Maternity ad Infant Welfare Exhibition', File 90/1920 Part B, Education Department, Series: Chief Commissioner, DSA.
15 *The Countess of Dufferin's Fund 1885 1935 Fifty Years' Retrospect India 1885–1935*, p. 15. The League united with the Maternity and Child Welfare Branch of the Indian Red Cross Society. Ibid. p. 15.
16 Sehrawat, Colonial Medical Care in North India, pp. 142, 139–40n171.
17 See Sehrawat, *Colonial Medical Care in North India Gender, State and Society*, pp. 105, 118–128, 183–184.
18 'Maternity and Infant Welfare Exhibition To be held in Delhi in February 1920' in 'Infant Welfare Exhibition in Delhi during the year 1919–1920 Minutes Proceedings of a Meeting held at Nicholson Road, Delhi on? 20th March to consider the question of organising a Maternity and Infant Welfare Exhibition in Delhi in 1920', File 12/1919, Deputy Commissioner Department, DSA.
19 Ibid.
20 Balfour and Young, *The Work of Medical Women in India*, pp. 145–146.
21 Ibid., p. 146.
22 Ibid.
23 Ibid.
24 'Maternity and Infant Welfare Exhibition To be held in Delhi in February 1920' in 'Infant Welfare Exhibition in Delhi during the year 1919–1920 Minutes Proceedings of a Meeting held at Nicholson Road, Delhi on? 20th March to consider the question of organising a Maternity and Infant Welfare Exhibition in Delhi in 1920', File 12/1919, Deputy Commissioner Department, DSA.
25 Ibid. The words in italics were underlined in the original version – see Ranjana Saha, 'Modern Maternities: Discourses on Breastfeeding and Child Development in Colonial Bengal', PhD Thesis, 2017, University of Delhi, pp. 76–77. Also, in December 1920, there was the Exhibition in Medical, Sanitary and Allied Subjects Including Maternity & Infant Welfare in Connection with the Fifteenth Annual Conference of the All-India Sub-Assistant Surgeons' Association Delhi 17th to 20th December 1920. It also had an elaborate section on Maternity and Infant Welfare organised by Dr. Megh Raj Chaddah (M.P.L.) and assisted by Dr. Ruth Young, Miss Griffin, and Miss. Graham. See *Handbook of the Exhibition in Medical, Sanitary and Allied Subjects Including Maternity & Infant Welfare in Connection with the Fifteenth Annual Conference of the All-India Sub-Assistant Surgeons' Association Delhi 17th to 20th December 1920*. (Delhi: Ratan Press, 1920), n.p., in File 217/1920 Part B, Subject: All India Sub-Assistant Surgeon's Association and Opening of the Medical, Sanitary, Maternity and Infant Welfare Exhibition in Delhi by H. E. The Viceroy, Department Home, Chief Commissioner Series, Delhi State Archives. Such exhibitions were said to have been organised in Madras, Agra and Calcutta in 1916, 1917, and 1918 respectively. For details on organisation, see correspondence papers included in the same file.
26 *Health and Child Welfare Exhibition*, p. 15.
27 Ibid., p. 18.
28 Ibid., p. 24.
29 Ibid., p. 17.
30 Ibid., p. 6.
31 Ibid., p. 26.
32 Ibid., p. 19.
33 Ibid., p. 18.

34 Ibid., p. 20. On Glaxo advertisement, also see chapter 3.
35 Balfour and Young, *The Work of Medical Women in India*, p. 148.
36 See Alison Blunt, *Domicile and Diaspora Anglo-Indian Women and the Spatial Politics of the Home* (Oxford: Blackwell Publishing, 2005), Satoshi Mizutani, *The Meaning of White Race, Class, and the 'Domiciled Community' in British India 1858–1930* (New York: Oxford University Press, 2011), among others.
37 Fitzroy Collection Typescript of Copy of Yvonne Fitzroy's Diary of the Activities of the Viceroy and the Vicereine, Lord and Lady Reading, January-December 1922, Diary entry Calcutta December 19th 1921, MSS Eur E.312/8b, British Library.
38 Mrs. Arthur Page (ed), *Bengal Baby Week 1924 With a Foreword by the Countess of Lytton* (Calcutta: Caledonian Printing Co, Ltd., 1924), p. 17. For The Best Baby image, permission has also been obtained from the WSIF journal.
39 Lady Pamela F. Lytton,'Foreword' in Ibid., p. 3.
40 *Bengal Baby Week 1924*, p. 7.
41 Milton Lewis, 'The Problem of Infant Feeding: The Australian Experience from the Mid-Nineteenth Century to the 1920s', *Journal of the History of Medicine and Allied Sciences*, vol. 35, no. 2, 1980, p. 187.
42 See Maneesha Lal, "The ignorance of women is the house of illness". Gender, Nationalism, and Health Reform in Colonial North India', in Mary P. Sutphen and Bridie Andrews (eds), *Medicine and Colonial Identity* (London: Routledge, 2003), pp. 14–40.
43 Rima D. Apple, *Perfect Motherhood Science and Childrearing in America* (New Brunswick: Rutgers University Press, 2006); and Rima D. Apple, *Mothers and Medicine A Social History of Infant Feeding, 1890–1950* (Madison, WI: The University of Wisconsin Press, 1987), Part III Scientific Motherhood, pp. 95–132.
44 Davin, 'Imperialism and Motherhood', *History Workshop*, p. 33.
45 Margaret Jolly, 'Introduction Colonial and postcolonial plots in histories of maternities and modernities', in Kalpana Ram and Margaret Jolly (eds), *Maternities and Modernities Colonial and Postcolonial Experiences in Asia and the Pacific* (Cambridge: Cambridge University Press, 1998), p. 4.
46 Ibid.
47 Andrea Major, 'Mediating Modernity: Colonial State, Indian Nationalism, and the Renegotiation of the 'Civilizing Mission', in the Indian Child Marriage Debate of 1927–1932', in Carey A. Watt and Michael Mann (eds), *Civilizing Missions in Colonial and Postcolonial South Asia* (Delhi: Anthem Press, 2012), p. 185.
48 Srirupa Prasad, *Cultural Politics of Hygiene in India, 1890–1940 Contagions of Feeling* (New York: Palgrave Macmillan., 2015), p. 17.
49 *Bengal Baby Week 1924*, pp. 20–21.
50 Page, *Bengal Baby Week 1924*, p. 50.
51 Page, *Bengal Baby Week 1924*, p. 47.
52 Ibid.
53 Ibid., pp. 49–50.
54 Shudha Mazumdar, *A Pattern of Life The Memoirs of an Indian Woman*, ed. by Geraldine H. Forbes (New Delhi: Manohar, 1977), p. 193. Siobhan Lambert-Hurley's work highlights the success of baby shows in Bhopal organised by elite Muslim women in Bhopal through their use of Unani medicine. She, however, contrasts its success with the 'unsuccessful' baby shows in colonial Bengal. See Siobhan Lambert-Hurley, 'Subtle Subversions and Presumptuous Interventions: Reforming Women's Health in Bhopal State in the Early Twentieth Century', in

Anindita Ghosh (ed), *Behind the Veil Resistance, Women and the Everyday in Colonial South Asia* (Basingstoke: Palgrave Macmillan, 2008), p. 135. My aim is to nuance this particular argument on Bengal here.

55 Mazumdar, *A Pattern of Life*, pp. 193–194.

56 Dagmar Engels, *Beyond Purdah? Women in Bengal 1890–1939* (Delhi: Oxford University Press, 1996), pp. 147–148.

57 'Improvement of Health: Propaganda Need', *Amrita Bazar Patrika*, 1 January 1941, n.p. cited in Ambalika Guha, *Colonial Modernities Midwifery in Bengal, c. 1860–1947* (London: Routledge, 2018), p. 125.

58 Guha, *Colonial Modernities*, p. 125.

59 Ibid., pp. 7–8.

60 See, Ishita Pande, *Medicine, Race and Liberalism in British Bengal Symptoms of Empire* (London: Routledge, 2010), pp. 2–3, 6, 13, 22.

61 Michel Foucault, *The History of Sexuality* Volume I: An Introduction Translated from the French by Robert Hurley (New York: Pantheon Books, 1978). pp. 67–69, 100.

62 Projit Bihari Mukharji, *Nationalizing the Body The Medical Market, Print and Daktari Medicine* (Delhi: Anthem Press, 2012), p. 77. Also see Dipesh Chakrabarty, *Provincializing Europe Postcolonial Thought and Historical Difference* (Princeton: Princeton University Press, 2000); and Pande, *Medicine, Race and Liberalism in British Bengal*, pp. 6–7.

63 For details about the Bengal Social Service League see Guha, *Colonial Modernities*, p. 171.

64 *Health and Child Welfare Exhibition*, p. 25.

65 He also used arguments from Michel Foucault, "Two Lectures." In *Power/Knowledge: Selected Interviews and Other Writings, 1972–1977*, edited by Colin Gordon, 78–108. Toronto: Random House, 1980., p. 105 paraphrased in Projit Bihari Mukherjee, 'Munisipal Darpan: Imagining the Embodied State and Subaltern Citizenship in 1890s Calcutta', *South Asian History and Culture*, vol. 4, no. 1, 2013, p. 40.

66 Mukharji, 'Munisipal Darpan', p. 34.

67 Ibid., p. 38.

68 Ibid., p. 37.

69 Ibid., p. 36.

70 Ibid., p. 44.

71 Ibid., p. 37.

72 Ibid., p. 36.

73 Lantern lectures were conducted with the help of magic lantern (or projector) slides. For details see John Hannavy ed. *Encyclopedia of Nineteenth-Century Photography* Volume I A-I Index (Routledge: New York, 2008), p. 826.

74 *Dai* or *dhatri* refers to both the traditional midwife and wet nurse, see endnote 4 in Introduction.

75 Partha Chatterjee, 'The Nationalist Resolution of the Women's Question', in Kumkum Sangari and Sudesh Vaid (eds), *Recasting Women. Essays in Colonial History* (New Delhi: Kali for Women, 1989), p. 248.

76 *Putana* was also regarded as one among the several gr*ahas* which 'means both "seizing" or "laying hold of" and simply "planet,"' and also redescribed as *matrikas* or "mothers" or *graha-matrikas* (planet-mothers). Ayurvedic traditions and their connections with religion, astrology, and other areas incorporated these 'intangible agencies' believed to threaten human health, particularly

specific periods of infant life. For details, see Projit Bihari Mukharji, *Doctoring Traditions Ayurveda, Small Technologies, and Braided Sciences* (Chicago, IL: The University of Chicago Press, 2016), pp. 261–263.

77 For instance, Dr. Y. Sen, F.R.F.P. & S. (Glasgow), Women's Medical Service, Raj Dufferin Hospital, Bettiah. in 'Chapter VI. Papers Continued: Drs. G.J. Campbell, Wallace, Sen, George', in *Improvements of the Conditions of Childbirth in India*, p. 129; also Mridula Ramanna, *Health Care in Bombay Presidency 1896–1930* (Delhi: Primus, 2012), p. 123.

78 On so-called scientific, 'clean midwifery', caste, childbirth and related issues, see Margaret Ida Balfour and Ruth Young, *The Work of Medical Women in India* With a foreword by Dame Mary Scharlieb (London: Humphrey Milford Oxford University Press, 1929), pp. 123–140.

79 For details, see Chapter 2, the section – The 'dai question'.

80 Meredith Borthwick, *The Changing Role of Women in Bengal, 1849–1905* (Princeton, NJ: Princeton University Press, 1984), p. 153.

81 B.D. Mukharji, 'Child Welfare and Indigenous Dais', in *Health and Child Welfare Exhibition*, p. li. In Bengali.

82 Ibid., pp. l-lii

83 Ibid., p. liii.

84 Ibid., p. lii.

85 L.S.S. O'Malley, *Census of India, 1911*, Volume VI, Part 1, p. 30 cited in Dagmar Engels, *Beyond Purdah? Women in Bengal 1890–1939* (Delhi: Oxford University Press, 1996), p. 129 in Sujata Mukherjee, *Gender, Medicine, and Society in Colonial India Women's Health Care in Nineteenth- and Early Twentieth-Century Bengal* (New Delhi: Oxford University Press, 2017), p. 75.

86 Suhrawardy, 'The Care of the Expectant Mother and Newborn Infant', p. lxiii.

87 Ibid., lxv–lxvi.

88 Guha, '"The Best Swadeshi": Reproductive Health in Bengal, 1840–1940', in Sarah Hodges (eds), *Reproductive Health in India. History, Politics, Controversies* (Hyderabad: Orient Longman, 2006), p. 139.

89 Suhrawardy, 'The Care of the Expectant Mother and Newborn Infant', p. lxvii.

90 Ibid., pp. lxvii–lxviii.

91 Suhrawardy, 'The Care of the Expectant Mother and Newborn Infant', pp. lx–lxi; on merits of regular breastfeeding, Ibid., p. lxxvi also Ibid., pp. xii–xiii cited in Guha, 'The Best Swadeshi', p. 139.

92 Suhrawardy, 'The Care of the Expectant Mother and Newborn Infant', p. lxiii

93 Dr. J. Chakravarti, 'The Need of Fresh Air' *in Health and Child Welfare Exhibition*, pp. cii–ciii.

94 Rai Bahadur Dr. Chunilal Bose, 'Impure Air and Infant Mortality', *in Health and Child Welfare Exhibition*, pp. vii–viii.

95 Bose, 'Impure Air and Infant Mortality', *Health and Child Welfare Exhibition*, p. ix.

96 Ibid.

97 Supriya Guha, 'The Nature of Woman: Medical Ideas in Colonial Bengal', *Indian Journal of Gender Studies*, vol. 3, no. 1, 1996, p. 30.

98 Maneesha Lal, 'Purdah as Pathology: Gender and the Circulation of Medical Knowledge in Late Colonial India', in Sarah Hodges (ed), *Reproductive Health in India History, Politics, Controversies* (Hyderabad: Orient Longman, 2006), p. 109.

99 Guha, 'The Nature of Woman: Medical Ideas in Colonial Bengal', p. 30.

100 Charu Gupta, 'Hindu Wombs, Muslim Progeny: The Numbers Game and Shifting Debates on Widow Remarriage in Uttar Pradesh, 1890s–1930s', in Sarah Hodges (ed), *Reproductive Health in India History, Politics, Controversies* (Hyderabad: Orient Longman, 2006), p. 168.
101 W.H. Thompson, *Census of India 1921 Volume V Bengal Part I Report* (Calcutta: Bengal Secretariat Book Depot, 1923), p. 158.
102 See Pradip Kumar Datta, '"Dying Hindus": Production of Hindu Communal Common Sense in Early 20th Century Bengal', *Economic and Political Weekly*, vol. 28, no. 25, 1993, pp. 1317n27, 1305.
103 Ibid., p. 68.
104 Ibid., p. xi.
105 Sonia Nishat Amin, *The World of Muslim Women in Colonial Bengal, 1876–1939* (Leiden: E. J. Brill, 1996), pp. 12–13.
106 Mahua Sarkar, *Visible Histories, Disappearing Women Producing Muslim Womanhood in Late Colonial Bengal* (Durham: Duke University Press, 2008). p. 2.; Begum Sufia Kamal, personal communication, Dhaka, 1996 cited in Sarkar, *Visible Histories*, p. 186.
107 Sarkar, *Visible Histories*, p. 70.
108 Ibid., p. 72.
109 Amin, *The World of Muslim Women in Colonial Bengal*, p. 13
110 Mrs. R. S. Hossein, 'Care of Babies', in *Health and Child Welfare Exhibition*, p. lxxxv. On the Boer War and lessons for India, see Ibid., p. lxxxv. Besides this article which cites Dr. Bharat Chandra's argument on learned motherhood, similar argument is cited in subsection '*Santanpalan*' (or 'Childrearing') in article titled '*Sugrihini*'. In this article, she also asked the '*sugrihini*', or good wife and mother in contemporary nationalist discourses, to teach her family that they are '*bharatbasi*' or 'Indian' first, and their community identity came after that. She emphasised that with every drop of breast milk the mother's *manogato bhab* or mental state and inner feelings were passed into the child. She also quoted (in a slightly different order than that cited by Indira Chowdhury-Sengupta) a brief excerpt on breastfeeding and its connection with creation of patriotic sons. For details, see Rokeya Sakhawat Hossein, 'Sugrihini' cited in Syed, Abdul Mannan, Selina Hossein, Mohammad Shamshul Alam and Abdul Quadir (eds), *Rokeya Rachanabali* [Complete Works of Begum Rokeya Sakhawat Hossain] (Dhaka: Bangla Academy, 1971), pp. 31–40, mainly pp. 37–38. Her name has been spelt according to its spelling in the *Health and Child Welfare Exhibition* report. The aforesaid excerpt seems to be the same section of the song by Dwarkanath Ganguly, Brahmo Samaji who supported women's education and emancipation (husband of famous Dr. Kadambini Ganguly), from Yogindranath Sarkar, *Bande Mataram* (Calcutta: City Book Society, sixth ed., 1908) translated and cited in Indira Chowdhury-Sengupta, 'The Effeminate and the Masculine: Nationalism and the Concept of Race in Colonial Bengal', in Peter Robb (ed), *The Concept of Race in South Asia* (New Delhi: Oxford University Press, 1995), pp. 292–293. For further reading, see mainly Bharati Ray, *Early Feminists of Colonial India Sarala Devi Chaudhurani and Rokeya Sakhawat Hossain* (Oxford: Oxford University Press, 2002), among others.
111 Hossein, 'Care of Babies', p. lxxxv.
112 Ibid., p. lxxxii.
113 Ibid.
114 Ibid., p. lxxxiii.
115 Miss H. Bose, 'Flies' in, *Health and Child Welfare Exhibition*, pp. xiii–xvi.
116 Hossein, 'Care of Babies', p. lxxxii.

117 Ibid., p. lxxxv.

118 'Child-Wives' in Extracts from the *Indian Medical Gazette* for September and October 1890 in Home Department, Judicial Branch, October 1890 Proceeding, File 211, National Archives of India (hereafter NAI). Also, see Ishita Pande, *Medicine, Race and Liberalism in British Bengal Symptoms of Empire* (London: Routledge, 2010), p. 163; Mrinalini Sinha, *Colonial Masculinity: The 'Manly Englishman' and the 'Effeminate Bengali' in the Late Nineteenth Century* (Manchester: Manchester University Press, 1995), p. 158.

119 He was a member of the Calcutta Medical Society, Licentiate in Medicine and Surgery (L.M.S.), Assistant-Surgeon and Teacher of Medicine at the Campbell Medical School, Calcutta.

120 A very similar discussion by Keshub Chunder Sen in Pande, *Medicine, Race and Liberalism in British Bengal*, p. 158.

121 Mrinalini Sinha (ed), *Mother India* by Katherine Mayo. Edited with an Introduction by Mrinalini Sinha (Ann Arbor, MI: University of Michigan Press, 2000, 1998), p. 24.

122 Mrinalini Sinha, 'Refashioning Mother India: Feminism and Nationalism in Late-Colonial India', *Feminist Studies*, Points of Departure: India and the South Asian Diaspora, vol. 26, no. 3, 2000, p. 630.

123 Durba Mitra *Indian Sex Life Sexuality and the Colonial Origins of Modern Social thought*, (Princeton: Princeton University Press, 2020), p. 6.

124 Ishita Pande, 'Time for Sex: The Education of Desire and the Conduct of Childhood in Global/Hindu Sexology', in Veronika Fuechtner, Douglas E. Haynes, and Ryan M. Jones (eds), *A Global History of Sexual Science, 1880–1960* (Berkeley: University of California Press, 2018), p. 287.

125 Ibid., p. 284; as also mentioned in Chapter 1, on lack of 'coevalness' and 'allochronism', see mainly Johannes Fabian, *Time and the Other: How Anthropology Makes Its Object* (New York: Columbia University Press, 1983, reprint edition), pp. 35, 202n13.

126 Ibid., p. 280.

127 Ibid.

128 Kaviraj Harnam Das, *Sachitra Vivahit Anand* (Lahore: Harnam Singh, 1929) cited in Pande, 'Time for Sex', p. 279.

129 On Truby King's childcare methods mainly see Philippa Mein Smith, *Mothers and King Baby. Infant Survival and Welfare in an Imperial World: Australia 1880–1950* (London: Macmillan Press, 1997); Linda Bryder, 'New Zealand's Infant Welfare Services and Maori, 1907–60', *Health and History*, vol. 3, no. 1, Maori Health, 2001, pp. 65–86, among others.

130 Samita Sen, *Women and Labour in Late Colonial India The Bengal Jute Industry* (Cambridge: Cambridge University Press, 1999), p. 149.

131 Frederic Truby King, *Feeding and Care of Baby* (London and Calcutta: Macmillan and Co., 1913).

132 Robbie P. Kahn, 'Women and Time in Childbirth and During Lactation', in Frieda Johles Forman and Caoran Sowton (eds), *Taking Our Time Feminist Perspectives on Temporality* (New York: Pergamon Press, 1988), pp. 27–29; Fiona Dykes, *Breastfeeding in Hospital Mothers, Midwives and the Production Line* (New York: Routledge, 2006), pp. 96–97, 126.

133 Judith E. Walsh, *How to Be the Goddess of Your Home. An Anthology of Bengali Domestic Manuals* (New Delhi: Yoda Press, 2005), p. 2–3. On colonialism, the self-image of the *bhadralok* and fears of 'racist humiliation, and clock time and the appeal of *Kaliyuga*, see Sumit Sarkar, *Writing Social History* (Delhi: Oxford University Press, 1997), pp. 188–190.

134 Ruth Young, 'Preface to the First Edition', *Maternity and Infant Welfare A Handbook for Health Visitors, Parents, and Others in India* (Calcutta: The Lady Chelmsford All-India League for Maternity and Child Welfare, second ed. 1922), p. iii.
135 Young, *Maternity and Infant Welfare*, p. 96–97. In the above excerpt, the emphasis on 'can' in the sentence 'The baby *can* be trained in good habits.' has been given by Young (1922). Rest of emphases are mine. Reference to the male child was also common in women's magazines like the *Bamabodhini Patrika*, for example, ShriHemantakumari Debi, 'Santan-Palan', *Bamabodhini Patrika*, Sraban-Kartik 1323 Bengali year, 1916 in Pradip Basu (ed), *Samayiki*, pp. 779–793.
136 Milton Lewis, The "Health of the Race" and Infant Health in New South Wales: Perspectives on Medicine and Empire', in Roy Macleod and Milton Lewis (eds), Disease, Medicine and Empire Perspectives on Western Medicine and the Experience of European Expansion (New York: Routledge, 1988), p. 310.
137 Ibid.
138 Cathy Urwin and Elaine Sharland, 'From Bodies to Minds in Childcare Literature: Advice to Parents in Inter-war Britain', in Roger Cooter (ed), *In the Name of the Child Health and Welfare 1880 to 1940* (New York: Routledge, 1992), p. 177.
139 Mein Smith, *Mothers and King Baby*, p. 112
140 Ibid.
141 Urwin and Sharland, 'From Bodies to Minds in Childcare Literature', p. 177. Here they refer to King, *Feeding and Care of Baby* (revised ed. 1925), p. 3.
142 Mary Barfield, 'In the Tropics', *Mothercraft Training Society Half-Yearly Magazine* (9), February 1929, pp. 247–249. Source: Records of the Mothercraft Training Society, Highgate Literary and Scientific Institution, Highgate, London, United Kingdom.
143 Miss Carleton, 'Extracts from Letters', *Mothercraft Training Society Half-Yearly Magazine*, No. 9, February 1929, p. 251. Source: Records of the Mothercraft Training Society, Highgate Literary and Scientific Institution, Highgate, London, United Kingdom. For a discussion on the rearing European infants in tropical India, see Sen, *Gendered Transactions*, pp. 144–171.
144 Miss Carleton, 'Extracts from Letters', p. 251.
145 Sundari Mohan Das, *Saral Dhatri-Sikkha o Kumar-Tantra* (Calcutta: Shri Premananda Jogananda Das, seventh ed. 1935), n.p., Title Translation: Simple Education in Midwifery and Doctrines of Childrearing; Saha, 'Milk, 'Race' and Nation', pp. 155–156.
146 See Dipesh Chakrabarty, 'The Difference: Deferral of (A) Colonial Modernity: Public Debates on Domesticity in British Bengal', *History Workshop*, vol. 36, Colonial and Post-Colonial History, Autumn 1993, pp. 1–34, especially pp. 7–13.
147 Sumathi Ramaswamy, *The Goddess and the Nation Mapping Mother India* (Durham: Duke University Press, 2010), p. 52.
148 Chakrabarty, The Difference', pp. 9–10.
149 Sundari Mohan Das, 'Resurrection of Motherhood and Fatherhood', *The Modern Review*, vol. XXVI, no. 2, 1919, pp. 189–192; also see Maneesha Lal, '"The ignorance of women is the house of illness". Gender, Nationalism, and Health Reform in Colonial North India', in Mary P. Sutphen and Bridie Andrews (eds), *Medicine and Colonial Identity* (London: Routledge, 2003), pp. 27–28, p39n64.

150 Rameshwari Nehru was invited to the Age of Consent Committee in 1927 to examine public opinion surrounding social legislation on the age of consent issue which ultimately became the Child Marriage Restraint Act (CMRA) of 1929, see Lal, 'The ignorance of women is the house of illness', p. 17.
151 Ibid., p. 27.
152 Sundari Mohan Das, 'Mātā kā Navjīvan', 'New Life for Mother', *Stri Darpan*, 1919 in Lal, 'The ignorance of women is the house of illness', pp. 27–28. In this article, he also praises infant welfare in New Zealand as having remarkable success in reducing infant mortality – symptomatic of contemporary popularity of New Zealand physician Frederic Truby King's centrality to infant welfare advice in New Zealand and Britain as well as Das' deployment of King's clocked schedules in his advice on infant feeding.
153 Das, 'Resurrection of Motherhood and Fatherhood', p. 189.
154 Lal, 'The ignorance of women is the house of illness', pp. 27–28; also Saha, 'Milk, "Race" and Nation', p. 155.
155 Also see Saha, Milk, "Race" and Nation, p. 155.
156 George L. Mosse, *Nationalism and Sexuality. Middle-Class Morality and Sexual Norms in Modern Europe* (Madison: University of Wisconsin Press, 1985), p. 93.
157 Ramaswamy, *The Goddess and the Nation*, p. 60.
158 Ibid., pp. 22–23, 60.
159 Sundari Mohan Das, *Saral Dhatri-Sikkha o Kumar-Tantra* (Calcutta: Oriental Enterprises Syndicate, third ed. 1922), Title Translation: Simple Education in Midwifery and Doctrines of Childrearing, pp. n.p., 102; also, see Saha, 'Milk, "Race" and Nation', p. 156. For Figure 5.7, permission has also been obtained from the WSIF journal. For Das' *Saral Dhatri Shikkha* and *Sishu Mangal*–translations are mine.
160 Borthwick, *The Changing Role of Women in Bengal*, p. 171.
161 Das, *Saral Dhatri-Sikkha*, p. 102; and Sundari Mohan Das, *Sishu Mangal Pratham Shikkha* Calcutta: Shri Premananda Das and Shri Jogananda Das, 1927), p. 43, Title Translation: Child Welfare First Education; also see Saha, 'Milk, "Race" and Nation', p. 156.
162 Ramaswamy, *The Goddess and the Nation*, p. 52.
163 Ibid., p. 52.
164 Jacques Derrida, 'That Dangerous Supplement', in *Of Grammatology* (Baltimore, Maryland: John Hopkins University Press, 1976), p. 144 in Ramaswamy, 'The Goddess and the Nation', p. 52.
165 Kajri Jain, *Gods in the Bazaar The Economies of Indian Calendar Art* (Durham, NC: Duke University Press, 2007) in Ramaswamy, *The Goddess and the Nation*, 309n24.
166 It is particularly relevant to note that King was the Medical Director at the Mothercraft Training Society (the Babies of the Empire Society) in London which was backed by the Overseas Club and the Patriotic League – together they published this particular manual. Saha, 'Milk, 'Race' and Nation', p. 156.
167 Frederic Truby King, *Natural Feeding of Infants* With an Introduction by J. S. Fairbairn. London: Whitcombe & Tombs Limited, 1918), n.p.
168 Petrina Brown, *Eve Sex, Childbirth and Motherhood through the Ages* (Chichester: Summersdale Publishers, 2004), p. 154; Saha, 'Milk, 'Race' and Nation', p. 156.
169 Guha, *Colonial Modernities*, p. 86.
170 Rames Chandra Ray, 'Prasutir Proti Kartabba', *Vishak-Darpan*, vol. 15, no. 11, 1905, p. 423. Article title translation: 'Duties Toward Parturient Women';

the journal title *Vishak-Darpan* translates as physician's mirror. Translation mine.

171 Ibid.

172 Ibid., pp. 423–4. Also see Rameshchandra Roy, 'Prasutir Proti Kartabya (Duty Towards a Parturient Women)', *Bhishak Darpan*, vol. 15, no. 11, November 1905, pp. 423–424 cited in Ambalika Guha, *Colonial Modernities*, p. 86.

173 Rames Chandra Ray, 'Child Welfare VIII (B) Mothercraft and Housewifery', *The Amrita Bazar Patrika*, 1 May, 1919, p. 7. Also see some parts of this excerpt cited as Ramesh Chandra Ray, 'Child Welfare', *Indian Medical Record*, vol. 39, September 1919, n.p. in Guha, *Modern Maternities*, p. 113.

174 Frederic Truby King, *Feeding and Care of Baby* (London and Calcutta: Macmillan and Co., 1913), p. 36, (Accessed 16 June 2016) http://wellcomelibrary.org/item/b21512115#c=0&m=0&s=0&cv=40&z=0.1797%2C0.6791%2C2.0422%2C1.0347.

175 Ibid., p. 96.

176 Ibid., p. 36.

177 Ibid., 96; also see Saha, 'Milk, mothering & meanings', p. 103.

178 Illustration: This clock is a schedule for feeding of the durbal sishu or weak infant. Translation of Caption at the bottom of the page: 'Picture Number 15 – Feeding by the clock of durbal sishu or weak infant. Ibid., 148.

179 Illustration: Right at the top, 'gharir daak'/'call of the clock' is followed by the caption below 'Nurse! Look in the direction of the clock; Must Feed at the Right Time'. The caption at the bottom of the page reads: 'Picture Number 16 – Feeding by the clock of the sabal sishu or strong infant'. [There are two Bengali words in the picture itself: Ghum or Sleep and Khaoya or Feeding]. Das, *Saral Dhatrisikkha*, p. 149; also see Saha, 'Milk, mothering & meanings', p. 104. For this image of the *sabal sishu*, permission has also been obtained from the WSIF journal.

180 Das, *Saral Dhatri-Sikkha* (ed. 1940), pp. 146–149, 153; also Das, *Sishu Mangal*; and Saha, 'Milk, Race and Nation', p. 156.

181 In Das' detailed table for artificial feeding for infants: The headers from left to right, horizontally at the top of the table, translate as 'Age' (age of the infant: third day, fourth day, fifth day, sixth day, seventh to the 14th day, third week, and fourth week of the infant respectively), 'How many times in a day' (6 times is the standard cited in the table), 'Frequency' (every three hours throughout), Amount in Each Feed' (amount in each feed in relation to the age of the infant: 2, 3, 4, 5, 6, 7, and 8 respectively), 'Amount in 24 Hours' (amount varied in relation to age of the infant:12, 18, 24, 30, 36, 42 and 48 teaspoons respectively in the different stages), 'Proportion of Cow's Milk' (3, 6, 10, 15, 12, 18 and 36 teaspoons respectively), and 'Proportion of Water' (9, 12, 14, 15, 14, 14 and 12 spoons respectively). The amount of each feed every three hours, the total food in 24 hours, and the proportions of milk and water were all determined by the requirements of the infant by age cited in the extreme left hand side of the table vertically. Das, *Sishu Mangal*, p. 51.

182 'Advertisement for New South Wales first baby week, "Long Live King Baby?", Sunday News, Sydney, 24 March 1920' in Davin, 'Imperialism and Motherhood', p. 14 cited in Mein Smith, *Mothers and King Baby*, p. 63; also see Saha, 'Milk, "Race" and Nation', p. 160n19.

183 Sundari Mohan Das, 'Ravages of Putana', in *Health and Child Welfare Exhibition*, pp. lvii–lix.

184 Saha, 'Milk, "Race" and Nation', p. 157.

185 Ibid.
186 Borthwick, *The Changing Role of Women in Bengal*, p. 151; also see Saha, 'Milk, "Race" and Nation', p. 157.
187 Das, 'Ravages of Putana', pp. lvii–lix; also some parts of the excerpt cited in Guha, 'The Best Swadeshi', pp. 148–149.
188 Das, 'Ravages of Putana', pp. lvii-lviii.
189 Ibid., pp. lix–lx. A similar argument in Das, 'Resurrection of Motherhood and Fatherhood', pp. 189–192.
190 Das, 'Ravages of Putana', p. lix.
191 Das, *Saral Dhatrisikkha*, p. 149; also see Saha, 'Milk, mothering & meanings', p. 104.
192 Das, *Saral Dhatrisikkha*, p. 148.
193 Das, *Saral Dhatri-Shikkha* (ed. 1940), pp. 146–149, 153; also Das, *Sishu Mangal*; also see Saha, 'Milk, Race and Nation', p. 156.
194 Lewis, 'The health of the race and infant health in New South Wales', p. 310.
195 Mein Smith, *Mothers and King Baby*, p. 34.
196 Urwin and Sharland, 'From Bodies to Minds in Childcare Literature', p. 178.
197 Saul Dubow, *Scientific Racism in Modern South Africa* (Cambridge, Cambridge University Press, 1995), p. 145
198 Ibid., p. 148.
199 On Miss. Silvia de la Place, see M. Miles, 'Disability Care and Education in 19th Century India: Some Dates, Places and Documentation', *ActionAid Disability News: The Newsletter of Disability Division, ActionAid, India*, vol. 5 (2 supplement), January 1, 1994, pp. 1–22. Miss. de la Place, 'Feeble-Mindedness in India (Paper prepared for the Child Welfare Exhibition by Miss de la Place, Lady Superintendent, the Children's House, Kurseong.)', in *Health and Child Welfare Exhibition, Calcutta, 1920*, Appendix II, pp. cxxxi–cxlii. She was unable to present the paper in person, however. It was included in the official Exhibition report.
200 de la Place, 'Feeble-Mindedness in India', pp. cxxxiii–cxli,
201 Ibid., p. cxli.
202 Luzia Savary, *Evolution, Race and Public Spheres in India Vernacular Concepts and Sciences (1860–1930)* (London: Routledge, 2019), pp. 10–11, 120–121.
203 de la Place, 'Feeble-Mindedness in India', p. cxxxviii.
204 Ibid.
205 For details, see Bejoyketu Bose, 'Mental Hygiene Movement in India', *The Modern Review*, vol. LXXVII, no. 3, 1945, pp. 123–124.
206 J. A. Richey, *Progress of Education in India, 1917–1922 Eighth Quinquennial Review Vol. I* (Calcutta: Superintendent of Government Printing, India, 1923), p. 221.
207 For an interesting discussion on the subject, see Shilpi Rajpal, 'Psychiatrists and Psychiatry in late colonial India', *The Indian Economic and Social History Review*, vol. 55, (4), 2018, pp. 23–25.
208 A. D. Stewart, 'Exhibits Committee Report', in *Indian Red Cross Society Bengal Provincial Branch Bengal Health Welfare Week 1931* With a Foreword by Hon'ble Lady Jackson (Calcutta: 1931), pp. 12–13.

CONCLUSION

My book aimed to address an excitingly new and wide range of issues concerning medical advice about breastfeeding in colonial Calcutta. The rationale behind the book was to problematise and analyse previously underexplored medical instruction about mothering of infants, imbued with 'scientific' and moralising rhetoric, as a key entry point into the social histories of medicine, maternities and childcare in colonial Calcutta. One of the most distinguishing features of this volume is that it brought to light rare textual and visual materials on medical opinions about breastfeeding across diverse social milieus namely: the *bhadramahila* ('respectable' Bengali-Hindu women), memsahibs (European women) and *dais* (indigenous midwives and/or wet nurses). Medical handbooks and periodicals, governmental medical and judicial proceedings and reports on native newspapers, national and international child welfare exhibition and conference reports, personal correspondence and memoirs, illustrations and advertisements have provided enormous information on the subject. While the topics covered are varied, at the same time, these are thematically interconnected throughout the book. Infant feeding like maternal breastfeeding, wet nursing and/or artificial feeding of infants were often integral to defining different kinds of maternities. In colonial India, ideals of 'good' versus 'bad' maternities were tied up with anxieties about infant feeding and the future health and manly vigour of the wider community, 'race' and/or nation. I located breastfeeding advice at the centre of the very making of modern maternities in nineteenth and twentieth century Calcutta. 'Pure'/'polluting' and 'good'/'bad' biocultural qualities believed to have been constituted by 'race', gender, community, class and/or caste, and age and considered transmissible through milk and blood were central to my interrogation of the crisscrossing perceptions of colonial modernity, medicine and motherhood.

As breastfeeding was central to 'ideal' mothering of infants as prescribed and proscribed by various medical practitioners from different medical systems – it explored the centrality of medical print media in the modernisation and medicalisation of motherhood in colonial Calcutta. This volume, therefore, began by giving a glimpse of how 'race' and gender were central

DOI: 10.4324/9781003327837-7

to the colonial medical gaze on European and 'native' maternal bodies in the 'tropics'. It also provided an alternative perspective to the dominant historiographical trend of placing the detailed examination of the wet nurse's body entirely within the purview of *colonial difference* and racism. My research provided a nuanced argument highlighting that even Bengali *daktars* offered similarly harsh medical checklists for hiring a wet nurse or *dai*. 'Science' was also meant to discipline, replace or reconfigure beliefs and practices of 'dirty' indigenous *dais*/untrained midwives, Hindu ritual pollution of touch associated with caste hierarchies, confinement and childbirth; and Indian mother love often associated with the customary breastfeeding practices like 'over-nursing' of infants. My research also attempted to illustrate that it is not always clear as to who/what exactly counted as a 'healthy' and 'good' mother and child. Was anyone eligible to become a 'good' mother? Explorations of newspaper advertisements to medical manuals and periodical essays on 'ideal' baby foods and the problem of infant mortality also brought up the question – could '[a] bottle mother . . . still be a perfect mother'[1]?

Moreover, representations of the *bhadramahila* as the 'traditional' and 'modern' literate 'new woman' whose main duty was to become a *sugrihini* or 'good' wife and mother had to confront the fact that she was usually the problematic figure of the 'girl-child/woman'.[2] Colonial and nationalist writings on child marriage, mainly the problematic area of breastfeeding in early motherhood, have largely been ignored by earlier studies. An in-depth study of medical advice on child marriage and 'premature maternity' revealed the urgent need doctors felt at the time to differentiate between the bodily makeup of the girl child and woman. Medical advice on breastfeeding and early motherhood, therefore, provided novel entry points into colonial and indigenous representations of 'Indian mothers' and their childrearing practices in late nineteenth and early twentieth century colonial Bengal, mainly Calcutta.

This volume closed with the global resonances of 'maternal ignorance' and medicalised motherhood popularised as 'mothercraft', 'clean'/'dirty' midwifery, and the *bhadramahila* 'ideal' central to the early twentieth-century child welfare drive in Calcutta, often imbued with highly racialised and gendered, classed and caste-ridden overtones within the broader colonial framework. 'Mothercraft' and feeding by the clock aimed to clock 'Indian mothers' and their 'child's cries' for the breast are previously underexplored recurring themes in colonial and indigenous maternal and infant care manuals. It also explored in detail, earlier overlooked, transnational connections – renowned Calcutta *daktar* Sundari Mohan Das' clocks for feeding 'weak' and 'strong' babies alongside his tables for clocked feeding in several ways closely resemble the most influential proponent of 'mothercraft', famous New Zealand physician Truby King's 'Clock Faces'. Motherhood under medical supervision popularised as 'mothercraft' in the early twentieth century primarily involved medical knowledge and supervision of 'ignorant' mothers and their newborn babies. Such childcare 'by the clock' involved global precepts of disciplined and well-ordered domesticity and motherhood which came to be medically crafted and tied to variegated imperial, colonial and nationalist agendas. Das' understandings of Hinduism, western medicine and Ayurveda influenced his deification of the breastfeeding 'Indian mother' figure as *Ma Lakkhi* as well as her pathologisation and medicalisation with the help of modern clocks as anti-colonial nation-building.

However, this study has been far from comprehensive. To begin with, the study primarily focused on motherhood and the mother figure, the child as such did not get much attention beyond analysing the fact that the 'male' child was usually central to the medical print media in colonial India. Ideas about 'good'/'bad' child and varied perceptions of childhood in Bengal at the time have been ignored as it goes beyond the purview of my current research. The significance of everyday interactions in early childhood in the nursery,[3] and Pierre Bourdieu's ideas about the embodiment of 'cultural capital' and the psychological implications of tastes and markets would offer important entry points into childhood memories.[4] In the context of Bengal, Sibaji Bandyopadhyay's arguments on the 'good'/'bad' (male) child and the invisibility of the girl child and her lack of girlhood explored through an investigation of Bengali children's literature would certainly have to be included.[5] Further unexplored questions which I might like to look into at a later stage include: What were the pre-colonial ideas about childhood? How were maternal breastfeeding, wet-nursing and 'milk kinship' perceived in the Mughal period? What were the prescriptions and proscriptions on breastfeeding in the Unani? How did ideas about childrearing and childhood travel primarily between intersections of gender, class and/or caste, and community? How do we move beyond colonial modernity and the colonial frameworks to understand the variegated perceptions of motherhood and childhood? Global connections drawn have been primarily based on ideas of 'mothercraft' and clocked feeding in Britain, New Zealand and Australia. Therefore, the exploration of ideas about 'race' in relation to breastfeeding has been rather limited. Even though 'vernacularization' has been a useful category here, it has not been critically engaged with at the theoretical level. It has also risked possible essentialisation of ideas translated and exchanged across socio-economic and political disparities between Britain and colonial Bengal. This study, dependent on transcultural exchanges of 'mothercraft' and medicine, has also focused primarily on mainstream ideas of clocked feeding across regional boundaries instead of, for instance, exploring actual experiences of breastfeeding in greater detail. It traced the historical trajectories of clocked medical regimen for breastfeeding and mother love. The affective ties from maternal breastfeeding and wet nursing often carefully tucked away in the pages of memoirs and personal letters have only been briefly touched upon and left largely unexplored. Was there an emotional price and piety that mothers or wet nurses expected from the children they have breastfed? What about the 'emotional labour'[6] costs of paid caregivers?

What about its 'exchange value'?[7] Here Gayatri Chakravorty Spivak refers to an aspect of such close mother/wet nurse-child bonding, or lack thereof, that is, the 'psycho-social affect' on the child, and the emotional piety/gifts expected in return for '(professional) motherhood'.[8] Furthermore, possibly our 'selfish gene' has had an important role to play as a large amount of physical investment on the part of the mother occurs due to her biological design? As Richard Dawkins points out, her 'large, food-rich egg' to nurture and protect the foetus and then the baby means that she is supposed to be already 'committed', more than the father, especially from the point of conception through to the weaning period.[9] I aspire to incorporate some of these problems, which have been outside the scope of this study, in future research endeavours to develop a global historical perspective for a broader contextualisation of maternal and infant health connecting colonial India with Britain and the rest of the British empire, and beyond.

Notes

1 L. E. Holt, *The Good Housekeeping Book of Baby and Child Care* (New York, Popular Library, Inc., 1957), p. 65 cited in S. M. Crowther, L. A. Reynolds and E. M. Tansey (eds), *The Resurgence of Breastfeeding, 1975–2000*. Wellcome Witnesses to Twentieth Century Medicine, vol. 35 (London: Wellcome Trust Centre for the History of Medicine at UCL, 2009), p. xxiii.

2 Ruby Lal, 'Recasting the Women's Question The Girl-Child/Woman in the Colonial Encounter', *Interventions*, vol. 10, no. 3, 2008, p. 321.

3 On the everyday, see for example, Henri Lefebvre, *Everyday Life in the Modern World* Translated by Sacha Rabinovitch (London: Allen Lane The Penguin Press, 1968).

4 Pierre Bourdieu, 'The forms of capital', in J. Richardson (ed), *Handbook of Theory and Research for the Sociology of Education*. Translation by Richard Nice (New York: Greenwood, 1986), pp. 46–58; on 'habitus'/disposition and tastes, see Pierre Bourdieu, *Distinction A Social Critique of the Judgement of Taste* Translated by Richard Nice (Cambridge: Harvard University Press, 1984).

5 See Sibaji Bandyopadhyay, *Gopal-Rakhal Dwandasamas, Upanibeshbad o Bangla Sishusahitya* (Calcutta: Papyrus, 1999); *Aabar Shishushikha* (Kolkata: Anustup, 2005); and *Bangla Shishusahityer Chhoto Meyera by Sibaji Bandyopadhyay* (Kokata: Ganghil, 2007).

6 On 'emotional labour', see, for example, Arlie Russell Hochschild, *The Managed Heart Commercialization of Human Feeling* (Berkeley: University of California Press, 1983); also Mithreyi Krishnaraj (ed), *Motherhood in India Glorification without Empowerment* (New Delhi: Routledge, 2010), p. 23; among others.

7 On exchange value of wet nursing, see Mahasweta Devi, *Breast Stories* Translated with introductory essays by Gayatri Chakravorty Spivak (London: Seagull, 2016, first printing 1997), pp. 79–80, 84. Also significant, Gayatri Chakravorty Spivak, 'Can the Subaltern Speak?' in *Marxism and the Interpretation of Culture* Edited and with an Introduction by Cary Nelson and Lawrence Grossberg (London: Macmillan, 1988), pp. 271–313.

8 Ibid., p. 84.

9 Cf. Richard Dawkins, *The Selfish Gene* (Oxford: Oxford University Press, 1989, 1976 first ed.), p. 146.

BIBLIOGRAPHY

Primary Sources

National Archives of India (New Delhi)

Home Department, Medical Branch Proceedings
Home Department, Judicial Branch Proceedings
Education Department, Sanitary Branch Proceedings
Native Newspaper Reports, Bengal Presidency

Delhi State Archives (New Delhi)

Chief Commissioner's Office Proceedings.
Deputy Commissioner's Office Proceedings

West Bengal State Archives (WBSA, Kolkata, West Bengal)

Finance Department, Medical Branch Proceedings
General Department Proceedings

British Library (London, U.K.)

Administration Reports of the Commissioners of Calcutta
Reports on the Municipal Administration of Calcutta
Reports of the Sanitary Commissioners for Bengal
Bengal Public Health Reports
Private papers of Marchioness of Reading as Vicereine of India 1921–26
Private papers of Yvonne Alice Gertrude Fitzroy (1891–1971), chiefly as Private Secretary to Alice, Marchioness of Reading, Vicereine 1921–26 from the Fitzroy Collection

Highgate Literary and Scientific Institution (London, U.K.)

Records of the Mothercraft Training Society

Wellcome Library (London, U.K.)

Private Papers of Margaret Ida Balfour

The Countess of Dufferin's Fund 1885–1935 Fifty Years' Retrospect India 1885–1935 (London: The Women's Printing Society, 1935).

Select Journals and Newspapers (English)

The British Gynaecological Journal
The Calcutta Journal of Medicine
The Indian Journal of Pediatrics
The Indian Medical Gazette
The Indian Medical Record
The India Review and Journal of Foreign Science and the Arts
The Modern Review
The Statesman and Friend of India (Calcutta)
Transactions of the Obstetrical Society of London

Select Journals (Bengali)

Ayurved
Bamabodhini Patrika
Chikitsak Bandhab
Chikitsa-Prokash
Chikitsa Sammilani
Janmabhumi
Sakhi
Swasthya Samachar
Vishak-Darpan

Published Primary Sources (Books, Official Publications and Reports)

'Address of John Marshall, F.R.S. President At the Annual Meeting, March 1st, 1883' in *Medico-Chirurgical Transactions* Published by The Royal Medical Chirurgical Society of London Second Series Volume The Forty-Eighth, (London: Longmans, Green, Reader, and Dyer, Paternoster Row, 1883), pp. 1–37.

Ally, Meer Ushruff, *Diseases of Children in Bengalee Balchikitsa* (Calcutta: Das and Sons, 1870).

——, *Handbook of Midwifery in Bengalee* (Calcutta: Das and Sons, 1869).

Anonymous, *A Domestic Guide to Mothers in India Containing Particular Instructions on the Management of Themselves and Their Children* (By A Medical Practitioner of Several Years' Experience in India; Bombay: American Mission Press, 1836).

Atkinson, Edwin T., *Statistical Descriptive and Historical Account of the North-Western Provinces of India Volume III Meerut Division Part II* (Allahabad: North Western Provinces Government Press, 1876).

Balfour, Margaret Ida, *Bharater desi daider jonno dhatrisikkha* (Calcutta, Printed at the Baptist Mission Press, 1922). [Title Translation: Midwifery for the Indian indigenous midwives].

_____, and Ruth Young, *The Work of Medical Women in India* (With a foreword by Dame Mary Scharlieb; London: Humphrey Milford and Oxford University Press, 1929).

Barfield, Mary, 'In the Tropics', *Mothercraft Training Society Half-Yearly Magazine*, 9 February 1929, pp. 247–249 (Source: Records of the Mothercraft Training Society, Highgate Literary and Scientific Institution, Highgate, London).

Basu, Mrs Latika, 'Oral Evidence of Mrs. Latika Basu, Chittaranjan Seva Sadan, 148, Russa Road (South Calcutta) (Calcutta 19th December 1928)', in *Age of Consent Committee Evidence 1928–1929 Volume VI Oral Evidence and Written Statements of Witnesses from Bengal Presidency* (Calcutta: Government of India Central Publication Branch, 1929), pp. 67–69.

Basu, Sri Manindralal, 'Bongey Sishu Mrittyur Karon', *Swasthya Samachar*, vol. 8, no. 6, 1919, p. 139 (Title translation: 'Causes of Infant Mortality in Bengal').

Belnos, Mrs Sophie Charlotte, and Alexandre-Marie Colin, *Twenty Four Plates Illustrative of Hindoo and European Manners in Bengal Drawn on the Stone by A. Colin from the Sketches by Mrs. Belnos* (London: Smith and Elder Cornhill, 1832).

Bhishagratna, Kaviraj Kunja Lal M.R.A.S., *An English Translation of the Susruta Samhita* (With a Full and Comprehensive Introduction, Additional Texts, Different Readings, Notes, Comparative Views, Index, Glossary and Plates in Three Volumes Vol. II) *Nidána-Sthána, S'árira-Sthána, Chikitsita-Sthána and Kalapa-Sthána* (Calcutta: Published by the Author, No. 10, Kashi Ghose's Lane, 1911).

Bose, Bejoyketu, 'Mental Hygiene Movement in India', *The Modern Review*, vol. LXXVII, no. 3, 1945, pp. 123–125.

Bose, Dr. Bidhu Mukhi, 'Chapter VIII. – Extracts From Papers Written by Qualified Doctors and Nurses', in *Improvements of the Conditions of Childbirth in India Including a Special Report on the Work of the Victoria Memorial Scholarships Fund during the past Fifteen Years and Papers Written by Medical Women and qualified Midwives* (Calcutta: Superintendent Government Printing, India, 1918), pp. 150–151.

Bose, Dr. Juggobandhu, 'Appendix B Note by Dr. Juggobandhu Bose, M. D. on the "Age of Consent Bill" Showing that it is uncalled for even on physiological grounds', in *An Appeal to England to Save India from the Wrong and the Shame of the "Age of Consent" Act* (Calcutta: Published by Báli Sádharáni Sabhá, 1891), pp. 1–19.

Bose, Kumudini, 'Sishu Palan', *Ayurbed*, vol. 4, no. 1, Bengali Year 1326, c. 1919, pp. 18–23.

_____, 'Sishu Palan', *Ayurbed*, vol. 4, no. 2, Bengali Year 1326, c. 1919, pp. 66–72.

Bose, Nripendra Kumar, and Aradhana Debi, *NarNarir Jounobodh Jouno Khudha o Jounojiban* (Calcutta: Katyani Book Stall, 1934) (Title Translation: Sexual Awareness, Sexual Appetite and Sexual Life of Men and Women).

Bose, Rai Bahadur Dr. Chunilal, 'Impure Air and Infant Mortality', in *Health and Child Welfare Exhibition, Calcutta, 1920* (Calcutta: Bengal Secretariat Book Depot, 1921), pp. vii–xiii.

——, *The Milk Supply of Calcutta* (Calcutta: H. W. B. Moreno at the Central Press, 1918).

Bose, Shib Chunder, *The Hindoos as They Are. A Description of the Manners, Customs and Inner Life of Hindoo Society in Bengal* (With a Prefatory Note by The Rev. W. Hastie, B. D. Principal of the General Assembly's Institution; Calcutta: W. Newman & Co., 1881)

Carleton, Miss, 'Extracts from Letters', *Mothercraft Training Society Half-Yearly Magazine*, 9 February 1929, p. 251 (Source: Records of the Mothercraft Training Society, Highgate Literary and Scientific Institution, Highgate, London).

Central Advisory Board of Health, *Report on Maternity and Child Welfare Work in India* by Special Committee, (Simla: n.p., First Reprint, 1940, 1938).

Chakraberty, Chandra, *National Problems* (Calcutta: Ram Chandra Chakraberty, 1923).

——, *Infant Feeding and Hygiene* (Calcutta, Ramchandra Chakraberty, MA, 1923).

Chakravarti, Dr. J., 'The Need of Fresh Air', in *Health and Child Welfare Exhibition, Calcutta, 1920* (Calcutta: Bengal Secretariat Book Depot, 1921), pp. c–cv.

Chatterjee, Captain H. (L.R.C.P.S, Edin), 'Saishobiyo Aparipushtota', *Chikitsa-Prokash*, vol 17, no. 10, Bengali Year 1331, pp. 396–399.

Chatterjee, J. C., *An Introduction to the Study of Midwifery* (Calcutta, 1930).

Chattopadhyay, Kshirodaprasad, L.M.S., *Dhatribidya Subikhyato Daktar W. S. Playfair Sahiber A Treatise on the Science and Practice of Midwifery*. Granther Anubad. (Two Volumes) (Bhowanipur: Authorised and selected by the Vernacular Textbook Committee, and Printed at Oriental Press, 1886). [Title Translation: *Midwifery Famous Doctor W. S. Playfair Sahib's A Treatise on the Science and Practice of Midwifery*. Book Translation].

Chevers, Norman *A Manual of Medical Jurisprudence for India Including the History of Crime against the Person in India* (Calcutta: Thacker, Spink & Co., 1870)

Choudhuri, ShriBasantakumar, 'Sishu Khaddya', *Swasthya Samachar*, vol. 14, no. 1, Bengali Year 1332, c. 1925, pp. 8–21.

Chowdhri, Mrs., Sub-Assistant Surgeon, 'Barabanki cited in "Chapter VIII. – Extracts From Papers Written by Qualified Doctors and Nurses', in *Improvements of the Conditions of Childbirth in India Including a Special Report on the Work of the Victoria Memorial Scholarships Fund during the Past Fifteen Years and Papers Written by Medical Women and Qualified Midwives* (Calcutta: Superintendent Government Printing, India, 1918), pp. 151–152.

Cooper, Elizabeth, *The Harim and the Purdah Studies of Oriental Women* (New York: The Century Company, 1915).

Corbyn, Frederick, *Management and Diseases of Infants under the Influence of the Climate of India Being Instructions to Mothers and Parents in Situations Where*

Medical Aid Is Not to Be Obtained and a Guide to Medical Men, Inexperienced in the Nursery and the Treatment of Tropical Infantile Disease (Illustrated By Coloured Plates; Calcutta: Thacker and Co., 1828).

——, 'Preface' in Frederick Corbyn (ed), *The India Review and Journal of Foreign Science and the Arts* (Calcutta), vol I, pp. i–iv, (Accessed 10 November, 2016). http://dli.serc.iisc.ernet.in/scripts/FullindexDefault.htm? path1=/data2/upload/0048/5968&first=1&last=745&barcode=4990010194444.

Crooke, William, *An Introduction to the Popular Religion and Folklore of Northern India* (Allahabad: Printed at the Government Press, North-Western Provinces and Oudh, 1894).

Curjel, Dagmar F., M.D. (Glas), W.M.S., 'The Weight at Birth of Infants in India', *Indian Journal of Medical Research*, 1920–21 in Margaret Ida Balfour and Ruth Young, *The Work of Medical Women in India* With a foreword by Dame Mary Scharlieb (London: Humphrey Milford Oxford University Press, 1929), pp. 174–175.

Das, Kedarnath, *A Text-book of Midwifery for the Medical Schools and Colleges in India* (Calcutta: Thacker Spink & Co., 1921).

Das, SriNarendrakumar (M.B., M.C.P.S.), 'Sishu Mangal O Sishu Chikitsa' Part 1, *Chikitsa-Prokash*, vol.19, nos. 6 and 7, Bengali year 1333, pp. 224–227.

——, 'Sishu-Mangal O Sishu-Chikitsa' Parts 1 and 2, *Chikitsa-Prokash*, vol. 19, no. 9, Bengali Year 1333, pp. 355–356.

Das, Dr. SriNarendranath (L.M.S.), 'Saishabiyo Atisar – Infantile Diarrhea', *Chikitsa-Prokash*, vol 10, no. 11, Bengali Year 1324, pp. 413–19.

Das, Sundari mohan, 'Resurrection of Motherhood and Fatherhood (Illustrated)', *The Modern Review*, vol. XXVI, no. 2, 1919, pp. 189–92.

de la Place, Miss, 'Feeble-Mindedness in India (Paper prepared for the Child Welfare Exhibition by Miss de la Place, Lady Superintendent, the Children's House, Kurseong.)' in *Health and Child Welfare Exhibition, Calcutta, 1920* (Calcutta: Bengal Secretariat Book Depot, 1921), Appendix II, pp. cxxxi–cxlii.

——, 'Ravages of Putana' in *Health and Child Welfare Exhibition, Calcutta, 1920* (Calcutta: Bengal Secretariat Book Depot, 1921) pp. lvii–lx.

——, *Saral Dhatri-Sikkha o Kumar-Tantra* (Calcutta: Oriental Enterprises Syndicate, third ed. 1922). [Title Translation: Simple Education in Midwifery and Doctrines of Childrearing].

——, *Sishu Mangal Pratham Sikkha* (Calcutta: Shri Premananda Das and Shri Jogananda Das, 1927). [Title Translation: Child Welfare First Education].

——, *Saral Dhatri-Sikkha o Kumar-Tantra* (Calcutta: Shri Premananda Jogananda Das, seventh ed. 1935). [Title Translation: Simple Education in Midwifery and Doctrines of Childrearing].

——, *Saral Dhatri-Sikkha Kumar-Tantra O Stri-Rog* (Calcutta: Shri Premananda Das and Shri Jogananda Das, ninth ed. 1940). [Title Translation: Simple Education in Midwifery, Doctrines of Childrearing and Diseases of Women].

Dasgupta, Kabiraj Sri Harimohan, *Ayurvediyo Dhatribidya Sangraha.* Pratham Khando *A Compilation of Ayurvedic Midwifery Part 1* (Berhampur: Kabiraj Srinikhilranjan Sengupta Kabibhushan Berhampur Dhanantari Pharmacy, Bengali Year 1324, c.1917).

Datt, Mr. Amar Nath, Written Statement of Mr. Amar Nath Datt, B.A., B.L., M.L.A., Advocate, High Court, dated 13th August 1928, and Oral evidence of Mr. Amar Nath Dutt, M.L.A., Advocate, High Court (Delhi, 11th October 1928) in *Age of*

Consent Committee Evidence 1928–1929 Volume VI Oral Evidence and Written Statements of Witnesses from Bengal Presidency (Calcutta: Government of India Central Publication Branch, 1929), pp. 1–11.

Davies, W. L., *Indian Indigenous Milk Products* (Calcutta: Thacker, Spink & Co., 1940).

Deb, Shib Chunder, *The Infant Treatment First Part Sishu Palan Pratham Bhag* (Calcutta: reprint 1864; First Edition, 1857).

Debi, ShriHemantakumari, '*Santan-Palan*', *Bamabodhini Patrika* (Sraban-Kartik, 1323 Bengali year, 1916; cited in Pradip Basu (ed), *Samayiki Purano Samayik Patrer Prabondho Sankalan Ditiyo Khanda: Griha o Paribar*; Kolkata, Ananda Publishers Private Limited, 2009), pp. 779–793. [Title Translation: Journal on Current Topics Collection of Old Essays from Periodicals Second Volume: Home and Family].

Directory of the City Health and Baby Week 1931 (Madras: The City Health and Baby Week Committee, 1931)

Dutt, S. P., 'Susantaner Asha', *Chikitsak Bandhab*, vol. 1 no. 3, Chaitra 1330 (1924), pp. 9–10.

English-Speaking Conference on Infant Mortality Report of the Proceedings of the English-Speaking Conference on Infant Mortality, held at Caxton Hall, Westminster, on August 4 and 5, 1913 (London: National Association for the Prevention of Infant Mortality and for the Welfare of Infancy, 1913).

Gangooly, Hurrish Chunder, (L. M. S. Assistant Surgeon, Nawadi), 'Infant's Food To The Editor of the Indian Medical Gazette', 4th May 1876, *Indian Medical Gazette*, vol. XI, no. 6, 1876, p. 164.

Ganguli, Miss Jyotirmoyi, 'Written Statement of Miss Jyotirmoyi Ganguli, M.A., 6, Guru Prosad Chaudhuri Lane, Calcutta and Oral Evidence of Miss Jyotirmoyi Ganguli, M.A., 6, Guru Prosad Chaudhuri Lane, Calcutta (Calcutta, 18th December 1928)', in *Age of Consent Committee Evidence 1928–1929 Volume VI Oral Evidence and Written Statements of Witnesses from Bengal Presidency* (Calcutta: Government of India Central Publication Branch, 1929), pp. 11–18.

Ghose, S. B., M.B. Chemical Analyst, Municipal Corporation, Calcutta, 'Food Adulteration in Calcutta', *Calcutta Medical Journal*, 1907, n.p., [in Kabita Ray, *Public Health in Colonial Calcutta and the Calcutta Corporation 1923–1947* Selections from Journals and Newspapers (Kolkata: Corpus Research Institute, 2010), pp. 119–121].

Ghosh, Mrs Edith, 'Oral Evidence of Dr. (Mrs) Edith Ghosh Representative of Bengal Presidency Council of Women (Calcutta 19 December 1928)', in *Age of Consent Committee Evidence 1928–1929 Volume VI Oral Evidence and Written Statements of Witnesses from Bengal Presidency* (Calcutta: Government of India Central Publication Branch, 1929), pp. 38–45.

Goswami, Surendranath, *Arya Dhatribidya. A Treatise on the Ayurvedic System of Midwifery* (With Sanskrit text and English translation. Part I; Kumarkhali: Author, 1899).

Greenwood, Alfred. 'Some Conditions under which infants are nursed away from home', *The Hospital*, 1908, vol 44, no. 1133, 171–174.

Griffin, E., 'Nursing Sister, Health Visitor, Delhi, in Chapter VII. – Papers Written by qualified midwives – Miss Patch, Miss Griffin, Mrs. Vonwein', in *Improvements of the Conditions of Childbirth in India Including a Special Report on the Work of the Victoria Memorial Scholarships Fund during the past Fifteen Years and Papers Written by Medical Women and qualified Midwives* (Calcutta: Superintendent Government Printing, 1918), pp. 142–146.

Halliday, Sir Frederick. *Annual Report on the Police Administration of the Town of Calcutta and Its Suburbs for the Year 1912* (Calcutta: The Bengal Secretariat Book Depot, 1913).

Hansraj, Dr. Jadavji, 'Written Statement, dated 12th August 1928, of Dr. Jadavji Hansraj, D.O.M.S., (Eng.), J.P. President, and Mr. Premji Chaturbhuj, Honororary Secretary of the Bhatia Mitra Mandal, 203–5, Horby Road, Fort, Bombay', in *Age of Consent Committee Evidence, Volume III Oral Evidence and Written Statements of Witnesses from the Bombay Presidency (Continued – Bombay and Poona) and the Central Provinces and Berar* (Calcutta: Government of India Central Publication Branch, 1929), pp. 149–150.

Headwards, Dr. A., 'Ante-Natal Work', in *Report of Maternity and Child Welfare Conference Held at Delhi. February 4th – 8th 1927* (Delhi: The Lady Chelmsford All-India League for Maternity and Child Welfare, 1927), pp. 101–103

Hogg, Francis R., *Practical Remarks Chiefly Concerning the Health and Ailments of European Families in India, with Special Reference to Maternal Management and Domestic Economy* (Benares: Medical Hall Press, 1877).

———, 'Notes on Infantile Diseases of India', *Indian Medical Gazette*, vol 11, no. 10, 1876, pp. 258–263.

———, 'Notes on Infantile Diseases of India', *Indian Medical Gazette*, vol. 12, no. 7, 1877, pp. 179–181.

Hossein Mrs. Rokeya Sakhawat (1921) 'Care of Babies', in *Health and Child Welfare Exhibition, Calcutta, 1920* (Calcutta: Bengal Secretariat Book Depot, 1921), pp. lxxxi–lxxxv [Recorded as Mrs. R. S. Hossein in this source].

———, 'Sugrihini' in Syed, Abdul Mannan, Selina Hossein, Mohammad Shamshul Alam and Abdul Quadir (eds), *Rokeya Rachanabali* [Complete Works of Begum Rokeya Sakhawat Hossain] (Dhaka: Bangla Academy, 1971), pp. 31–40.

Improvements of the Conditions of Childbirth in India Including a Special Report on the Work of the Victoria Memorial Scholarships Fund during the past Fifteen Years and Papers Written by Medical Women and qualified Midwives (Calcutta: Superintendent Government Printing, India, 1918).

Jackson, J., M.D., 'On Midwifery in the East (Communicated by Dr. Metcalfe Babington)', *Transactions of the Obstetrical Society of London*, vol. II, 1860, pp. 37–47.

Joshi, Lemuel Lucas, *The Milk Problem in Indian Cities* (With Special Reference to Bombay With A Forward by John A. Turner; Bombay: D. B. Taraporevala Sons & Co., 1916).

Khastagir, Annadacharan, *A Treatise on the Science and Practice of Midwifery with Diseases of Children and Women Manab-Jatna Tattva, Dhatribidya, Nabaprasuto Sishu o Stri Jatir Byadhi-Sangraha* (Calcutta: Author, 1878 second ed., first ed. 1868).

King, Frederic Truby, *Feeding and Care of Baby* (London and Calcutta: Macmillan and Co., 1913), (Accessed 1 May, 2016). http://wellcomelibrary.org/item/b21512115 #c= 0&m=0&s=0&cv=40&z=0.1797%2C0.6791%2C2.0422%2C1.0347

———, *Natural Feeding of Infants* (With an Introduction by J. S. Fairbairn; London: Whitcombe & Tombs Limited, 1918).

Kingscote, Mrs. H., *The English Baby in India and How to Rear It* (London: J. & A. Churchill, 1893).

Kipling, John Lockwood, *Beast and Man in India A Popular Sketch of Indian Animals in their Relations with the People* (London: Macmillan, 1891).

Mayo, Katherine, *Volume II* (London: Jonathan Cape, 1931).

Mazumdar, Shudha, *A Pattern of Life The Memoirs of an Indian Woman* (Edited by Geraldine H. Forbes; New Delhi: Manohar, 1977).

Mcleod, K. 'Nubile Age of Females in India' cited in 'Transactions of Medical Societies', *Indian Medical Gazette*, vol. 25, no. 9, 1890, pp. 278–280.

Mellin, G., *The Care of Infants in India A Work for Mothers and Nurses Upon the Feeding and Rearing of Infants* (London: G. Gill & Sons, second ed. 1895).

Mitra, Charu Chandra, 'Written Statement of Mr. Charu Chandra Mitra, Attorney at law, 5 Hastings Street, Calcutta and Oral Evidence of Mr. Charu Chandra Mitra, Attorney-at-law, Calcutta. (*Calcutta, 18th December 1928*)', in *Age of Consent Committee Evidence 1928–1929 Volume VI Oral Evidence and Written Statements of Witnesses from Bengal Presidency* (Calcutta: Government of India Central Publication Branch, 1929), pp. 18–37.

Mody, Cooverjee Rustomjee, *An Essay on Female Infanticide: To Which the Prize Offered by the Bombay Government, for the Second Best Essay against Female Infanticide among the Jadajas and other Rajpoot Tribes of Guzerat, was Awarded* (Bombay: Printed by order of Government, at the Bombay Education Society's Press, 1849).

Moore, William James, *A Manual of Family Medicine for India* (London: J. & A. Churchill, 1874).

Morton, Edward, *Remarks on the Subject of Lactation: Containing Observations on the Healthy and Diseased Conditions of the Breast-milk, the Disorders Frequently Produced in Mothers by Suckling: And Numerous Illustrative Cases, Proving That, When Protracted, it is a Common Cause, in Children, of Hydrencephalus, or Water in the Brain and Other Serious Complications* (London: Longman, Rees, Orme, Brown, and Green, 1831).

Muhammad, Munshi Waazuddin, *Islamiya Mantra*, vols. I and II (Calcutta: Muhammad Soleman and Brothers, 1910).

Mukerje, Jodu Nath, *Dhatri Sikkha A Guide to the Dhaees or Native Midwives and to the Mothers Written in the Form of a Dialogue in Two Parts Part 1* (Chinsura: Printed by Greesh Chunder Bhuttacharje, Chitsaprokash Press; third ed. 1875, first ed. 1867).

Mukhopadhyay, Bipradas, *Jubati Stri-Jibaner Aadorsho* (Calcutta: Sanyal and Brothers, Bengali year 1296). Title Translation: Young Woman The Purpose of a Woman's Life.

Mukhopadhyay, Gangaprasad, *Matrisiksha Arthat Garbhabasthay o Sutikagrihey Matar ebong Ballabastha Porjonto Santaner Sasthyarakkha Bishayak Upodesh* (Calcutta: United Press, second ed. 1902). [Title Translation: Educating the Mother Meaning Healthcare Advice During Pregnancy and in the Lying-Room for the Mother and the Infant Till Childhood.

Neal Edwards, M. I., *Report of an Enquiry into the Causes of Maternal Mortality in Calcutta* [Field Investigators: I. M. Massick, M.R.C.P., W.M.S., S. Pandit,

M.B., B.S., D.M.C.W., W.M.S., F.M. Shaw, M.B., B.S. and Two Statistical Notes by Satya Swaroop M.A]. (Delhi: Manager of Publications, 1940).

O'Malley, L. S. S., *Census of India, 1911. Volume VI City of Calcutta. Part I: Report* (Calcutta: Bengal Secretariat Book Depot, 1913).

Page, Mrs. Arthur (ed), *Bengal Baby Week 1921* (With a Foreword by the Countess of Lytton; Calcutta: Caledonian Printing Co, Ltd., 1924).

Platt, Kate, *The Home and Health in India and the Tropical Colonies* (London: Baillière, Tindall and Cox, 1923).

Playfair, William Smoult, *A Treatise on the Science and Practice of Midwifery* (With Notes and Additions by Robert P. Harris, M.D., Philadelphia: Henry C. Lea, Second American edition, 1878, first ed. 1876).

Pritchard, Eric. *Infant Education* (London: Marylebone Health Society, 1907).

Pughe, Colonel J. R., *Report on the Police of the Lower Provinces of the Bengal Presidency for the Year 1873* (Calcutta: Bengal Secratariat Press, 1874).

Ranade, Dr. N. L., 'Is There Need for an Enquiry into the Causes of Infant Mortality?', in *Report of the Maternity and Child Welfare Conference held at Delhi. February 4th-8th, 1927* (Delhi: Printed for The Lady Chelmsford All-India League for Maternity and Child Welfare by the Delhi Printing Works, 1927), pp. 45–48.

Ray, Daktar Srijukta J. N. Ray, 'Saishabiyo Khaddya O Pattha Prodan', *Chikitsa-Prokash*, Bengali Year 1324, vol. 10, no. 9, pp. 358–372.

Ray, Rames Chandra, 'Kochi Cheleder Khabar', in *Swasthya Samachar*, vol. 8, 1919, pp. 204–206.

_____, 'Prasutir Proti Kartabba', *Vishak Darpan*, vol. 15, no. 11, p. 423–4.

_____, 'Rogi O Sishudiger Khadya', *Chikitsa-Prokash*, vol. III, no. 9, Bengali Year 1317, pp. 248–55.

Ray Sengupta, Kabiraj Srijukta Girijabhushan, 'Sishu-Palan' (Child-Rearing), *Janmabhumi*, Ashar Bengali Year 1317, c. 1910 in Pradip Basu (ed), *Samayiki Purano Samayik Patrer Prabondho Sankalan Ditiyo Khanda: Griha o Paribar* (Kolkata, Ananda Publishers Private Limited, 2009), pp. 713–718. [Title Translation: Journal on Current Topics Collection of Old Essays from Periodicals Second Volume: Home and Family].

Raya, Hurro Nath, Letter '5, Sukeas Street, February 1891', in the section 'Homeopathic Practitioners' (Appendix B) 'Medical Opinions on the Alleged Cruelty to Tender-Aged Wives by Their Husbands'. Appended to *The Full Proceedings of a Public Meeting held on the 22nd January, 1891, at the Residence of the late Maharajah Kamal Krishna Deb, Bahadur, Sabhabazar Rajbati, Calcutta, to Protest against the Age of Consent Bill* (Calcutta: The Sabhabazar Standing Committee, 1891), p. 48.

_____, *Midwife's Vade-Mecum. Dhatrishiksha Sangraha Ba Garbha Chikitsa Bishaya Pancha Bingshoti batsarer pariksha o adhayaner fal Chikitsak, chatra, dhatri, sikkhita strilok o gribaswamidiger nimitto sangribito o birochito* (Calcutta: Shri Binod Kishore Ray, 1887). [His name was spelt as Haranth Ray in his book]. Title Translation: Midwife's Vade-Mecum. An Anthology on Midwifery Obstetrics. Or A Result of Twenty-Five Years of Examination and Deep Study About Obstetrics. Compiled and Composed for the Doctor, Student, Midwife, Educated Women and Married Men.

Remfry, C. I., (Mrs. Douglas Remfry), Written Statement, dated 11th August 1928, of C. I. Remfry (Mrs. Douglas Remfry), Acting Honorary Secretary, Bengal

Presidency Council of Women, for and on behalf of the Committee, 2, Victoria Terrace, Calcutta" in *Age of Consent Committee Evidence 1928–1929 Volume VI Oral Evidence and Written Statements of Witnesses from Bengal Presidency* (Calcutta: Government of India Central Publication Branch, 1929) pp. 37–38.

Report of Cases Determined in the Court of Nizamut Adawlut, From July to December 1853. With an Index. Volume III, Part I (Calcutta: Thacker, Spink & Co., 1855).

Review of *Management and Diseases of Infants Under the Influence of the Climate of India Being Instructions to Mothers and Parents in Situations Where Medical Aid Is Not to Be Obtained and a Guide to Medical Men, Inexperienced in the Nursery and the Treatment of Tropical Infantile Disease*. Illustrated By Coloured Plates. *By* Frederick Corbyn, Esq., Surgeon on the Bengal Establishment; and Author of a Treatise on the late Epidemic Cholera and Taraii Fever, M.R.C.S.L. Calcutta, Thacker and Co. Royal 8 vo. Pp. 463.1828; in Thomas Wakley (ed), *The Lancet* MDCCCXXVIII-IX In Two Volumes, vol. II, 1829, pp. 757–762.

Richey, J. A., *Progress of Education in India, 1917–1922* Eighth Quinquennial Review Vol. I (Calcutta: Superintendent of Government Printing, India, 1923).

Risley, Herbert Hope, *The People of India* Edited by W. Crooke (Calcutta, Thacker, Spink & Co., 1915 second ed.)

Rousseau, Jean Jacques, *Emile, or On Education* Translated by Barbara Foxley and Introduction by André Boutet de Monvel (London: J. M. Dent & Sons Ltd., 1911, first ed. 1762)

Roy, Devendranath, L.M.S., *Garhastha Sastharakkha ebong sachitro Dhatrisikkha Domestic Hygiene and Guide to Bengali Midwives (with illustrations)* (Calcutta: S. K. Lahiri & Co, 1904).

Sankaran, G., 'Physiological bases of infant nutrition. *Indian Journal of Pediatrics*, vol. VIII, no. 29, 1941, pp. 1–20.

Sanyal, Shri Pulinchandra (M.B.), 'Striloker Mashik Rajahsrab ba Ritu', *Chikitsa Sammilani*, 1294 Bengali year, c. 1887, pp. 101–103.

———, 'Bibaha Bichar', *Chikitsa Sammilani*, 1294 Bengali year, c. 1887, pp. 193–197.

Sen, Bolye Chunder, 'The Nubile Age of Females in India Physiologically Treated', *British Gynaecological Journal*, vol. VI, no. 24, 1891, pp. 605–21.

Sen, Keshub Chunder, 'Marriageable Age of Native Girls', *Calcutta Journal of Medicine: A Monthly Record of the Medical and Auxiliary Sciences*, vol. 4, no. 7, 1871, pp. 258–273.

Sen, Dr. Y. Sen, F.R.F.P. & S. (Glasgow), Women's Medical Service, Raj Dufferin Hospital, Bettiah. in 'Chapter VI. Papers Continued: Drs. G.J. Campbell, Wallace, Sen, George' in *Improvements of the Conditions of Childbirth in India Including a Special Report on the Work of the Victoria Memorial Scholarships Fund During the past Fifteen Years and Papers Written by Medical Women and Qualified Midwives* (Calcutta: Superintendent Government Printing, 1918), pp. 126–134.

Seth, Nripendranath, L.M.S., 'Amader Sishu' or 'Our Children', *Sakhi*, Chaitra, Bengali Year 1307, c. 1900; cited in Pradip Basu, *Samayiki Purano Samayik Patrer Prabondho Sankalan Ditiyo Khanda: Griha o Paribar* (Kolkata: Ananda Publishers Private Limited, 2009), pp. 684–687.

Sircar, Mahendralal, 'The Earliest Marriageable Age', *Calcutta Journal of Medicine*, vol. IV, no. 7, 1871, pp. 251–256

Sirkar, Sarasi Lal, M.A., Civil Surgeon, Chittagong Hill Tracts; 'Some Observations on Infant Feeding', *Indian Medical Record*, vol. XXXVII, 1917, pp. 3–4.

Sprawson, Cuthbert Allan, *Moore's Manual of Family Medicine and Hygiene for India* Eighth edition, re-written by the editor. Foreword by Charles Pardey Lukis. (London: J.&A. Churchill, 1916)

Staley, Mildred, *Handbook for Wives and Mothers in India* (Calcutta: Thacker, Spink & Co., 1908).

Steel, Flora Annie, and Grace Gardiner, *The Complete Indian Housekeeper & Cook* (London: William Heinemann, 1909, first ed. 1888).

Stewart, A. D. 'Exhibits Committee Report' in Indian Red Cross Society Bengal Provincial Branch Bengal Health Welfare Week 1931 With a Foreword by Hon'ble Lady Jackson (Calcutta, 1931), pp. 12–18.

Suhrawardy, Hasan, M.D., F.R.C.S.I., L.M. (Rotunda), District Medical Officer Lillooah, E.I.R., 'The Care of the Expectant Mother and Newborn Infant' in *Health and Child Welfare Exhibition, Calcutta, 1920* (Calcutta: Bengal Secretariat Book Depot, 1921), pp. lx–lxxx.

———, *Child Welfare with Reference to the Care of the Expectant Mother and the New Born Infant* (Printed at the Indian Railway Press and Published by Dr. H. Suhrawardy, n.d.)

Summaries of Some Essays, etc Relating to Census and Caste (Calcutta: The Govt Printing, 1911), [Rare Books, West Bengal State Archives, Kolkata].

Tavernier, Jean Baptiste, *Travels in India* (In Two Volumes Volume II. Translated from the original French edition of 1676 with a biographical sketch of the Author, Notes, Appendices, Etc. by V. Ball) (London: Macmillan and Co, 1889).

'The Infantile Mortality in Calcutta' in *The Calcutta Municipal Gazette*, 1932, vol. 16, no. 23, n.p. in Kabita Ray, *Public Health in Colonial Calcutta and The Calcutta Corporation 1923–1947 Selections from Journals and Newspapers* (Kolkata: Corpus Research Institute, 2010), pp. 195–197).

Thompson, W. H., *Census of India 1921. Volume V Bengal Part I Report* (Calcutta: Bengal Secretariat Book Depot, 1923).

United States Bureau of Foreign and Domestic Commerce, Henry D. Baker, American Consul at Bombay and Other Consular Officers, *British India with Notes on Ceylon, Afghanistan, and Tibet* (Washington, DC: Government Printing Office, 1915).

Ward, William, *A View of the History, Literature, and Religion, of the Hindoos: Including a Minute Description of their Manners and Customs and Translations from their Principal Works* [In Two Volumes Volume II The Second Edition: Carefully Abridged and Greatly Improved (Serampore: Mission Press, 1815)].

Waters, Lt. Col. E. E. (1918) in 'Chapter II. Opinions of provinces. I. – Bengal presidency' *Improvements of the Conditions of Childbirth in India Including a Special Report on the Work of the Victoria Memorial Scholarships Fund during the Past Fifteen Years and Papers Written by Medical Women and Qualified Midwives* (Calcutta: Superintendent Government Printing, India, 1918), pp. 10–11.

Wilkins, William Joseph. *Modern Hinduism Being An Account of the Religion and Life of the Hindus in Northern India* (London: T. Fisher Unwin, 1887).

Wilson, Lt.-Colonel R. P. I.M.S., Superintendent, Campbell Medical School Calcutta in *Improvements of the Conditions of Childbirth in India Including a Special Report on the Work of the Victoria Memorial Scholarships Fund during the past Fifteen Years and Papers Written by Medical Women and qualified Midwives* (Calcutta: Superintendent Government Printing, India, 1918), pp. 9–10.

Wilson, W. H., *Markets of Empire* (London: Effingham Wilson, 1930).

Yacoob, Munshi Mohamed, *The Cry of The Child & The Calf* (Ellore: 1908).

Yeo, Burney. 'A Discussion on Foods for Invalids and Infants' (In the Section of Pharmacology and Therapeutics at the Annual Meeting of the British Medical Association, held in Leeds, August, 1889), *British Medical Journal*, vol. 2, no. 1510, 1889, pp. 1261–1266.

Young, Ruth, *Maternity and Infant Welfare A Handbook for Health Visitors, Parents, and Others in India* (Calcutta: The Lady Chelmsford All-India League for Maternity and Child Welfare, second ed. 1922)

——, *Antenatal Work in India A Handbook for Nurses, Midwives, and Health Visitors* [Indian Red Cross Society Maternity and Child Welfare Bureau (Incorporating the Lady Chelmsford All-India League for Maternity and Child Welfare, and the Victoria Memorial Scholarships Fund), 1930]

Secondary Sources

Agnew, Éadaoin *Imperial Women Writers in Victorian India Representing Colonial Life, 1850–1910* (Cham: Palgrave Macmillan, An Imprint of Springer Nature, 2017).

Ahluwalia, Sanjam, *Reproductive Restraints Birth Control in India 1877–1947* (Ranikhet: Permanent Black, 2008).

Ahmed, Rafiuddin. *The Bengal Muslims, 1871–1906 A Quest for Identity* (Delhi: Oxford University Press, 1981).

Alexander, Kristine. *Guiding Modern Girls Girlhood, Empire and Internationalism in the 1920s and 1930s* (Vancouver: UBC Press, 2017).

Alter, Joseph S., *The Wrestler's Body Identity and Ideology in North India* (Berkeley: University of California Press, 1992).

Amin, Sonia Nishat, *The World of Muslim Women in Colonial Bengal, 1876–1939* (Leiden: E. J. Brill, 1996).

Anagol-McGinn, Padma, 'The Age of Consent 1891 Reconsidered Women's Perspectives and Participation in in the Child-Marriage Controversy in India', *South Asia Research*, 1992, vol. 12 no. 2, pp. 100–118.

Apple, Rima D., *Perfect Motherhood Science and Childrearing in America* (New Brunswick: Rutgers University Press, 2006).

——, *Mothers and Medicine A Social History of Infant Feeding, 1890–1950* (Madison: The University of Wisconsin Press, 1987).

Arnold, David, '"An ancient race outworn": malaria and race in colonial India, 1860–1930', in Waltraud Ernst and Bernard Harris (eds), *Race, Science and Medicine, 1700–1960* (London: Routledge, 1999), pp. 123–143.

——, *Colonizing the Body State Medicine and Epidemic Disease in Nineteenth-Century India* (Berkeley: University of California Press, 1993).

_____, *The Problem of Nature Environment, Culture and European Expansion* (Oxford: Blackwell Publishers Ltd., 1996).

_____, *The Tropics and the Traveling Gaze India, Landscape, and Science 1800–1856* (Delhi: Permanent Black, 2005).

Bagchi, Jasodhara, 'Representing Nationalism: Ideology of Motherhood in Colonial Bengal', *Economic and Political Weekly*, vol. 25, no. 42/43, 1990, pp. WS65–WS71.

Baird, Julia, *Victoria The Queen An Intimate Biography of the Woman Who Ruled an Empire* (New York: Random House, 2016)

Bala, Poonam, *Imperialism and Medicine in Bengal A Socio-Historical Perspective* (New Delhi: Sage Publications, 1991).

Bandopadhyay, Sekhar, *Caste, Culture and Hegemony Social Dominance in Colonial Bengal* (New Delhi: Sage Publications, 2004).

Bandyopadhyay, Sibaji, *Gopal-Rakhal Dwandasamas Upanibeshbad o Bangla Sishusahitya* (Calcutta: Papyrus, 1999)

_____, *Aabar Sishushikkha* (Kolkata: Anustup, 2005)

_____, *Bangla Shishusahityer Chhoto Meyera* (Kolkata: Ganghil, 2007)

Banerjee, Swapna M., 'Blurring Boundaries, Distant Companions: Non-kin Female Caregivers for Children in Colonial India (Nineteenth and Twentieth centuries)', *Paedagogica Historica*, vol. 46, no. 6, 2010, pp. 775–788.

_____, *Fathers in a Motherland Imagining Fatherhood in Colonial India* (New Delhi: Oxford University Press, 2022).

Bannerji, Himani, 'Fashioning a Self: Educational Proposals for and by Women in Popular Magazines in Colonial Bengal', *Economic and Political Weekly*, vol. 26, no. 43, 1991, pp. WS50–WS62.

_____, *Inventing Subjects Studies in Hegemony, Patriarchy and Colonialism* (New Delhi: Tulika, 2001).

Bartlett, Alison, 'Babydaze: Maternal Time', *Time & Society*, vol. 19, no. 1, 2010, pp. 120–132.

Bates, Crispin, 'Race, Caste and Tribe in Central India: The Early Origins of Indian Anthropometry' in Peter Robb, *The Concept of Race in South Asia* (Delhi: Oxford University Press, 1995), pp. 219–259.

Bayly, Susan, 'Caste and "Race" in the Colonial Ethnography of India', in Peter Robb (ed), *The Concept of Race in South Asia* (New Delhi: Oxford University Press, 1995); pp. 165–218.

Benzaquén, Adriana S. 'The Doctor and the Child: Medical Preservation and Management of Children in the Eighteenth Century', in Anja Müller (ed), *Fashioning Childhood in the Eighteenth Century Age and Identity* (Aldershot: Ashgate Publishing, 2006), pp. 13–24.

Berger, Rachel, *Ayurveda Made Modern Political Histories of Indigenous Medicine in North India 1900–1955* (New York: Palgrave MacMillan, 2013).

Bhattacharji, Sukumari, 'Motherhood in Ancient India', *Economic and Political Weekly*, vol. 25, no. 42/43, 1990, pp. WS50–WS57.

Bhattacharya, Sabyasachi, *The Defining Moments in Bengal 1920–1947* (New Delhi: Oxford University Press, 2014).

Biswas, Shri Sailedra, *Samsad Bengali-English Dictionary* Revised by Sri Subodhchadra Sengupta (Calcutta: Sahitya Samsad, 1968).

Blunt, Alison, *Domicile and Diaspora Anglo-Indian Women and the Spatial Politics of the Home* (Oxford: Blackwell Publishing, 2005).

——, 'Embodying War: British Women and Domestic Defilement in the Indian 'Mutiny', 1857–8', *Journal of Historical Geography*, vol. 26, no. 3, 2000, pp. 403–428.

Borthwick, Meredith, *The Changing Role of Women in Bengal, 1849–1905* (Princeton: Princeton University Press, 1984).

Bose, Sugata, *The Nation as Mother and Other Visions of Nationhood* (Gurgaon: Penguin Viking, An imprint of Penguin Random House, 2017)

Bourdieu, Pierre, *Distinction A Social Critique of the Judgement of Taste* (Cambridge: Harvard University Press, 1984).

——, 'The forms of capital', in J. Richardson (ed), *Handbook of Theory and Research for the Sociology of Education*. Translation by Richard Nice (New York: Greenwood, 1986), pp. 46–58.

Brown, Petrina, *Eve Sex, Childbirth and Motherhood through the Ages* (Chichester: Summersdale Publishers, 2004).

Bryder, Linda, 'Mobilising Mothers: The 1917 National Baby Week', *Medical History*, vol. 63, no. 1, 2019, pp. 2–23.

——'Breastfeeding and Health Professionals in Britain, New Zealand and the United States, 1900–1970', *Medical History*, vol. 49, no. 2, 2005, pp. 179–196.

——, 'New Zealand's Infant Welfare Services and Maori, 1907–60', *Health and History*, vol. 3, no. 1, Maori Health, 2001, pp. 65–86.

Buettner, Elizabeth, *Empire Families Britons and Late Imperial India* (New York: Oxford University Press, 2004).

Burton, Antoinette, 'From Child Bride to "Hindoo Lady": Rukhmabai and the Debate on Sexual Respectability in Imperial Britain', *The American Historical Review*, vol. 103, no. 4, 1998, pp. 1119–1146.

Carol A. Breckenridge and Peter van der Veer, 'Orientalism and the Postcolonial Predicament' in Carol A. Breckenridge and Peter van der Veer (eds), *Orientalism and the Postcolonial Predicament Perspectives on South Asia* (Philadelphia: University of Pennsylvania Press, 1993), pp. 1–19.

Carty, T. J., *A Dictionary of Literary Pseudonyms in the English Language* (New York: Routledge, 2014, published in 2000 in the U.K. by Mansell Publishing).

Chakrabarti, Pratik, *Western Science in Modern India Metropolitan Methods, Colonial Practices* (Delhi: Permanent Black, 2004).

Chakrabarty, Dipesh, *Provincializing Europe Postcolonial thought and Historical Difference* (Princeton: Princeton University Press, 2000).

——, 'The Difference: Deferral of (A) Colonial Modernity: Public Debates on Domesticity in British Bengal', *History Workshop*, vol. 36, 1993, pp. 1–34.

Chakrabarty, Rachana, 'Women's Education and Empowerment in Colonial Bengal', in Hans Hägerdal (ed), *Responding to the West Essays on Colonial Domination and Asian Agency* (Amsterdam: Amsterdam University Press, 2009), pp. 87–102.

Chandra, Sudhir 'Rukhmabai: Debate over Woman's Right to Her Person' *Economic and Political Weekly*, vol. 31, no. 44, 1996, pp. 2937–2947.

Chatterjee, Partha, *Our Modernity* (Rotterdam/Dakar: SEPHIS CODESRIA, 1997).

——, 'The Nationalist Resolution of the Women's Question', in Kumkum Sangari and Sudesh Vaid (eds), *Recasting Women. Essays in Colonial History* (New Delhi: Kali for Women, 1989), pp. 233–253.

Chatterjee, Sukla, *Women and Literary Narratives in Colonial India Her Myriad Gaze on the 'Other'* (New York: Routledge, 2019).

Chattopadhyay, Swati, *Representing Calcutta Modernity, Nationalism and the Colonial Uncanny* (London: Routledge, 2005).

Chaudhuri, Nupur, 'Memsahibs and Motherhood in Nineteenth-Century Colonial India', *Victorian Studies*, vol. 31, no. 4, 1988, pp. 517–535.

_____, 'Shawls, Jewelry, Curry and Rice in Victorian Britain', in Nupur Chaudhuri and Margaret Strobel (eds), *Western Women and Imperialism Complicity and Resistance* (Bloomington and Indianapolis: Indiana University Press, 1992), pp. 231–246.

Chowdhury, Indira, *The Frail Hero and Virile History Gender and the Politics of Culture in Colonial Bengal* (Delhi: Oxford University Press, 1998)

Chowdhury-Sengupta, Indira, 'The Effeminate and the Masculine: Nationalism and the Concept of Race in Colonial Bengal', in Peter Robb (ed), *The Concept of Race in South Asia* (New Delhi: Oxford University Press, 1995), pp. 282–303.

Choudhury, Ishani, 'In Search of Proper Diet for Kids: Concerns Regarding Children's Food As Reflected in Bengali Periodicals of the Early Twentieth Century', *The International Journal of Social Sciences and Humanities Invention*, vol. 3, no. 1, 2016, p. 1794.

Cohen, Michèle, *Fashioning Masculinity: National Identity and Language in the Eighteenth Century* (New York: Routledge, 1996).

Cohn, Bernard S., *Colonialism and Its Forms of Knowledge The British in India* (Princeton: Princeton University Press, 1996).

_____, 'Representing Authority in Victorian India', In Eric Hobsbawm and Terence O. Ranger (eds), *The Invention of Tradition* (Cambridge: Cambridge University Press, 1983), pp. 165–210.

Conrad, Peter, *Deviance and Medicalization: From Badness to Sickness* (Philadelphia: Temple University Press, 1992, expanded ed.).

Cooper, Frederick, and Ann Laura Stoler (eds), *Tensions of Empire Colonial Cultures in a Bourgeois World* (Berkeley: University of California Press, 1997).

Crowther, S. M., L. A. Reynolds and E. M. Tansey (eds), *The Resurgence of Breastfeeding, 1975–2000* (Wellcome Witnesses to Twentieth Century Medicine), vol. 35 (London: Wellcome Trust Centre for the History of Medicine at UCL, 2009).

Darby, Robert. 'Pathologizing Male Sexuality: Lallemand, Spermatorrhea, and the Rise of Circumcision', *Journal of the History of Medicine and Allied Sciences*, vol. 60, no. 3, 2005, pp. 283–319.

Das, Rahul Peter, *The Origin of the Life of a Human Being Conception and the Female According to Ancient Medical and Sexological Literature* (Delhi: Motilal Banarsidass Publishers Private Limited, 2003).

Das, Shinjini, 'Debating Scientific Medicine: Homoeopathy and Allopathy in Late Nineteenth-century Medical Print in Bengal', *Medical History*, vol. 56, no. 4, 2012, pp. 463–480.

Datta, Pradip Kumar, '"Dying Hindus": Production of Hindu Communal Common Sense in Early 20th Century Bengal', *Economic and Political Weekly*, 1993, vol. 28, no. 25, pp. 1305–1319.

Davenport-Hines, R. P. T., and Judy Slinn, *Glaxo A History to 1962* (Cambridge: Cambridge University Press, 1992).

Davin, Anna, 'Imperialism and Motherhood' *History Workshop*, vol. 5, no. 1, 1978, pp. 9–65.

Dawkins, Richard, *The Selfish Gene* (Oxford: Oxford University Press, 1989, first ed. 1976).

Devi, Mahasweta, *Breast Stories* Translated with introductory essays by Gayatri Chakravorty Spivak (London: Seagull, 2016, 1997).

Dirks, Nicholas, *Castes of Mind Colonialism and the Making of Modern India* (Princeton: Princeton University Press, 2001).

Douglas, Mary, *Purity and Danger An Analysis of the Concepts of Pollution and Taboo* (London: Routledge, ARK ed. 1984, first ed. 1966).

Dubow, Saul, *Scientific Racism in Modern South Africa* (Cambridge: Cambridge University Press, 1995).

Dykes, Fiona, *Breastfeeding in Hospital Mothers, Midwives and the Production line* (New York: Routledge, 2006).

Engels, Dagmar, *Beyond Purdah? Women in Bengal 1890–1939* (Delhi: Oxford University Press, 1996).

——, 'The Age of Consent Act of 1891: Colonial Ideology in Bengal', *South Asia Research*, 1983, vol. 3, no. 2, pp. 107–131.

Falconer, John, 'Photography in Nineteenth Century India', in C. A. Bayly (ed), *The Raj India and the British 1600–1947* (London: Pearson National Portrait Gallery Publications, 1990), pp. 278–304.

Fildes, Valerie A., *Breasts, Bottles and Babies A History of Infant Feeding* (Edinburgh: Edinburgh University Press, 1986).

——, *Wet Nursing A History from Antiquity to the Present* (Oxford: Basil Blackwell, 1988).

Forbes, Geraldine, *Women in Colonial India. Essays in Politics, Medicine, and Historiography* (New Delhi: Chronicle Books, 2005).

——, *Women in Modern India* (Cambridge: Cambridge University Press, 1996).

——, and Tapan Raychaudhuri (eds), *The Memoirs of Dr. Haimabati Sen From Child Wife to Lady Doctor* Translated by Tapan Raychaudhuri. Introduced by Geraldine Forbes (New Delhi: Lotus Collection, Roli Books, 2000).

Foucault, Michel, *Discipline and Punish The Birth of the Prison* Translated from the French by Alan Sheridan (New York: Vintage Books, second ed. 1991).

——, *The History of Sexuality Volume I: An Introduction* (Translated from the French by Robert Hurley; New York: Pantheon Books, 1978).

George, Rosemary Marangoly, *The Politics of the Home Postcolonial Relations and Twentieth-Century Fiction* (Berkeley: University of California Press, 1999).

Gibson, Rebecca, *The Corseted Skeleton A Bioarchaeology of Binding* (Cham: Palgrave Macmillan imprint published by Springer Nature Switzerland AG, 2020).

Goswami, Tinni, *Sanitising Society Public Health and Sanitation in Colonial Bengal 1880–1947* (Delhi: B. R. Publishing Corporation, 2011).

Goswami Bhatacharya, Tinni, 'Femininity and Imperialism Women and Raj in Colonial Bengal (1880–1930)', Conference Paper Ecole Normale Superieure Paris, 2011, pp. 1–20, (Accessed 1 February, 2014), https://caluniv.academia. edu/ TinniGoswami/Conference-Presentations.

Guha, Ambalika, *Colonial Modernities Midwifery in Bengal, c. 1860–1947* (London: Routledge, 2018).

Guha, Supriya, 'Midwifery in Colonial India The Role of Traditional Birth Attendants in Colonial India', *Wellcome History*, vol. 28, no. 2–3, 2005, pp. 2–3.

_____, '"The Best Swadeshi": Reproductive Health in Bengal, 1840–1940', in Sarah Hodges (eds), *Reproductive Health in India. History, Politics, Controversies* (Hyderabad: Orient Longman, 2006), pp. 139–166.

_____, 'The Nature of Woman: Medical Ideas in Colonial Bengal', *Indian Journal of Gender Studies*, vol. 3, no. 1, 1996, pp. 23–38.

Gupta, Charu, 'Hindu Wombs, Muslim Progeny: The Numbers Game and Shifting Debates on Widow Remarriage in Uttar Pradesh, 1890s–1930s', in Sarah Hodges (ed), *Reproductive Health in India History, Politics, Controversies* (Hyderabad: Orient Longman, 2006), pp. 167–198.

_____, *The Gender of Caste. Representing Dalits in Print* (Ranikhet: Permanent Black, 2016).

_____, 'The Icon of Mother in Late Colonial North India, "Bharat Mata", "Matri Bhasha" and "Gau Mata"', *Economic and Political Weekly*, vol. 36, no. 45, 2001, pp. 4295–4297.

Gupta, Jayati, *Travel Culture, Travel Writing and Bengali Women, 1870–1940* (London: Routledge, 2021).

Hancock, Mary 'Home Science and the Nationalization of Domesticity in Colonial India', *Modern Asian Studies*, vol. 35, no. 4, 2001, p. 871–903.

Hannavy, John, ed. *Encyclopedia of Nineteenth-Century Photography Volume I A-I Index* (Routledge: New York, 2008).

Hareven, Tamara K., *Family Time and Industrial Time The Relationship between the Family and Work in New England Industrial Community* (Cambridge: Cambridge University Press, 1982).

Harrison, Mark, *Climates and Constitutions Health, Race, Environment and British Imperialism in India 1600–1850* (Oxford: Oxford University Press, 1999).

_____, 'Differences of Degree: Representations of India in British Medical Topography, 1820-c.1870', in Nicolaas A. Rupke (ed), *Medical Geography in Historical Perspective* (London: Wellcome Trust Centre for the History of Medicine, 2000), pp. 51–69.

Hassan, Narin, 'Feeding Empire: Wet Nursing and Colonial Domesticityin India' in Poonam Bala ed. *Medicine and Colonial Engagements in India and Sub-Saharan Africa* (Newcastle Upon Tyne: Cambridge Scholars Publishing, 2018) pp. 69–81.

Haynes, Douglas E. 'Vernacular Capitalism, Advertising, And the Bazaar in Early Twentieth-Century Western India', in Ajay Gandhi, Barbara Harris-White, Douglas E. Hayne, and Sebastian Schwecke (eds), *Rethinking Markets in Modern India Embedded Exchange and Contested Jurisdiction* (Cambridge: Cambridge University Press, 2020), pp. 116–146.

Headrick, Daniel R., *The Tools of Empire Technology and European Imperialism in the Nineteenth Century* (New York: Oxford University Press, 1981).

Hochschild, Arlie Russell, *The Managed Heart Commercialization of Human Feeling* (Berkeley: University of California Press, 1983).

Hodges, Sarah, *Contraception, Colonialism and Commerce Birth Control in South India, 1920–1940* (New York: Routledge, 2016, 2008 Ashgate ed.).

_____, 'Towards a History of Reproduction in Modern India', in Sarah Hodges (ed), *Reproductive Health in India History, Politics, Controversies* (Hyderabad: Orient Longman Private Ltd, 2006), pp. 1–21.

Hunt, Nancy Rose, '"Le bébé en brousse": European Women, African Birth Spacing, and Colonial Intervention in Breast Feeding in the Belgian Congo', in Frederick

Cooper and Ann Laura Stoler (eds), *Tensions of Empire Colonial Cultures in a Bourgeois World* (Berkeley: University of California Press, 1997), pp. 287–321.

Illich, Ivan, *Medical Nemesis The Expropriation of Health* (New York: Pantheon Books, 1976, Great Britain ed. 1975).

Jacob, Sharon. *Reading Mary Alongside Indian Surrogate Mothers Violent Love, Oppressive Liberation, and Infancy Narratives* (New York: Palgrave Macmillan, 2015).

Jayawardena, Kumari, *The White Woman's Other Burden Western Women and South Asia During British Rule* (New York: Routledge, 1995).

Jeffery, Patricia, Roger Jeffery, and Andrew Lyon, *Labour Pains and Labour Power. Women and Childbearing in India* (New Delhi: Manohar, 1989).

Jolly, Margaret, 'Introduction Colonial and Postcolonial Plots in Histories of Maternities and Modernities', in Kalpana Ram and Margaret Jolly (eds), *Maternities and Modernities Colonial and Postcolonial Experiences in Asia and the Pacific* (Cambridge: Cambridge University Press, 1998), pp. 1–25.

Jones, Colin and Roy Porter, (eds), *Reassessing Foucault Power, Medicine and the Body* (New York: Routledge, 1994).

Kahn, Robbie P., 'Women and Time in Childbirth and During Lactation', in Frieda Johles Forman and Caoran Sowton (eds), *Taking Our Time Feminist Perspectives on Temporality* (New York: Pergamon Press, 1988), pp. 20–36.

Kakar, Sudhir, *Shamans, Mystics and Doctors A Psychological Inquiry Into India and Its Healing Traditions* (New York: Alfred A. Knopf, 1982).

Karmakar, Bikas and Ila Gupta, 'Unraveling the Social Position of Women in Late-Medieval Bengal: A Critical Analysis of Narrative Art on Baranagar Temple Facades', *Rupkatha Journal on Interdisciplinary Studies in Humanities*, vol. 12, no. 5, 2020, pp. 1–18.

Kapur, Malavika, *Psychological Perspectives on Childcare in Indian Indigenous Health Systems* (With a foreword by B. V. Subbarayappa; New Delhi: Springer, 2016).

Kennedy, Dane, *The Magic Mountains Hill Stations and the British Raj* (Berkeley: University of California Press, 1996).

Krishnaraj, Mithreyi (ed), *Motherhood in India Glorification without Empowerment* (New Delhi: Routledge, 2010).

Krishnaswamy, Revathi, *Effeminism: The Economy of Colonial Desire* (Ann Arbor, MI: University of Michigan Press, 1998).

Kumar, Deepak, *Science and the Raj 1857–1905* (Delhi: Oxford University Press, 1995).

Lal, Maneesha, 'Purdah as Pathology: Gender and the Circulation of Medical Knowledge in Late Colonial India', in Sarah Hodges (ed), *Reproductive Health in India History, Politics, Controversies* (Hyderabad: Orient Longman, 2006), pp. 85–114.

_____, ' "The ignorance of women is the house of illness". Gender, Nationalism, and Health Reform in Colonial North India', in Mary P. Sutphen and Bridie Andrews (eds), *Medicine and Colonial Identity* (London: Routledge, 2003), pp. 14–40.

_____, 'The Politics of Gender and Medicine in Colonial India: The Countess of Dufferin' Fund, 1885–1888', *Bulletin of the History of Medicine*, vol 68, no. 1, 1994, pp. 29–66.

Lal, Ruby, 'Recasting the Women's Question The Girl-Child/Woman in the Colonial Encounter', *Interventions*, vol. 10, no. 3, 2008, pp. 321–339.

Lambert-Hurley, Siobhan, *Muslim Women, Reform and Princely Patronage Nawab Sultan Jahan Begum of Bhopal* (New York: Routledge: 2007)

_____, 'Subtle Subversions and Presumptuous Interventions: Reforming Women's Health in Bhopal State in the Early Twentieth Century', in Anindita Ghosh (ed), *Behind the Veil Resistance, Women and the Everyday in Colonial South Asia* (Basingstoke: Palgrave Macmillan, 2008), pp. 116–138.

Lang, Sean, 'Drop the Demon Dai: Maternal Mortality and the State in Colonial Madras, 1840–1875', *Social History of Medicine*, vol. 18, no. 3, 2005, pp. 357–378.

Latour, Bruno, *We Have Never Been Modern* Translated by Catherine Porter (Cambridge: Harvard University Press, 1993).

Lears, Jackson, *Fables of Abundance: A Cultural History of Advertising in America* (New York: Basic Books, 1994).

Lefebvre, Henri, *Everyday Life in the Modern World* Translated by Sacha Rabinovitch (London: Allen Lane The Penguin Press, 1968).

Leong-Salobir, Cecelia, *Food Culture in Colonial Asia: A Taste of Empire* (London: Routledge, 2011).

Levine, Philippa, *Prostitution, Race and Politics Policing Venereal Disease in the British Empire* (New York and London: Routledge, 2003)

Lewis, Milton, 'The "Health of the Race" and Infant Health in New South Wales: Perspectives on Medicine and Empire', in Roy Macleod and Milton Lewis (eds), *Disease, Medicine and Empire Perspectives on Western Medicine and the Experience of European Expansion* (New York: Routledge, 1988).

_____, 'The Problem of Infant Feeding: The Australian Experience from the Mid-Nineteenth Century to the 1920s', *Journal of the History of Medicine and Allied Sciences*, vol. 35, no. 2, 1980, pp. 174–187.

Lock Margaret, and Vinh-Kim Nguyen, *An Anthropology of Biomedicine* (Chichester: Wiley-Blackwell, 2010).

Major, Andrea, 'Mediating Modernity: Colonial State, Indian Nationalism, and the Renegotiation of the 'Civilizing Mission' in the Indian Child Marriage Debate of 1927–1932', in Carey A. Watt and Michael Mann (eds), *Civilizing Missions in Colonial and Postcolonial South Asia* (Delhi: Anthem Press, 2012), pp. 165–189.

Malhotra, Anshu, 'The Body as a Metaphor for the Nation Caste, Masculinity, and Femininity in the *Satyarth Prakash* of Swami Dayananda Sarasvati', in Avril A. Powell and Siobhan Lambert-Hurley (eds), *Rhetoric and Reality Gender and the Colonial Experience in South Asia* (Oxford: Oxford University Press, 2006), pp. 121–153.

Marks, Shula, 'What is Colonial about Colonial Medicine? And What has Happened to Imperialism and Health?', *Social History of Medicine*, vol. 10, 1997, pp. 205–219.

McClintock, Anne, *Imperial Leather Race, Gender and Sexuality in the Colonial Contest* (New York: Routledge, 1995).

Mein Smith, Philippa, *Mothers and King Baby. Infant Survival and Welfare in an Imperial World: Australia 1880–1950* (London: Macmillan Press, 1997).

Miles, M. 'Disability Care and Education in 19th Century India: Some Dates, Places and Documentation', *ActionAid Disability News: The Newsletter of Disability Division, ActionAid, India*, Vol. 5 (2 supplement), January 1, 1994, pp. 1–22.

Mishra, Saurabh, *Beastly Encounters Livelihoods, Livestock and Veterinary Health in North India* (Manchester: Manchester University Press, 2015).
Mitra, Durba, *Indian Sex Life Sexuality and the Colonial Origins of Modern Social thought* (Princeton: Princeton University Press, 2020).
Mizutani, Satoshi, *The Meaning of White Race, Class, and the 'Domiciled Community' in British India 1858–1930* (New York: Oxford University Press, 2011).
Morris, David B. *Illness and Culture in the Postmodern Age* (Berkeley: University of California Press, 1998).
Mosse, George L., *Nationalism and Sexuality. Middle-Class Morality and Sexual Norms in Modern Europe* (Madison: University of Wisconsin Press, 1985).
Mukharji, Projit Bihari, *Doctoring Traditions Ayurveda, Small Technologies, and Braided Sciences* (Chicago, The University of Chicago Press, 2016).
_____, 'Munisipal Darpan: Imagining the Embodied State and Subaltern Citizenship in 1890s Calcutta', *South Asian History and Culture*, vol. 4, no. 1, 2013, pp. 31–47.
_____, *Nationalizing the Body The Medical Market, Print and Daktari Medicine* (Delhi: Anthem Press, 2012).
_____, 'Symptoms of Dis-Ease: New Trends in the Histories of "Indigenous" South Asian Medicines', *History Compass*, vol. 9/12, 2011, pp. 887–899.
Mukherjee, Sujata. *Gender, Medicine, and Society in Colonial India Women's Health Care in Nineteenth- and Early Twentieth-Century Bengal* (New Delhi: Oxford University Press, 2017).
_____, 'Medical Education and Emergence of Women Medics in Colonial Bengal', Occasional Paper 37, Institute of Development Studies Kolkata, August 2012, pp. 1–32.
Mukherjee, Sumita, 'Using Legislative Assembly for Social Reform: The Sarda Act of 1929', *South Asia Research*, vol. 26, no. 3, 2006, pp. 219–33.
Müller, Anja (ed), *Fashioning Childhood in the Eighteenth Century Age and Identity* (Aldershot: Ashgate Publishing, 2006).
Naono, Atsuko, 'Educating Lady Doctors in Colonial Burma Missionaries, the Lady Dufferin Hospital, and the Local Government in the Making of Burmese Medical Women' in Poonam Bala (ed), *Contesting Colonial Authority Medicine and Indigenous Responses in Nineteenth- and Twentieth Century India* (New York: Lexington Books, 2012), pp. 97–114.
Nathoo, Tasnim and Aleck Ostry, *The One Best Way? Breastfeeding History, Politics, and Policy in Canada* (Waterloo: Wilfrid Laurier University Press, 2009)
Pande, Anupa, and Parul Pandya Dhar (eds), *Cultural Interface of India with Asia Religion, Art and Architecture* (New Delhi: D. K. Printworld (P) Ltd and National Museum Institute, 2004).
Pande, Ishita, 'Coming of Age: Law, Sex and Childhood in Late Colonial India', *Gender & History*, vol. 24, no. 1, 2012, pp. 205–30.
_____, *Medicine, Race and Liberalism in British Bengal Symptoms of Empire* (London: Routledge, 2010).
_____, 'Phulmoni's Body: The Autopsy, the Inquest and the Humanitarian Narrative on Child Rape in India', *South Asian History and Culture*, vol. 4, no. 1, 2013, pp. 1–22.
_____, *Sex, Law, and the Politics of Age Child Marriage in India, 1891–1937* (Cambridge: Cambridge University Press, 2020)

_____, 'Sorting Boys and Men: Unlawful Intercourse, Boy-Protection and the Child Marriage Restraint Act in Colonial India', *The Journal of the History of Childhood and Youth*, vol. 6, no. 2, 2013, pp. 332–58.

__, 'Feeling Like a Child: Narratives of Development and the Indian Child/Wife', in Stephanie Olsen (ed), *Childhood, Youth and Emotions in Modern History: National, Colonial and Global Perspectives* (Basingstoke, Hampshire: Palgrave Macmillan, 2015), pp. 35–55.

_____, 'Time for Sex: The Education of Desire and the Conduct of Childhood in Global/Hindu Sexology', in Veronika Fuechtner, Douglas E. Haynes, and Ryan M. Jones (eds), *A Global History of Sexual Science, 1880–1960* (Berkeley: University of California Press, 2018), pp. 279–302.

Paranjape, Makarand R., *Making India: Colonialism, National Culture and the Afterlife of Indian English Authority* (London: Springer, 2013).

Pati Biswamoy, and Mark Harrison (eds), *The Social History of Health and Medicine in Colonial India* (London: Taylor and Francis, 2011).

_____, Biswamoy Pati and Mark Harrison, 'Introduction Health, Medicine and Empire: Perspectives on Colonial India' in Biswamoy Pati and Mark Harrison (eds), *Health, Medicine and Empire Perspectives on Colonial India* (New Delhi: Orient Longman, 2001), pp. 1–36.

Perry, Ruth, (1991) 'Colonizing the Breast: Sexuality and Maternity in Eighteenth-Century England', *Journal of the History of Sexuality, Special Issue, Part 1: The State, Society, and the Regulation of Sexuality in Modern Europe*, vol. 2, no. 2, 1991, pp. 204–34.

Pinney, Christopher, 'Colonial Anthropology in the Laboratory of Mankind', in C. A. Bayly (ed), *The Raj India and the British 1600–1947* (London: Pearson National Portrait Gallery Publications, 1990), pp. 252–263.

Prakash, Gyan, *Another Reason: Science in the Making of Modern India* (Princeton: Princeton University Press, 2000).

Prasad, Srirupa. *Cultural Politics of Hygiene in India 1890–1940 Contagions of Feeling* (New York: Palgrave Macmillan, 2015).

Pratt, Mary Louise, *Imperial Eyes. Travel Writing and Transculturation* (New York: Routledge, 1992; Taylor & Francis e-Library, 2003).

Radhakrishna, Meena, 'Of Apes and Ancestors: Evolutionary Science and Colonial Ethnography', *The Indian Historical Review*, vol. XXXIII, no. 1, 2006, pp. 1–23.

Raina, Dhruv, and Habib, S. Irfan, *Domesticating Modern Science A Social History of Science and Culture in Colonial India* (New Delhi: Tulika, 2004).

Ram, Kalpana, and Jolly, Margaret (eds), *Maternities and Modernities Colonial and Postcolonial Experiences in Asia and the Pacific* (Cambridge: Cambridge University Press, 1998).

Ramanna, Mridula, *Health Care in Bombay Presidency 1896–1930* (Delhi: Primus, 2012).

Ramaswamy, Sumathi, *The Goddess and the Nation Mapping Mother India* (Durham: Duke University Press, 2010).

Ramusack, Barbara N., 'Cultural missionaries, maternal imperialists, feminist allies British women activists in India 1865–1945', in Nupur Chaudhuri and Margaret Strobel (eds), *Western women and Imperialism Complicity and*

Resistance (Bloomington and Indianapolis: Indiana University Press, 1992), pp. 119–136.

Ray, Bharati, *Early Feminists of Colonial India Sarala Devi Chaudhurani and Rokeya Sakhawat Hossain* (Oxford: Oxford University Press, 2002).

Ray, Kabita *Public Health in Colonial Calcutta and The Calcutta Corporation 1923–1947 Selections from Journals and Newspapers* (Kolkata: Corpus Research Institute, 2010).

Ray, Sukhendu, Bharati Ray and Malavika Karlekar (eds), *The Many Worlds of Sarala Devi: A Diary & The Tagores and Sartorial Style: A Photo Essay* (London: Routledge, 2017).

Ray, Utsa, *Culinary Culture in colonial India, A Cosmopolitan Platter and the Middle-Class* (Cambridge: Cambridge University Press, 2015).

Rendich, Franco, *Comparative Etymological Dictionary of Classical Indo-European Languages Indo-European – Sanskrit – Greek – Latin* (Trans. by Gordon Davis; n.p., 2013).

Richell, Judith, 'Ephemeral lives: The unremitting infant mortality of colonial Burma, 1891–1941', in Valerie Fildes, Lara Marks and Hilary Marland (eds), *Women and Children First International Maternal and Infant Welfare 1870–1945* (New York: Routledge, 1992), pp. 133–153.

Robb, Peter (ed), *The Concept of Race in South Asia* (Oxford: Oxford University Press, 1995).

Roy, Anupama, *Gendered Citizenship Historical and Conceptual Explorations* (Hyderabad: Orient Longman Private Limited, 2005).

Roy, Parama, *Alimentary Tracts Appetites, Aversions, and the Postcolonial* (Durham: Duke University Press, 2010)

_____, 'Women, Hunger and Famine: Bengal, 1350/1943', in Bharati Ray (ed), *Women of India: Colonial and Post-Colonial Periods* (New Delhi: Published by Professor Bhuvan Chandel, 2005) [General Editor D.P. Chattopadhyaya, Series on History of Science, Philosophy and Culture in Indian Civilization Volume IX, Part 3].

Roy, Tapti, 'Disciplining the Printed Text: Colonial and Nationalist Surveillance of Bengali Literature', in Partha Chatterjee (ed), *Texts of Power, Emerging Disciplines in Colonial Bengal* (Minneapolis: University of Minnesota Press, 1995), pp. 30–62.

Rozario, Santi 'The Dai and the Doctor: Discourses on Women's Reproductive Health in Rural Bangladesh', in Kalpana Ram and Margaret Jolly (eds), *Maternities and Modernities Colonial and Postcolonial Experiences in Asia and the Pacific* (Cambridge: Cambridge University Press, 1998), pp. 144–176.

Saha, Ranjana, 'Infant Feeding: Child Marriage and "Immature Maternity"', in Colonial Bengal, 1890s–1920s', *Proceedings of the Indian History Congress* Platinum Jubilee (75th) Session 2014, 2015, p. 708–715.

_____, 'Milk, "Race" and Nation: Medical Advice on Breastfeeding in Colonial Bengal', *South Asia Research*, vol. 37, no. 2, 2017, pp. 147–165.

_____, 'Milk, Mothering & Meanings: Infant Feeding in Colonial Bengal', *Women's Studies International Forum*, vol. 60, 2017, pp. 97–110

_____, 'Motherhood on Display: The Child Welfare Exhibition in Colonial Calcutta', *The Indian Economic and Social History Review*, vol. 58, no. 2, 2021, pp. 249–277.

Said, Edward W., *Orientalism* (New York: Vintage Books, 1979; reprint of Pantheon Books edition 1978).

Sanders, Nichole, 'Mothering Mexico: The Historiography of Mothers and Motherhood in 20th-Century Mexico', *History Compass*, vol. 7, no. 6, 2009, pp. 1542–1553

Sarkar, Mahua, *Visible Histories, Disappearing Women Producing Muslim Womanhood in Late Colonial Bengal* (Durham: Duke University Press, 2008).

Sarkar, Sumit, *The Swadeshi Movement in Bengal 1903–1908* (New Edition with a Preface by the author and critical essays by Neeladri Bhattacharya and Dipesh Chakrabarty; Ranikhet: Permanent Black, 2010, first ed. 1973).

_____, 'The Women's Question in Nineteenth Century Bengal', in Kumkum Sangari and Sudesh Vaid (eds), *Women and Culture* (Bombay: Research Centre for Women's Studies, 1994), pp. 103–112.

_____, *Writing Social History* (Delhi: Oxford University Press, 1997).

Sarkar, Tanika, 'A Prehistory of Rights: The Age of Consent Debate in Colonial Bengal', *Feminist Studies* vol. 26, no. 3, 2000, pp. 601–622

_____, *Hindu Wife, Hindu Nation Community, Religion and Cultural Nationalism* (Delhi: Permanent Black, 2001).

_____, 'Rhetoric Against Age of Consent: Resisting Colonial Reason and Death of a Child-Wife', *Economic & Political Weekly*, vol. 28, no. 36, 1993, pp. 1869–1878.

_____, 'Nationalist Iconography: Image of Women in 19th Century Bengali Literature', *Economic & Political Weekly*, vol. 22, no. 47, 1987, pp. 2011–2015.

Sehrawat, Samiksha, *Colonial Medical Care in North India Gender, State and Society c. 1840–1920* (New Delhi: Oxford University Press, 2013)

_____, 'Colonial Domesticities, Contentious Interactions: Ayahs, Wet-Nurses and Memsahibs in Colonial India', *Indian Journal of Gender Studies*, vol. 16 no. 3, 2009, pp. 299–328.

Sen, Indrani, 'Discourses of "Gendered Loyalty" Indian Women in Nineteenth-century "Mutiny" Fiction', in Biswamoy Pati (ed), *The Great Rebellion of 1857 in India Exploring Transgressions, Contests and Diversities* (London: Routledge, 2010), pp. 111–128.

_____, *Gendered Transactions The White Woman in Colonial India, c. 1820–1930* (Manchester: Manchester University Press, 2017).

_____, 'Memsahibs and Health in Colonial Medical Writings, c. 1840 to c.1930', *South Asia Research*, vol. 30, no. 3, 2010, pp. 253–274.

_____, *Memsahibs' Writings Colonial Writing on Indian Women* (New Delhi: Orient Longman, 2008).

_____, 'Resisting Patriarchy: Complexities and Conflicts in the Memoir of Haimabati Sen', *Economic and Political Weekly*, vol. 47, no. 12, 2012, pp. 55–62.

Sen, Samita, *Women and Labour in Late Colonial India: The Bengal Jute Industry* (Cambridge: Cambridge University Press, 1999).

Sen, Satadru, 'The Savage Family: Colonialism and Female Infanticide in Nineteenth-Century India', *Journal of Women's History*, vol. 14, no. 3, 2002, pp. 53–79.

Sharma, Kanika, Laura Lammasniemi, and Tanika Sarkar, 'Dadaji Bhikajiv Rukhmabai (1886) ILR 10 Bom 301: Rewriting Consent and Conjugal Relations in Colonial India', *Indian Law Review*, vol. 5, no. 3, pp. 265–287.

Sharma, Madhuri, 'Creating a Consumer Exploring Medical Advertisements in Colonial India', in Biswamoy Pati and Mark Harrison (eds), *The Social History of Health and Medicine in Colonial India* (London: Routledge, 2009), pp. 213–228.

Singh, Upinder, and Parul Pandey Dhar (eds), *Asian Encounters Exploring Connected Histories* (Delhi: Oxford University Press, 2014).

Sinha, Mrinalini, *Colonial Masculinity The 'Manly Englishman' and the 'Effeminate Bengali' in the Late Nineteenth Century* (Manchester: Manchester University Press, 1995).

——, 'Gender in the Critiques of Colonialism and Nationalism Locating the "Indian Woman"', in Sumit Sarkar and Tanika Sarkar (eds), *Women and Social Reform in Modern India Volume Two* (Ranikhet: Permanent Black, 2007), pp. 211–242.

—— (ed), *Mother India* by Katherine Mayo. Edited with an Introduction by Mrinalini Sinha (Ann Arbor, MI: University of Michigan Press, 2000, 1998).

——, 'Refashioning Mother India: Feminism and Nationalism in Late-Colonial India', *Feminist Studies* (Points of Departure: India and the South Asian Diaspora), vol. 26, no. 3, 2000, pp. 623–44.

Spivak, Gayatri Chakravorty 'Can the Subaltern Speak?' in *Marxism and the Interpretation of Culture* Edited and with an Introduction by Cary Nelson and Lawrence Grossberg (London: Macmillan, 1988), pp. 271–313.

Stokes, Patricia R., 'Purchasing Comfort: Patent Remedies and the Alleviation of Labour Pain in Germany between 1914 and 1933', in P. Betts, and G. Eghigianed (eds), *Pain and Prosperity Reconsidering Twentieth-century German History* (Stanford: California: Stanford University Press, 2003), pp. 61–87.

Stoler, Ann Laura, 'Making Empire Respectable: The Politics of Race and Sexual Morality in 20th-Century Colonial Cultures', *American Ethnologist*, vol. 16, no. 4, 1989, pp. 634–660.

——, *Carnal Knowledge and Imperial Power Race and the Intimate in Colonial Rule* (With a New Preface; Berkeley: University of California Press, 2002, 2010).

Suleri, Sara, *The Rhetoric of English India* (Chicago: University of Chicago Press, 1992).

Syed, Abdul Mannan, Selina Hossein, Mohammad Shamshul Alam and Abdul Quadir (eds), *Rokeya Rachanabali* [Complete Works of Begum Rokeya Sakhawat Hossain] (Dhaka: Bangla Academy, 1971).

Tarlo, Emma, *Clothing Matters Dress and Identity in India* (London: Hurst & Company, 1996).

Thomas, Nicola J., 'Embodying Imperial Spectacle: Dressing Lady Curzon, Vicereine of India 1899–1905', *Cultural Geographies*, vol. 14, no. 3, 2007, pp. 369–400.

Thompson, E. P., 'Time, Work-Discipline and Industrial Capitalism', *Past and Present*, vol. 38, no. 1, 1967, pp. 56–97.

Trautmann, Thomas R., *Aryans and British India* (New Delhi: Yoda Press, 2004).

Trouille, Mary Seidman, *Sexual Politics in the Enlightenment Women Writers Read Rousseau* (Albany: State University of New York Press, 1997).

Urwin, Cathy, and Elaine Sharland, "From Bodies to Minds in Childcare Literature: Advice to Parents in Inter-war Britain", in Roger Cooter (ed), *In the Name of the Child Health and Welfare 1880 to 1940* (New York: Routledge, 1992), pp. 174–199.

Valenze, Deborah, *Milk A Local and Global History* (New Haven: Yale University Press, 2011).

Van Esterik, Penny, 'The Politics of Breastfeeding: An Advocacy Update', in Carol Counihan and Penny Van Esterik (eds), *Food and Culture a Reader* (New York: Routledge, third ed. 2003), pp. 510–530.

Van Hollen, Cecelia, *Birth on the Threshold Childbirth and Modernity in South India* (Berkeley: University of California Press, 2003).

Wald, Erica, *Vice in the Barracks Medicine, the Military and the Making of Colonial India, 1780–1868* (New York: Palgrave Macmillan, 2014)

Walsh, Judith E., *Domesticity in Colonial India What Women Learned When Men Gave Them Advice* (New York: Rowman and Littlefield Publishers, Inc., 2004).

———, *How to Be the Goddess of Your Home. An Anthology of Bengali Domestic Manuals* (New Delhi: Yoda Press, 2005).

West, Emily, and R. J. Knight, 'Mothers' Milk: Slavery, Wet-Nursing, and Black and White Women in the Antebellum South', *The Journal of Southern History* vol. 83, no. 1, 2017, pp. 37–68.

Whitehead, Judy, 'Modernising the Motherhood Archetype: Public Health Models and the Child Marriage Restraint Act of 1929', *Contributions to Indian Sociology*, vol. 29, nos. 1 and 2, 1995, pp. 187–209.

Wolf, Jacqueline H., 'Low Breastfeeding Rates and Public Health in the United States', *American Journal of Public Health*, vol. 93, no. 12, 2003, pp. 2000–2010.

Worboys, Michael, 'Was There a Bacteriological Revolution in Late Nineteenth-century Medicine?', *Studies in History and Philosophy of Biological and Medical Sciences*, vol. 38, 2007, pp. 20–42.

Yalom, Marilyn, *A History of the Breast* (London: Pandora An Imprint of Rivers Oram Press, 1998).

Zuckerman, Molly K., and Debra L. Martin (eds), *New Directions in Biocultural Anthropology* (New Jersey: John Wiley & Sons, 2016).

Unpublished PhD Thesis

Guha, Supriya, 'A History of the Medicalisation of Childbirth in Bengal in the Late Nineteenth and Twentieth Centuries', Unpublished PhD Thesis, 1996, University of Calcutta.

INDEX

Made in the USA
Monee, IL
12 November 2026

30e10ec7-2a2f-471f-8dd0-d436f84362aaR01